Promoting Health and Safety

This book is printed on recycled paper.

Promoting Health and Safety

Skills for Independent Living

Edited by

Martin Agran, Ph.D.
Professor
Department of Special Education
Utah State University, Logan

Nancy E. Marchand-Martella, Ph.D.
Associate Professor
Department of Curriculum and Instruction
University of Montana, Missoula

Ronald C. Martella, Ph.D.
Visiting Assistant Professor
Department of Curriculum and Instruction
University of Montana, Missoula

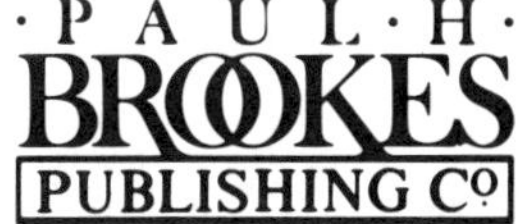

Baltimore • London • Toronto • Sydney

Paul H. Brookes Publishing Co.
Post Office Box 10624
Baltimore, Maryland 21285-0624

Typeset by Brushwood Graphics, Inc., Baltimore, Maryland.
Manufactured in the United States of America by
The Maple Press Company, York, Pennsylvania.

Names of individuals in case examples described in this book are pseudonyms.

Library of Congress Cataloging-in-Publication Data

Promoting health and safety : skills for independent living / edited by Martin Agran, Nancy E. Marchand-Martella, Ronald C. Martella.
p. cm.
Includes bibliographical references and index.
ISBN 1-55766-135-9
1. Developmentally disabled—United States—Life skills guides. 2. Handicapped—United States—Life skills guides. 3. Life skills—Study and teaching—United States. 4. Safety education—United States. I. Agran, Martin. II. Marchand-Martella, Nancy E. III. Martella, Ronald C.
HV1570.5.U65P76 1994
362.1'968–dc20 94-29719
CIP

British Library Cataloguing-in-Publication data are available from the British Library.

Contents

Contributors

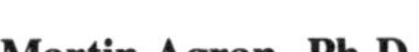

Martin Agran, Ph.D.
Professor
Department of Special Education
Utah State University
Logan, Utah 84322-2865

Belva Collins, Ed.D.
Assistant Professor
Department of Special Education
229 Taylor Education Building
University of Kentucky
Lexington, Kentucky 40506

David L. Gast, Ph.D.
Professor
Department of Special Education
577 Aderhold Hall
University of Georgia
Athens, Georgia 30602-7153

Alan E. Harchik, Ph.D.
Vice President
May Institute
150 Fearing Street
Amherst, Massachusetts 01002

Tecla Jaskulski
President
Jaskulski & Associates
6547 River Clyde Drive
Highland, Maryland 20777

Diane Bannerman Juracek, Ph.D.
Associate Director
Community Living Opportunities
2113 Delaware
Lawrence, Kansas 66046

Donna H. Lehr, Ph.D.
Associate Professor
Department of Special Education
School of Education
Boston University
605 Commonwealth Avenue
Boston, Massachusetts 02215

Sally Macurdy, M.S.
Consultant
233 Scraggy Neck Road
Cataumet, Massachusetts 02534

Nancy E. Marchand-Martella, Ph.D.
Associate Professor
Department of Curriculum and Instruction
University of Montana
Missoula, Montana 59812-1054

Ronald C. Martella, Ph.D.
Visiting Assistant Professor
Department of Curriculum and Instruction
University of Montana
Missoula, Montana 59812-1054

Christine Y. Mason, Ph.D.
Director, Grants & Innovations
National Association of Rehabilitation Facilities
P.O. Box 17675
Washington, D.C. 20041-0675

Daniel Morgan, Ph.D.
Associate Professor
Department of Special Education
Utah State University
Logan, Utah 84322-2865

Mary Ann Harvey Smith, Ph.D.
Professor and Coordinator
Clinical Nutrition Program
Department of Home Economics
Memphis State University
Memphis, Tennessee 38152

Dick Sobsey, Ed.D.
Professor
Department of Educational Psychology
University of Alberta
6-102 Education North
Edmonton, Alberta T6G 2G5
CANADA

Julie Wellons, M.S.
Coordinator
Preschool Exceptional Children Program
1400 North Graham Street
Charlotte, North Carolina 28206

Foreword

Security is mostly a superstition. It does not exist in nature, nor do the children of men as a whole experience it. . . . Avoiding danger is no safer in the long run than outright exposure. . . . Life is either a daring adventure, or nothing.

—Helen Keller (*The Open Door,* 1957, p. 17)

The above quotation from Helen Keller carries an important message to those working with people with disabilities. Historically, in many cases, people with disabilities have been denied access to certain environments and events in an effort to keep them secure, safe, and out of harm's way. Yet, without some element of risk, life does not hold the excitement of adventure.

Helen Keller spoke of the necessity of taking risks—precision, persistence, dignity, and risk are some of the underpinnings of a text about supporting people with disabilities to live safely in their communities. This volume utilizes behavior analysis as the instructional technology for teaching health and safety skills to persons with disabilities. Community-referenced instruction, as defined by Snell and Browder (1986), comprises two basic approaches: 1) the philosophy of normalization (Wolfensberger, 1972) and 2) the use of behavior analysis (Bijou & Baer, 1961). Living in the community is about dignity. Dignity for persons with disabilities is about risk. Perske (1972) has told us that there is dignity in risk, giving people the opportunity to live a fuller and more meaningful life. Yet, to send people with disabilities into the community unprepared and without the appropriate health and safety skills to combat hazards in both the physical and social environment, without appropriate information about nutrition and diet, job and personal safety skills, and appropriate education in human sexuality and substance use prevention would appear to be the wrong kind of risk. This is the technological frontier of the 1990s—applying behavioral-instructional strategies to alter the way that people live. These new applications should focus on developing functional measures of lifestyle quality (Horner, 1991). If people with disabilities are to live successfully in the community, the people who train them must provide them with a full armory of skills, including health and safety, and make taking risks a worthwhile adventure.

Through this seminal and inspiring text, Agran, Marchand-Martella, and Martella are taking the field to the next level of skill development for persons with disabilities. This book offers a comprehensive examination of health and safety needs for persons with disabilities and discusses curriculum, what to teach (e.g., self-medication skills, fire safety skills), and the methodological framework used to teach these curriculum areas. A full complement of effective behavioral-instructional strategies is offered, as well as guidelines for assessing an individual or the environment in which that individual is likely to function, generalizing specific skills to other environments or to other untrained skills of a similar nature, and maintaining those skills across time through self-monitoring procedures. The authors cover the full range of age levels and abilities. In total, the volume has something for everyone—from the young to the elderly and from those with severe disabilities to those who require less assistance.

The direction that Agran et al. have taken with the text parallels society's recent focus on prevention. As a society, we realize that our individual well-being is contingent upon how we live our lives. As we continue to take a preventive focus, our collective concern about health care issues increases. As more and more people with disabilities find their way into the community, they are gradually becoming an integral part of the community fabric. Their needs, specifically their health care needs, reflect the increased support of society in this critical area. As part of the continuum of community services for *all* persons, medical services (e.g., doctor's office visits, emergency room care) will continue to be an important component. The medical community will need to be further sensitized to the needs of persons with disabilities. For example, emergency room personnel, from secretaries to the physician on call, will need to be appropriately educated on the psychological, sociological, physiological, and anatomical needs of the person with a disability, in addition to attending to the medical emergency.

Good health and well-being have typically been associated with positive attitudes. However, a positive attitude may not always reflect changes in behavior. Baer, Wolf, and Risley (1968), both in their classic work on dimensions of applied behavior analysis and in their recent reiteration of the dimensions of applied behavior analysis (Baer, Wolf, & Risley, 1987), remind us about the benefits of *behavior* change over *attitude* change. Agran et al. contend that one of the best ways to teach health and safety skills in home and community environments is through the use of precise, replicable, data-based behavioral intervention.

In summary, Agran et al. have accomplished their purpose: to give the consumer illustrative case studies and up-to-date research findings on teaching health and safety skills to persons with disabilities. It is a book that can be used as a resource guide by direct care practitioners and parents, a book that most advocates and trainers should have on their shelves. This volume paves the way for the future. The training procedures offered increase the likelihood that more people with disabilities will live a satisfying and adventurous life, armed with the necessary skills to live in the community more successfully. Enjoy!

Fred Spooner, Ph.D.
Assistant Professor
Department of Teaching Specialties
University of North Carolina at Charlotte
Editor, TEACHING Exceptional Children

REFERENCES

Baer, D.M., Wolf, M.M., & Risley, T.R. (1968). Some current dimensions of applied behavior analysis. *Journal of Applied Behavior Analysis, 1,* 91–97.

Baer, D.M., Wolf, M.M., & Risley, T.R. (1987). Some still-current dimensions of applied behavior analysis. *Journal of Applied Behavior Analysis, 20,* 313–327.

Bijou, S.W., & Baer, D.M. (1961). *Child development: A systematic and empirical theory* (Vol. 1). New York: Appleton-Century-Crofts.

Horner, R.H. (1991). The future of applied behavior analysis for people with severe disabilities. In L.H. Meyer, C.A. Peck, & L. Brown (Eds.), *Critical issues in the lives of people with severe disabilities* (pp. 607–611). Baltimore: Paul H. Brookes Publishing Co.

Keller, H. (1957). *The open door.* Garden City, NY: Doubleday.

Perske, R. (1972). The dignity of risk. In W. Wolfensberger (Ed.), *Normalization: The principle of normalization in human services* (pp. 194–200). Toronto, Ontario, Canada: National Institute on Mental Retardation.

Snell, M.E., & Browder, D.M. (1986). Community-referenced instruction: Research and issues. *Journal of The Association for Persons with Severe Handicaps, 11,* 1–11.

Wolfensberger, W. (1972). *The principle of normalization in human services.* Toronto, Ontario, Canada: National Institute on Mental Retardation.

Preface

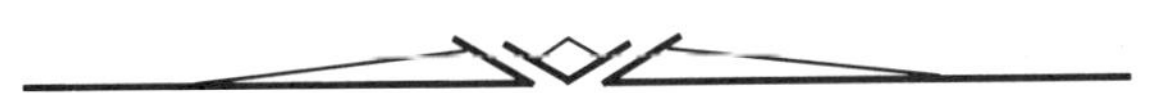

This book presents a comprehensive examination of various health and safety skills that can be taught to persons with disabilities. Although not specifically designed as a curriculum, the text provides teachers, service providers, parents, employers, and others working with people with disabilities a useful list of skills to teach students and young adults. (The words *teacher* and *instructor* are used throughout this book to refer to anyone working with or caring for individuals with disabilities who is interested in teaching these critical skills.) Acquisition of these skills will provide individuals with a functional repertoire of behaviors with which to respond adaptively or avoid or prevent any of a number of potentially risky situations across school, home, work, or community environments, thus promoting good health and general well-being.

One of the most fundamental changes in our culture has been an increased concern with health issues and how our well-being is dependent upon how we live our lives. As a result, we have learned to modify what we eat and what medications we consume; to exercise on a systematic and consistent basis; to use various procedures to reduce stress; to identify potential risk situations in our homes, at our jobs, and in the community; and to use a number of procedures to protect us from criminal assault, physical and/or sexual abuse, and injury. Rather than continue to follow a reactive orientation in which we respond only to problems as they occur, we have selected a proactive, preventive focus in which we learn ways to circumvent the negative consequences of unsafe health practices.

Few persons with disabilities have learned these health and safety practices. All too often, professionals decide what persons with disabilities should eat, how their medications should be administered, how their injuries should be treated, how to administer their health care procedures, and how much, if any, sex education they should receive. Additionally, our approach to ensuring their safety has been to place them in settings where there are minimal risks and to make sure that there are always adequate staff available to intervene if a potential problem arises.

Implicit in teaching functional community living and work skills to individuals with disabilities is risk taking. By its nature, community-based instruction exposes students to a variety of risks not present in classroom or school-based training settings. Thus, when providing community-based instruction, trainers need to address the following questions:

1. What are the risks involved in conducting such training?
2. Where should such training be provided?
3. Should in vivo training wait until the individual can perform the skill at some criterion level in a simulated condition?

Robert Perske (1972) stressed the importance of risk taking for persons with disabilities and indicated that "there can be such a thing as human dignity in risk. And there can be dehumanizing indignity in safety!" (p. 200). Persons with disabilities must be allowed the dignity to make errors, to experience the consequences when inappropriate decisions are made, and to learn that there will not always be someone there to offer guidance or provide assistance when they need help. To prepare persons with disabilities for normative functioning in the community, they must not be shielded from the risks of daily life, but taught to handle such risks adaptively.

Fortunately, a change in our field is occurring. As we assume more responsibility for our own health and well-being, we are beginning to realize that persons with disabilities are capable of exerting more control over their own health and well-being. This realization has prompted many of us to identify and teach critical health and safety skills. Additionally, we are beginning to realize that many of the procedures routinely assumed by service providers can be performed by persons with disabilities themselves. Teaching health and safety skills to these individuals represents a positive means to break the chain of dependence and allow them to become more independent. We, as professionals, need to shift our instructional focus. It is our hope that this book will help to promote this change.

Typically, we have associated good health or the avoidance of accidents with a person's positive attitudes. For example, if someone has a "good" attitude about work safety, he or she will be "aware" of work hazards and, consequently, avoid injury. Measuring positive attitudes may not, however, reflect any actual changes in an individual's behavior. That is, there may be no correspondence between what someone *says* and what he or she actually *does*. Thus, instruction should be focused on teaching specific, demonstrable skills for each health need (e.g., nutrition, self-medication) or risk situation (e.g., home fire, intruder), not on changing someone's attitude. To ensure effective responding to actual or potentially harmful situations, persons with disabilities need to be able to discriminate risk situations and respond appropriately.

It is our belief that health and safety skills can only be acquired and mastered if a precise, replicable, and data-based behavioral intervention is used. Consequently, the first chapter, "Effective Behavioral-Instructional Strategies," presents a basic introduction to behavioral-instructional techniques and provides general suggestions on how behavioral technology can be used to teach the various skills discussed throughout the book. Failure to provide such training runs counter to our efforts to promote full participation of persons with disabilities in their communities and leaves these individuals exposed to danger and dependent on their care and service providers in matters relating to their health and safety.

Chapter Two provides recommendations on teaching home and community safety skills to students with disabilities. Sample lesson plans and specific recommendations are presented for teaching safety skills as part of a functional curriculum. Chapter Three discusses problems persons with disabilities may experience that prevent them from obtaining optimal nutrition; also, guidelines for teaching food selection and preparation are presented. Chapter Four discusses issues relating to teaching persons with developmental disabilities to participate either partially or fully in administering their own medications safely. Chapter Five discusses the provision of quality care in school settings for children who have developmental disabilities and special health care needs. Chapter Six reviews existing practices in first-aid training and presents guidelines for teaching selected skills. Chapter Seven describes procedures for teaching individuals with disabilities living in the community to respond appropriately to various fire emergencies. Chapter Eight reviews practices for teaching work safety skills. Chapter Nine examines the substance use problem among students with disabilities and forwards recommendations for substance use prevention. Chapter Ten discusses the incidence of HIV/AIDS among people with disabilities and suggests educational programs to minimize the potential for transmission by promoting healthy sexual practices. Finally, Chapter Eleven discusses the incidence of and ways to minimize crimes against people with disabilities.

Given the exigencies of these times and rapidly evolving sociological, cultural, and medical changes in our society, the curricular domains we have formerly taught remain important, but, ultimately, inadequate. There is no question that an individual unprepared to take responsibility for his or her health and safety represents an individual ill-equipped for contemporary living. This book is designed to provide professionals, parents, and others with recommendations on how to teach individuals with disabilities the skills they need to face the challenges of living responsibly and safely across a variety of risky or less than accommodating situations. We believe that we owe the individuals we serve nothing less.

REFERENCE

Perske, R. (1972). The dignity of risk. In W. Wolfensberger (Ed.), *Normalization: The principle of normalization in human services* (pp. 194–200). Toronto, Ontario, Canada: National Institute on Mental Retardation.

Acknowledgments

We would like to thank the Department of Special Education at Utah State University for allowing us the opportunity to conduct our health and safety research. In particular, we would like to thank Susan Nash for her tireless secretarial (and grammatical) support. Our thanks are also extended to Kristle and Hailey Agran (M.A.) and Amédee Marchand Martella and our families for their love, support, and caring (N.M-M., R.M.).

Promoting Health and Safety

Chapter One

Effective Behavioral-Instructional Strategies

Ronald C. Martella,
Nancy E. Marchand-Martella, and Martin Agran

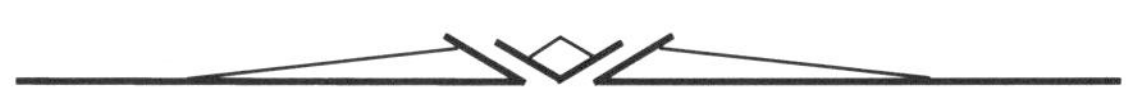

The health and safety issues discussed in this book reflect an important theme—improving the responses of individuals to their environment in order to ensure the overall health and well-being of those individuals and to strengthen their independence. To achieve these goals, educators and service providers must teach people with disabilities how to respond effectively when they are faced with challenging situations. Teaching these individuals a verbal classroom response as to how they should handle these types of situations is not enough; real changes in behavior must be learned and implemented.

An effective behavioral technology of instruction is available to promote new behavioral responses. This technology represents a tangible means by which people with disabilities can lessen their vulnerability to the harmful risks present in contemporary society. This chapter provides general explanations as to how the technology of behavioral instruction can be employed to teach the health and safety skills discussed in this book, as well as other related living skills that teachers and service providers may find appropriate.

BEHAVIORAL-INSTRUCTIONAL TECHNIQUES

Behavioral instruction is based on the fact that changes in behavior can be produced by manipulating the environment in which the behavior occurs. Educators who teach behavioral skills by using data-based instructional techniques are able to determine the situations (or antecedents) that give rise to a particular behavior and provide certain environmental changes (or consequences) for the behavior exhibited.

Behavioral-instructional techniques are well-suited to teaching health and safety skills. For example, a teacher targets a needed skill, such as treating a wound, and breaks the skill down into task-analyzed steps as illustrated in the following example:

1. Cover the wound with cloth or a sterile gauze pad.
2. Apply pressure to the wound.
3. Maintain pressure and elevate the injury above the heart.
4. Continue with steps 2 and 3 and show or tell a responsible adult what has happened.

The teacher decides to use a backward-chaining procedure to teach the skill; therefore, he or she demonstrates the first three steps and then actively instructs the learner on how to complete step 4 independently. After the learner has successfully demonstrated step 4, the teacher then performs the first two steps, leaving the third step for training, and so on, until all four steps have been taught.

The teacher then structures the antecedents or the occasion in which the individual's learned behavior will occur (e.g., a simulated injury). The learner then engages in the prescribed task, thereby exhibiting the acquired behavior. Finally, the teacher provides certain consequences for the exhibited behavior, including feedback that is positive (e.g., "Good job applying pressure.") or constructive (e.g., "You need to apply pressure like this.").

ADVANTAGES TO USING BEHAVIORAL INSTRUCTION

One of the most important advantages to using behavioral instruction is that it is well-grounded in decades of experimental research. Out of this research, some general laws of behavior have emerged:

1. It is commonly accepted that if a particular behavior is reinforced, the likelihood of that behavior being displayed in the future is increased. For example, if learners receive praise for preparing nutritious meals, they may be more likely to prepare nutritious meals in the future.
2. If a particular behavior is punished, the future likelihood of the same behavior occurring is reduced. For example, if students lose their privileges because of taking drugs, they may be less likely to take drugs in the future.
3. The effects of reinforcement are temporary. Therefore, if learners are no longer reinforced for a particular behavior, the behavior will return to preintervention levels. For example, if individuals no longer receive supervisor attention for following safe work procedures, they will be less likely to continue working in a careful manner. Such extinction of praise may even produce counterproductive results.
4. Like reinforcement, the effects of punishment are also temporary. If a person's behavior no longer meets with punishment, the behavior will return to preintervention levels. For example, if students are no longer punished for taking drugs, and they are not reinforced for remaining drug-free, they will be more likely to return to their prior level of drug use. The term for this type of phenomenon is *recovery.*

A second advantage to using behavioral instruction is that its methods define procedures based on their function or their effects on behavior. Thus, a *stimulus* (e.g., an object, event) is not a *reinforcer* unless it *increases* the future likelihood of a behavior occurring following either the presentation of a positive stimulus/event or the removal of a negative stimulus/event immediately after the behavior. For example, if students learn how to self-medicate and are praised for doing so, but then later exhibit decreased self-medication behavior, praise is no longer considered to be an effective reinforcer.

Similarly, a functional definition is used for punishment; a stimulus is not a *punisher* unless it *decreases* the future probability of a behavior. Thus, if students are reprimanded for talking to strangers, but continue to speak to them regardless, reprimands cannot be considered an effective punisher. Basing instruction on how it affects behavior over time is critical to effective teaching.

A third advantage to behavioral instruction is its emphasis on observable behavior. Health and safety skills lend themselves well to this advantage because their use can be directly observed and measured. In other words, behavior change is determined by an actual observable change in behavior, rather than a nonobservable change in some inferred theoretical construct such as perceptions or attitudes. If, for example, an instructor wishes to teach an individual to respond appropriately in an emergency situation, the instructor should target observable differences in that person's behavior, rather than attempt to change the person's attitude.

In the same vein, rather than trying to alter a person's perceptions of unsafe sex or drug use, we must ultimately change the person's actual behavior. Thus, students may report that they would "say no" to drugs because drugs are dangerous, but they may go ahead and buy drugs when approached by someone selling them. Although there may indeed be a correspondence between what a person *says* and what he or she actually *does,* it is clear that intervention must focus on the behavior itself (i.e., buying drugs), rather than on the verbal reports (i.e., saying no). Changes in behavior will result from environmental manipulations (structured antecedents and consequences) that serve to support the instructed behavior.

Assessment of observable changes in behavior is critical when instructing all learners; however, when an instructor begins to attribute changes in an individual's behavior to the person's internal mental processes, the value of good instruction is hidden. For example, an instructor may report that the student is engaging in safe sexual practices because of a perceived attitudinal change; yet attitudinal changes do not alter sexual behavior—effective behavioral-instructional programs do. Inferences do not provide the instructor with any more factual information than what has already been observed and may even lead to the wrong conclusions regarding what an individual has actually learned (Skinner, 1976).

The final advantage to behavioral instruction is that its methods and achievements can be replicated. The procedures are described in such a manner that those responsible for carrying out instructional programs can achieve success if they follow the procedures correctly, allowing for adjustments in instruction based on the effects observed in the student's behavior. Given the dire consequences that can result when health and safety skills are not taught, it seems especially prudent for those teaching these necessary skills to use a technology demonstrated to produce consistent outcomes.

METHODS OF BEHAVIORAL INSTRUCTION

Behavioral instruction offers a myriad of effective instructional strategies. These strategies include:

- Reinforcement
- Stimulus control
- Discrimination training
- Fading
- Shaping
- Chaining

Each of these methods is described in the sections that follow as they relate to training in health and safety skills.

Reinforcement

Reinforcement is the fulcrum for behavioral instruction. If a behavior is to be displayed in the future, it must be reinforced in the present, or it must have been reinforced in the past. A number of things must occur in order for reinforcement to be effective:

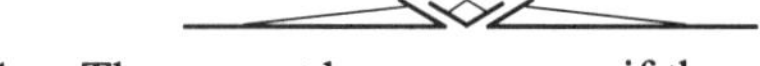

1. There must be a response; if there is no response, there is nothing to consequate.
2. The consequence should follow the response as soon as possible. For example, after an individual learns to self-catheterize, he or she should be immediately praised.
3. Reinforcers should fit the behavior. For instance, it would be less appropriate to reinforce a worker's safe behavior on the job with a candy bar at the end of the month than to reinforce the person with an "Employee of the Month" award.
4. The reinforcer should appear as natural as possible; if the current reinforcers are artificial, there should be an attempt to switch to natural reinforcers (stimuli that normally occur and are not foreign to the particular environment). For example, money given to students by their teachers is an artificial consequence, whereas grades or points are natural reinforcers. Similarly, grades provided by a manager for an employee's improved work behavior are artificial, whereas money is natural.

5. A variety of possible reinforcers should be available. Variety prevents the learner from becoming overexposed to a single reinforcer, causing a loss in its effectiveness (a process known as *satiation*). For example, if an individual leaves a building within a certain time frame during a fire drill, he or she can select his or her preference from a list of possible activities.
6. After a behavior has been learned and is being demonstrated at an adequate level, the reinforcers should be provided on an intermittent basis. For instance, instead of reinforcing a student for every demonstration of first-aid skills, reinforcement may be provided after every fourth or fifth demonstration on average (i.e., a *variable ratio schedule*). Thus, the educator will be actively programming for the maintenance of behavioral gains.

Stimulus Control

Stimulus control is defined as an increased likelihood that an individual will respond in a given way to a particular situation and will not respond in the absence of the situation. This training is usually accomplished by reinforcing the behavior in the presence of a particular stimulus and not reinforcing the behavior when the particular stimulus is absent. The behavior is said to be *extinguished* in the presence of any other stimulus except the one being trained. Two shortcut tactics of planning for stimulus control involve *modeling* the desired behavior in the presence of the desired controlling stimulus (e.g., dialing 911 in the presence of a simulated emergency) or *instructing* (teaching the individual to dial 911 only when there is an emergency situation).

Modeling Modeling is defined as demonstrating a given behavior in front of learners to induce them to engage in similar behavior. This is a simple, but extremely effective, instructional technique. The advantage to modeling is that it is used regularly throughout people's lives, and one often learns by example. The major concern with modeling, however, is whether or not learners can perform the necessary prerequisite skills. If they do not already possess these skills, they must first learn them through other instructional methods before stimulus control can be achieved.

Instruction Like modeling, instruction is also a regular part of everyone's lives. Depending on one's learning history, effective instructions are rules or guidelines in which three general categories of information are presented: 1) the behavior to be displayed, 2) when it is to be displayed, and 3) what will happen after it is displayed. For example, consider the following instruction: "If you smell smoke," (when) "get on the floor and feel if the door is hot" (behavior) "in order to avoid serious injury during a fire" (consequence).

However, also as with modeling, instructions will not work if students do not already have the prerequisite skills in their repertoires or if they lack the necessary receptive language skills. For example, if one of the editors of this book was told to rebuild his or her car engine as soon as possible or a great deal of money would have to be spent on car repairs, it is highly likely that person would end up paying a great deal of money. In other words, it does not matter what a person is told to do if he or she cannot respond to the instruction or does not have the necessary skills for performing the behavior. In such a case, other teaching methods should be utilized before instruction could be used as a short-cut method to stimulus control.

Discrimination Training

Discrimination training involves reinforcing an individual's response to a particular stimulus and not reinforcing his or her response to another stimulus. In other words, an individual undergoing discrimination training will learn when to respond in a certain manner and when not to respond. When teaching health and safety skills, it is critical that discrimination training is conducted, especially when teaching students how to distinguish an unsafe situation from a safe one. For example, in a course on crime prevention, the student must be taught to discriminate familiar people from strangers. If this goal is accomplished, students will refrain from responding to strangers in a manner that could make them susceptible to exploitation or abuse.

Fading

Fading is defined as the transfer of stimulus control from one stimulus or situation to another; as one stimulus is faded out, another is faded in. For example, when teaching an individual to self-medicate, the initial stimulus may be a verbal prompt from the teacher (e.g., "It's time to take your medication."). However, ultimately, the person must be able to respond to natural cues in the environment in the absence of the teacher's verbal prompt. Therefore, the verbal prompt may be gradually faded out and another prompt or cue faded in (e.g., time on the clock, time written on the medication bottle).

Fading of prompts can be accomplished in a number of ways. First, there may be a set or constant time delay (CTD) from the new desired cue (time on the clock) and the prompt to be faded out (verbal prompt). This delay permits the desired natural cue to be separated from the faded prompt, thus allowing the natural cue to acquire stimulus control over the same behavior. A progressive time delay (PTD) can also be utilized in which the time between the natural cue and the delivery of the teacher's prompt is increased in a graduated or progressive manner. The point at which the new prompt begins to control the response sooner than the unwanted verbal prompt is called the *moment of transfer.*

Second, graduated prompting, from least to most intrusive prompts, may be applied. For example, when teaching self-medication, the individual may be shown the time on the clock, followed by a verbal prompt only if the desired response does not occur. If the person does not respond to the verbal prompt, he or she is then given the medication. After a period of time, the individual may begin to respond to the less intrusive prompt. As the clock prompt is responded to more frequently, the more intrusive verbal prompts must be faded out.

Finally, graduated guidance can be used when the student is helped to take his or her medication by a hand-over-hand prompting procedure. After successive sessions, the amount of aid or physical guidance is gradually reduced until the student is taking the medication independently. The instructional strategies discussed thus far assume the preexistence of a given behavior in the learner's repertoire. The next two strategies, shaping and chaining, use reinforcement for teaching entirely new behaviors.

Shaping

Shaping involves reinforcing the successive approximations of behavior to achieve a desired behavioral goal. Cooper, Heron, and Heward (1987) illustrate this concept with the following example. A teacher is instructing a group of students in water safety. In a simulated situation, she teaches them to throw a life preserver a given distance to a person who appears to be struggling in the water. The desired goal of the lesson is to learn to throw the life preserver near the person "drowning." Therefore, the teacher reinforces the students for closer and closer throws. Thus, the criteria for the reinforcement of change in the behavior represents a systematic process of achieving closer approximations to the final desired behavior.

Chaining

Chaining teaches a new behavior by linking smaller component behaviors together to form one long sequence (or chain). For example, nutritional meal preparation involves a number of behaviors that are linked together in sequence to produce the desired product. If one were to prepare a cheese sandwich, a task analysis of the preparation would reveal a number of component actions. First, the individual would need to locate the bread, cheese, and mayonnaise. Second, the individual would need to take out two slices of bread, a slice of cheese, and open the mayonnaise jar. Also, the person may need to discriminate high fat or cholesterol bread, cheese, or mayonnaise from low fat products. Next, a knife would need to be taken out, and so on, until the sandwich is made.

Each individual step could then be taught in one of three ways. First, a forward chaining method could be used that involves teaching the first skill first (i.e., locating the bread, cheese, and mayonnaise) and the last skill last (i.e., putting away the bread, cheese, and mayonnaise). Thus, the first skill is taught; followed by the first and second; followed by the first, second, and third; and so on. The individual is usually prompted either verbally or physically through each successive step not being taught. Second, a backward chaining method could be used that involves teaching the last skill first and the first skill last. For example, the tenth skill is taught, then the ninth and eighth, and so on. As in forward chaining, the individual is usually prompted through each successive step until reaching the step being taught. Third, a total-task method could be used that involves teaching all of the steps at the same time. The individual is prompted through each step and receives concurrent feedback and training throughout the entire process.

Research has demonstrated that all three methods are effective, and no one method has consistently been shown to be more effective than the others. Therefore, when deciding how to teach a health or safety skill using a chaining procedure, a number of factors need to be considered: 1) the size or total number of steps involved to complete the task, 2) the language ability of the learner, and 3) the complexity of individual steps (Sulzer-Azaroff & Mayer, 1991).

Although there are no exact rules to be followed for each particular chaining method, there are some general recommendations. If a complex task is being taught, backward chaining may be the best option, as forward chaining does not begin with the ultimate reinforcer (i.e., task completed). The total-task method relies on all steps being taught together and is recommended because it involves the full sequence of responses for a given task. However, if the student is having difficulty with one or more responses in the chain, remediation may be difficult to provide. Similarly, if a student is faced with an extremely long chain of responses and reinforcement is not provided until the end of the task, backward chaining may again be the method of choice. If a student already has all of the component skills in his or her repertoire, is fluent in each, and simply requires the component skills to be placed in the correct sequence, total-task training may be the most efficient method. Finally, if the task is simple, but requires that new component skills be taught that can be individually reinforced, forward chaining may be the best option. Therefore, the choice is ultimately up to the educator and really depends upon the situation at hand.

PROGRAMMING FOR GENERALIZATION AND MAINTENANCE

It is generally agreed that educators should not entirely cease instruction after the teaching objectives have been met unless strategies for generalizing and maintaining the acquired behavior were incorporated into the instructional program. Educators often report that they teach skills to students only to find that the students are unable to exhibit these skills in the future. This problem is of particular concern in the areas of health and safety due to the serious consequences that can result from performing various components of a particular task incorrectly (e.g., picking up broken glass without wearing gloves) or not completing them at all (e.g., leaving broken glass on the floor). Therefore, ensuring that a new skill will be maintained by the learner and that he or she will be able to use the skill in a variety of situations is as important as teaching the skill itself.

Generalization of Learned Behaviors

Stokes and Osnes (1988) define generalization as the performance of learned behavior under conditions that are similar to those used in training (e.g., treating an actual burn in an emergency situation as compared to treating a simulated burn during training) or the performance of responses that are similar to the originally trained responses (e.g., treating a burn although the treatment of cuts was the skill that was originally taught). Stokes and Osnes recommend several methods for programming generalization. Those tactics specifically related to skill acquisition are discussed here. First, educators should teach relevant skills (i.e., skills that are both useful and adaptive). If relevant skills are being taught, learners will be more likely to encounter situations in their natural environment where their new skills can be utilized, and are thus more likely to receive positive consequences for their actions.

Health and safety skills fall into this domain, in that their successful completion in the learner's natural environment is likely to produce positive results (e.g., overcoming an illness because medication protocols were followed or lowering one's weight due to healthy eating). However, one caveat is in order here. Reinforcers must be immediate if they are to be effective. Unfortunately, most of the consequences of good health and safety behaviors are delayed for long periods of time (e.g., losing weight due to healthy eating). If this is the case, more immediate feedback must be planned (e.g., telling someone that he or she looks good, praising him or her for healthy eating, incorporating self-charting of nutritious meals) in order to bridge the temporal gap between the behavior and the ultimate reinforcer.

Second, educators should plan for naturally occurring reinforcers. For example, notifying a supervisor that you picked up a box that was sitting in the middle of a busy walkway may solicit his or her approval. ("Thanks, you prevented an accident.") This kind of feedback from the supervisor would be critical in maintaining the safety behavior; therefore, the educator should attempt to program ways for the student to receive positive feedback outside the training setting.

Third, educators need to include a variety of teaching examples during training to increase the likelihood that learners will exhibit generalized responding when faced with novel situations. For example, various sizes and brands of adhesive bandages should be used in teaching first aid so that students can use whatever bandages are available in an actual emergency situation. Albin and Horner (1988) noted that negative teaching examples should also be used "to teach the learner the conditions in which performance is not appropriate or in which some alternative response should be made" (p. 105). For example, teachers might incorporate cans of pet food as part of training to see if students can discriminate cans of food appropriate for human consumption from food that is appropriate for animals.

Fourth, when developing instructional programs, educators should target a multitude of behaviors that can produce the same results. For example, a burn can be treated by using a sterile pad or gauze and applying tape or by using a large adhesive bandage. These materials require differing procedures for application, but they serve the same function of keeping the wound clear of infection.

Fifth, educators should train "loosely." Training situations should vary (e.g., differing instructors or environments) to increase the likelihood that the correct behavior will occur in nontrained conditions. For example, individuals should be taught to shop in a variety of grocery stores to increase their success in finding and purchasing food in the different environments that they might encounter as they strive for greater independence.

Sixth, educators should reinforce unprompted generalizations. For example, if a learner observes an emergency and proceeds to dial 911 without any outside assistance, he or she should be reinforced as soon as possible. Also, educators should inform families of the value of immediate reinforcement should such an event occur at home.

Seventh, educators need to program for common social stimuli. If individuals learn to perform certain tasks in the presence of classroom staff, they should also be able to exhibit those skills in the presence of family, friends, or employers. However, some individuals, for example, might learn to take care of their own injuries while in the presence of a teacher, whereas they will not do so in front of a parent. Therefore, students need to learn to treat these injuries regardless of who is present, rather than relying on specific people to guide them.

Finally, educators should include self-management strategies (described in greater detail in the following section). Such procedures as self-instructions, self-monitoring, self-recording, self-charting, and self-reinforcement can all facilitate the occurrence of behaviors in varying settings and under varying circumstances. For example, students can talk themselves through treating an insect bite, monitor or record when their medications were taken, chart weight loss, or praise themselves for engaging in safe sex.

Strategies for Successful Maintenance

Sulzer-Azaroff and Mayer (1991) recommend several strategies for preventing relapse or skill atrophy over time. First, educators should strive to minimize learner errors when a skill is being taught. Every time that an error is made by the learner, there is an increased likelihood that the error will be repeated. Therefore, sound instructional procedures, such as those suggested here, should be utilized in order to maximize correct performance and minimize mistakes.

Second, educators should program for response fluency during training. West and Young (1992) noted that once skills have been acquired, they should be practiced to increase the speed or rate of correct responding, thereby increasing the likelihood of response maintenance over time. For example, if a young adult can treat a severe cut, but it takes him or her 30 minutes to do so, the teacher should focus on ways to decrease the amount of time that the student spends on treating the injury. Identifying the steps that are causing the most difficulties is a good place to start.

Third, educators should identify and utilize naturally occurring reinforcers within the learner's environment (e.g., classroom, work, home, group home). These may include ongoing feedback systems (e.g., notes at home, newsletter of accomplishments at work) and peer interactions (e.g., group discussion, cooperative learning, peer tutoring activities). Learners can present weekly health and safety reports to their peers and describe the various ways in which they are using what they have learned outside of the training setting.

Fourth, educators need to program for naturally maintained conditions in the environment. They should adjust when and how often they reinforce and the kinds of reinforcers that they use so that existing classroom and community conditions are approximated. For example, educators should fade from a continuous schedule of reinforcement for safe work behavior to an intermittent schedule of reinforcement or gradually increase the amount of time between safe work behavior and the reinforcer.

Educators should also program for group instructional activities that build upon peer support systems, instead of only relying on one-on-one instruction. For example, trained roommates can be used to cue other individuals to evacuate safely during a fire. Peers can also be very helpful in establishing supportive environments for refusing to experiment with alcohol or drugs.

Fifth, educators should reinforce correspondence between verbal responses (what learners say they are doing) and overt behaviors (what they actually are doing). For example, if an individual reports that he or she is eating nutritious meals, the teacher should observe what the person eats during lunch. If nutritious foods are consumed, the individual should be reinforced for the correspondence in his or her behavior.

Finally, educators should incorporate self-management strategies whenever possible. Learners can be taught to self-record or self-monitor their own safe behaviors (e.g., keep track of self-administered medication) and to chart their safe behavior (e.g., record on self-chart length of time for evacuation during simulated fire emergencies). Self-instructions may also be used to guide learners through the completion of health and safety skills (e.g., repeating the steps of dialing 911).

Individuals can also learn to self-manage their own lifestyles. Educators can help learners to modify their behavior and to maintain these changes by including them in their everyday activities (e.g., eating low-fat nutritious meals). Learners can be taught to manage their own health and safety behaviors by first teaching them the appropriate self-management skills; they should not be expected to manage their own behavior without these necessary skills. To accomplish the goal of self-management, educators will eventually need to transfer the control they have established with the learner during training to the naturally supportive reinforcers in the environment in which the individual interacts.

One method of training requisite self-management skills is teaching individuals how to problem-solve. D'Zurilla and Goldfried (1971) defined problem solving as "the process or technique by which one attempts to 'discover' a solution to a problem" (p. 109). That is, the individual generates a solution to a problem not previously encountered (Hale & Holt, 1986). It would be impossible to teach specific responses to every possible situation that an individual might encounter. At some point, the individual will have to be able to respond adaptively to the specific problem situation. Parsonson and Baer (1978) suggest that a problem only exists in the absence of an effective solution. Therefore, many problems can be dealt with by teaching skills that will help the person learn how to generate effective solutions.

CONCLUSIONS

Using behavioral-instructional strategies for teaching health and safety skills to persons with disabilities helps to ensure the acquisition, generalization, and maintenance of these necessary skills. Skinner (1992) indicated that all instructors should:

1. "Be clear about what is to be taught"(p. 22) (i.e., operationally define behaviors).
2. "Teach first things first" (p.23) (i.e., determine prerequisite skills before training is conducted).
3. "Stop making all students advance at essentially the same rate" (p. 24) (i.e., assess students individually).
4. "Program the subject matter" (p.24) (i.e., prime and prompt behavior until desired actions occur without outside assistance).

It is clear that if these strategies are used correctly, dramatic changes in the learner's health and well-being can take place.

Health and safety skills are critical components of learning to live independently. Once learned, these skills will allow people with disabilities to require little or no assistance from care providers, which we believe to be the ultimate goal of instruction. Failure to provide such training will leave many individuals ill-prepared to be responsible for their own health and safety and to deal with the many problems they will face as they strive for full participation in their communities. Community living and working can increase one's vulnerability to danger and risk, but we believe that this risk is a reasonable one.

REFERENCES

Albin, R.W., & Horner, R.H. (1988). Generalization with precision. In R.H. Horner, G. Dunlap, & R.L. Koegel (Eds.), *Generalization and maintenance: Life-style changes in applied settings* (pp. 99–120). Baltimore: Paul H. Brookes Publishing Co.

Cooper, J.O., Heron, T.E., & Heward, W.L. (1987). *Applied behavior analysis*. Columbus, OH: Merrill.

D'Zurilla, T., & Goldfried, M. (1971). Problem solving and behavior modification. *Journal of Abnormal Psychology, 78*, 107–126.

Hale, A., & Holt, A.S. (1986). Behavioral science. In J. Ridley (Ed.), *Safety at work* (2nd ed., pp. 229–318). London: Butterworths.

Parsonson, B.S., & Baer, D.M. (1978). The analysis and presentation of graphic data. In T.R. Kratochwill (Ed.), *Single-subject research: Strategies for evaluating change* (pp. 101–167). New York: Academic Press.

Skinner, B.F. (1976). *About behaviorism*. New York: Vintage Books.

Skinner, B.F. (1992). The shame of American education. In R.P. West & L.A. Hamerlynck (Eds.), *Designs for excellence in education: The legacy of B.F. Skinner* (pp. 15–30). Longmont, CO: Sopris West.

Stokes, T.F., & Osnes, P.G. (1988). The developing applied technology of generalization and maintenance. In R.H. Horner, G. Dunlap, & R.L. Koegel (Eds.), *Generalization and maintenance: Life-style changes in applied settings* (pp. 5–19). Baltimore: Paul H. Brookes Publishing Co.

Sulzer-Azaroff, B., & Mayer, G.R. (1991). *Behavior analysis for lasting change*. Fort Worth: Holt, Rinehart and Winston.

West, R.P., & Young, K.R. (1992). Precision teaching. In R.P. West & L.A. Hamerlynck (Eds.), *Designs for excellence in education: The legacy of B.F. Skinner* (pp. 113–146). Longmont, CO: Sopris West.

Chapter Two

Home and Community Safety Skills

David L. Gast, Julie Wellons, and Belva Collins

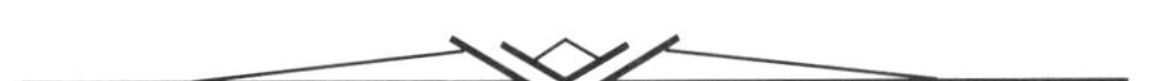

Physical dangers within the natural environment present an element of risk throughout the performance of everyday activities. Although several studies have demonstrated effective ways of teaching safety skills to persons without disabilities (Hillman, Jones, & Farmer, 1986; Jones, Ollendick, McLaughlin, & Williams, 1989; Lehman & Geller, 1990; Peterson & Mori, 1985; Rivera-Tovar & Jones, 1988; Sowers-Hoag, Thyer, & Bailey, 1987), few investigations have been conducted with persons with mental retardation. This chapter specifically addresses teaching people with developmental disabilities how to respond safely to potential physical and social dangers in the home and in the community.

The goal of education is to prepare individuals to function as independently as possible in society. The attainment of this goal for people with developmental disabilities and mental retardation has resulted in a commitment to community-referenced instruction; that is, instruction that is directly related to improving the ways in which individuals live, work, and recreate in community settings (Falvey, 1989; Janicki, Krauss, & Seltzer, 1988; Meyer, Peck, & Brown, 1991; Neel & Billingsley, 1989; Schleien & Ray, 1988; Wehman & Moon, 1988). Critical to this commitment is the importance of teaching individuals targeted skills in locations in which the learned skills will be used.

For example, if a student's individualized education program (IEP) includes teaching the student to deposit a weekly paycheck at a bank, shop for clothes, and eat at local restaurants, a community-based instructional approach might include teaching the individual how to take the city bus to the mall, where he or she would be taught to operate the computerized banker, select and purchase clothes at various apparel stores, and eat lunch at the mall cafeteria. The instruction would occur within the context of normal routines and in the natural settings in which the skills are to be performed. When community-based instruction is impractical, teaching the same community-referenced skills under simulation is recommended (Nietupski, Hamre-Nietupski, Clancy, & Veerhusen, 1986).

As students spend more time off school grounds learning functional skills, many parents, teachers, and administrators have expressed concerns regarding their safety (Jones & McDonald, 1986). These concerns may be a function of low expectations as to what individuals with mental retardation can actually learn and/or an unfamiliarity with school guidelines or policies for ensuring the safety of students. The former issue is often addressed by facilitating a meeting between the concerned parent, teacher, or administrator and other parents and professionals who can attest to the success of community-referenced and community-based instruction. Providing specific information about the types of materials and equipment to be used, the teaching procedures, teacher–student ratios, and the locations of instruction can also help to dispel safety concerns. In addition, it may be useful to provide appropriate readings or films that document the accomplishments of students with similar levels of ability.

In terms of school guidelines or policies concerning community-based instruction, there may not be a specific set of procedures different from those typically used for field trips, although this is strongly recommended. Safety guidelines and precautions should be more extensive for community-based instructional outings, not because students have been injured during functional curriculum activities, but because the potential for injury is greater. For example, during a field trip students may cross a street as a group in response to the teacher's direction, whereas during a community-based teaching trip each individual student would be taught to attend to environmental cues for crossing a street safely (e.g., no traffic in either direction, illuminated "Walk" signal).

The kinds of hazards or potential risks to students learning in the community appear to be of two types: those presented by the physical environment (e.g., knives, automobiles, electrical appliances) and those presented by the social environment (e.g., crime, strangers). (Further discussion of potential dangers in the social environment and ways to ensure personal safety is provided in Chapter 10 of this volume.) Examples of potentially dangerous physical situations include:

- Contact with poisons, toxins, and drugs (e.g., cleaning fluids, fertilizers, alcohol)
- Use of potentially dangerous tools, appliances, and equipment (e.g., knife, toaster oven, lawn mower)
- Emergency situations (e.g., fire caused by a sparking toaster)
- Exposure to situations where the risk of injury exists (e.g., crossing a street, approaching a stray animal).

To reduce the potential risk to students and to address the concerns of parents and families, teachers must prepare students to recognize potentially dangerous situations and to respond to them in a safe and appropriate manner. Specifically, students should be taught to: 1) discriminate safe from unsafe situations, 2) perform skills that have an element of risk in a safe manner, and 3) respond appropriately when confronted with a dangerous situation. Such skills should be taught to all students, regardless of age or abilities. As discussed in Chapter 1, it is important that instruction continue until students have consistently demonstrated that learned behaviors have generalized and maintained across various settings in the natural environment (Gast & Wolery, 1988). This chapter presents a model for safety skills instruction within the home and community, including specific recommendations and detailed lesson plans that may assist teachers in deciding what, where, when, and how to teach these important skills as part of a functional curriculum.

PREVENTION–REACTION MODEL FOR SAFETY SKILLS INSTRUCTION

There are two basic types of skills that all persons, regardless of ability, need to acquire if they are to function safely throughout the performance of daily activities. First, they must learn to perform skills in a manner that prevents or reduces the risk of injury. This is accomplished by teaching appropriate safety behaviors during the initial acquisition of a new skill. For example, unplugging an electrical appliance should involve teaching the learner to first make sure that his or her hands are dry and then to unplug the appliance by handling the heavy rubber plug end, rather than pulling on the cord itself. Similarly, students who are being taught to answer the telephone should be taught *not* to provide personal information over the phone. These two examples represent measures that are taken to prevent the likelihood of injury.

The second type of skill involves learning how to react appropriately when faced with a dangerous situation. Individuals should be taught the appropriate reaction behaviors immediately *following* their acquisition of the target skill. For example, the prevention–reaction model recommends teaching a student to cautiously handle plates, glasses, and silverware while learning how to wash dishes. The teacher needs to identify those steps in the task analysis in which there is a potential for injury (e.g., scalding one's hand while adjusting water temperature, cutting one's hand while handling a knife or other sharp utensil). Once the student can complete an accurate and fluent performance of dishwashing, the teacher should then instruct the student on how to react to a possible accident (e.g., how to clean up any broken glass) or injury (e.g., how to apply first aid if cut or scalded). (See chap. 6, this volume, for a discussion on teaching first-aid skills.) Teaching how to respond to an accident or injury should occur under simulated conditions.

Instructing a student on how to respond to a potentially dangerous social situation would be taught in a similar sequence. First the student would be taught to perform a community-referenced skill in a safe manner (e.g., walking on sidewalks, crossing streets) and to avoid dangerous situations (e.g., not walking alone at night). Once learned, the student would be taught to escape dangerous social situations that he or she may confront when walking in the community (e.g., the lure of a stranger).

Identifying Safety Skills for Instruction

In consultation with interdisciplinary team members, (e.g., teachers, occupational therapists, speech-language pathologists) educators should conduct an ecological inventory for each student, determine the types of activities in which the individual participates along with his or her family, assess the potential physical and social dangers associated with each environment and activity, and interview parents to identify their particular safety concerns. The ecological inventory is the basis for implementing a functional curriculum (Browder & Snell, 1993; Snell & Grigg, 1987). This inventory entails the following:

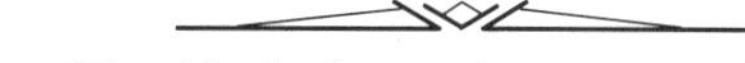

1. Identify the learner's present and possible future environments (e.g., home, school, work).
2. Divide each environment into component subenvironments (e.g., the home environment consists of kitchen, bedroom, bathroom, backyard).
3. Identify activities that take place in each subenvironment. For example, playing catch, swinging, and gardening are all backyard activities.
4. Complete a task analysis of skills used in each activity.
5. Teach skills in order of sequence or by priority.
6. Assess skill acquisition.

By analyzing each environment and activity, it is possible to pinpoint potentially dangerous situations associated with each. For example, during backyard home activities, a child will need to be taught to avoid standing too close behind a friend who is swinging a bat, to tell a parent or older sibling about a ball going into the street, to avoid a fire ant hill or wasp nest, to go inside if thunder is heard or lightning is seen, and any other associated safety precautions. The identified safety skills might also be applicable to activities performed in other subenvironments. Therefore, determining how often an individual might need a particular safety skill is one guideline for prioritizing a skill for instruction.

Families should be an integral part of this assessment process. Parents should be interviewed to identify those activities in which their child currently engages, as well as those activities in which he or she is likely to engage in the future based on the family's long-range residential plans. Activities in which family members participate should also be identified during the interview process because children are likely to imitate behaviors modeled by parents and other siblings.

Needless to say, the individual must be taught to avoid engaging in any activity that he or she has observed, but does not yet know how to perform (e.g., using a power saw, climbing a ladder, swimming). By identifying family activities it is possible for a teacher to instruct a student on the conditions under which he or she might be able to safely engage in a potentially dangerous activity. This will likely satisfy the person's curiosity, while simultaneously putting limits on when and where participation is appropriate.

As part of the family interview, it is important to identify parental concerns regarding the individual's participation in community-based instruction. By knowing of their concerns up front, the necessary precautions may be taken and the appropriate reassurances given. To help teachers identify these concerns, they may want to develop a "survey of safety concerns" similar to that used by Collins, Wolery, and Gast (1991). The list presented in Table 1 was identified by these investigators as areas of home safety in which parents were particularly concerned. (See chap. 10, this volume, for further information on protecting one's personal privacy.)

Prioritizing Skills for Instruction

Once safety concerns have been identified, based on the results of an ecological inventory, family activity survey, and family interview, the teacher and interdisciplinary team will need to prioritize skills for purposes of instruction. There are no established guidelines for deciding which skills should be taught first. Clearly, logic would lead one to begin by teaching those skills and behaviors that will prevent an immediate danger. For example, if an individual is currently permitted to walk alone to the corner grocery store to make small purchases, that person should be taught how to cross the street safely, conceal his or her money, and respond appropriately to an approach by a stranger. All three of these skills warrant immediate instruction because they are associated with a routine activity.

The possible consequences of current unsafe practices should be considered, especially if there is a potential for severe injury. For instance, if an individual currently uses a microwave oven, he or she should be instructed on the safe use of a microwave oven, including

Table 1. Safety concerns and related skills

HOME SAFETY

Kitchen
- Handling hot stove/oven
- Recognizing marked poisons
- Safe use of appliances
- Safe use of knives
- Detecting bad meat/food
- Not climbing into refrigerator/freezer
- Avoiding sharp corners on cabinets
- Reacting to cooking fires

Bathroom
- Recognizing marked poisons
- Shower/bathtub safety
- Adjusting water temperature
- Using hot hair appliances
- Care on wet floors

General Home Areas
- Picking up toys on stairs
- Electric sockets/cords
- Dialing emergency phone numbers
- Caution around glass doors/windows
- Safe tool/appliance use
- Cleaning up broken items
- Not using appliances during electric storm
- Safe use of scissors
- Changing light bulb
- Locking/unlocking doors
- Not playing with matches/lighters

OUTDOORS

Yard/Playground
- Safe use of tools (lawn mower)
- Not climbing trees
- Reacting to thunderstorms
- Keeping driveway clear
- Operating electric garage opener
- Safe use of gym equipment
- Staying inside boundaries
- Not pushing others
- Staying away from power sources
- Recognizing poisonous plants/berries
- Lighting a barbecue grill safely

Animals
- Reacting to dangerous animals
- Being careful around mother with young

(*continued*)

Table 1. (*continued*)

- Being careful around injured animals
- Not feeding strange animals
- Avoiding animals that are eating
- Calling humane society about strays
- Interacting with familiar animals

Bicycle
- Reflectors/lights when dark
- Not showing off
- Using bell/horn
- Staying aware of others
- Keeping to right of road
- Using turn signals
- Avoiding drain grates, gravel
- Avoiding parked cars
- Keeping hands/feet out of spokes

Walking Trips
- Informing others of one's destination
- Asking for directions
- Walking on sidewalk
- Facing traffic
- Carrying address, phone number, money
- Following traffic signs
- Using crosswalks
- Looking both ways before crossing

Car/Bus
- Using seat belts
- Not disturbing driver
- Keeping head/arms inside vehicle
- Knowing emergency exits
- Exiting vehicle away from traffic
- Not pushing on bus
- Staying calm in accident
- Proper bus stop behavior
- Sitting near bus driver when bus is uncrowded
- Moving if bothered by strangers
- Changing seats in moving bus
- Entering/exiting bus
- Standing in moving bus

Water Recreation
- Sunburn protection
- Swimming in pairs
- Communicating with lifeguard
- Not pushing others
- Using life jacket on boat
- Boat safety
- Aiding drowner
- Leaving water during storm
- Avoiding heat exhaustion
- Drinking fluids
- Wearing hat in hot sun

Camping/Hiking
- Recognizing poisonous plants
- Staying on trails
- Putting out campfires
- Thunderstorm safety
- Using whistle if lost
- Checking in with others
- Reacting to dangerous animals
- Using insect repellent

Cold Weather
- Dressing warmly
- Avoiding thin ice
- Aiding person who has fallen through ice
- Riding sleds
- Recognizing hypothermia or frostbite signs

Night
- Using flashlight
- Staying under street lights

CONCERNS ACROSS CATEGORIES

Fire
- Safe use of fire extinguisher
- Responding to fire/smoke alarms
- Awareness of exit signs
- Feeling doors for heat
- Leaving burning building
- Going to window for help
- Calling fire department
- Keeping gasoline away from heat
- Reacting to person on fire
- Not smoking in bed
- Safe use of matches/lighters

Disaster Procedures
- Reacting to floods
- Reacting to earthquakes
- Reacting to hurricanes

First Aid
- Treating injuries
- Treating burns
- Treating insect bites
- Removing objects from eye
- Removing splinters
- Calling ambulance/911
- Getting help from others
- Using first-aid kit
- Recognizing signs of illness

Meals
- Chewing before swallowing
- Using utensils properly
- Eating hot foods
- Choking procedures
- Serving hot liquids/foods
- Not eating on floor/ground

Strangers
- Recognizing strangers
- Responding to lures
- Caution in public bathrooms
- Avoiding dangerous areas
- Not talking to strangers
- Avoiding empty elevators
- Attracting attention when attacked

Personal Privacy
- Saying "no" to physical approaches
- Knowing one's private body parts
- Knowledge of safe sex
- Saying "no" to drugs

Adapted from Collins, Wolery, & Gast (1991).

how to avoid steam burns and how to treat them if necessary. Another consideration is the frequency with which an individual participates in an activity that exposes him or her to a potential danger; the more frequent the exposure, the more immediate the need for instruction. If a person rarely answers the door and is never left entirely alone, behaviors associated with the safe answering of the door may not be a priority. However, as the person becomes more independent, this type of behavior may become a priority, particularly if a transition plan includes an apartment living arrangement.

A final consideration in prioritizing the instruction of safety skills is the recommendation or request of a parent, teacher, or other individual who lives with, teaches, or supervises the person being taught. As previously mentioned, parental concerns and requests should be directly addressed to encourage cooperation and participation in the community-referenced curriculum. Failure to respond to parental concerns could jeopardize the frequency of the child's community outings with the family and possibly his or her community-based instruction at school.

TEACHING IN NATURAL CONTEXTS

Teaching in natural contexts entails teacher decisions regarding where, when, what, and how to teach targeted skills. Although community-based instruction should be the aim of all educational programs, it may not always be practical or safe. In the area of safety skills instruction, initial teaching may need to occur in more controlled environments. However, assessment of a learned safety skill should always be based on the individual's behavior under natural conditions.

This section forwards recommendations for teaching safety skills in as low-risk, but realistic, a setting as possible. The primary concept that should guide all decisions related to safety skills instruction is the *Principle of Least Dangerous Assumption* (Donnellan, 1984). This principle states that when two or more approaches are equally effective based on the most recent research or when there are no data available to support either approach under consideration, the approach that is believed to cause the least amount of harm should be chosen.

Where to Teach

As suggested earlier, the initial teaching of safety skills may need to occur in a simulated, rather than a natural, environment. Gast and Wolery (1988) present several reasons for teaching in simulation:

> First, simulations permit frequent instruction where repeated practice of target skills is possible; that is particularly important with safety skills since dangerous events may occur frequently in the natural environment. Second, simulations permit investigators to stage necessary environmental effects without exposing students to undue danger (e.g., use of dry ice to stage smoke, use of informed confederates to function as threatening strangers). Third, simulations permit investigators to modify materials (e.g., use of water rather than vodka in offering alcohol, use of dull knives in cutting), and task sequences (e.g., placement of casserole in cool oven prior to setting temperature, changing light bulbs with the lamp disconnected) to obtain functional effects of safe practices. Fourth, simulations permit investigators to program variations of tasks and conditions during acquisition that are similar to generalization situations (e.g., vary the appearance of persons who may lure them to unsafe situations). Fifth, simulations may reduce the costs of training (e.g., staff time, transportation, expenditure for materials). Sixth, simulations allow instruction to occur more easily with small groups and with non-handicapped peers serving as models. (pp. 4–5)

Although not specific to safety skills instruction, Nietupski et al. (1986) suggest the following guidelines for teachers interested in the development of effective simulations:

1. Inventory community settings to identify the range of behaviors that will need to be taught. Pay particular attention to the types of equipment, materials, and arrangements for which the individual should be prepared.
2. Pinpoint the range of behaviors that will allow the learner to prevent, escape, or avoid a dangerous situation.

3. Make the simulated environment as similar to the natural environment as possible by increasing the number of shared characteristics between the actual and simulated settings.
4. Regularly assess the learner's behavior in community settings to determine if the target skills have generalized. When possible, structure concurrent instruction under simulated and natural conditions.
5. Modify the simulated environment based on assessment of the learner's performance under natural conditions. It is not uncommon in the initial analysis of community settings to overlook subtle, yet critical, characteristics. This step recognizes that fact and advocates modifications based on a functional analysis of student behavior and a reassessment of the physical and social environments.
6. Even if instruction can occur in the natural environment, use the simulated setting for repeated practice.

A major drawback of some community-based instruction is that it typically does not allow for frequent learning opportunities. When this is the case, practice in the simulated environment can supplement the community-based instruction. Despite the logistical and control-related advantages of instruction under simulated conditions, the true test of success for safety skills training is based on performance under natural conditions in which the settings, persons, equipment, and materials are varied. Therefore, at minimum, weekly generalization tests are recommended to ensure that the safety skills being taught are functional for the learner.

When to Teach

Not only is the natural environment recommended for teaching functional safety skills, but teaching within the context of a learner's natural routine is also highly recommended. For example, the appropriate time for teaching how to clean up broken glass is during a dishwashing activity when dropping and breaking a glass is likely; not to leave with a stranger is best taught during community outings to the mall, park, or theater; and so on. Holvoet, Guess, Mulligan, and Brown (1980) describe this teaching method under what they refer to as the individualized curriculum sequencing (ICS) model. A basic tenet of this model is that "students should not be taught skills in isolation, but that skills should be taught in context of behavior clusters" (p. 340). Holvoet et al. (1980) advocate teaching target behaviors across the day, as well as in the context of natural routines, rather than during a conveniently scheduled mass trial session. In general, mass and spaced trial instructional sessions should be used when an individual requires repeated practice of a behavior that he or she is having difficulty learning or performing fluently (Bambara & Warren, 1993).

What to Teach

Specific safety skills to be taught are identified by the ecological inventory. In conducting this environmental and activity assessment, it is important to identify the range of stimuli or cues associated with each setting, activity, appliance, or material that may signal a dangerous or potentially dangerous situation. These natural cues should be recreated by the teacher in conditions that closely approximate natural conditions, while minimizing the risk to the student.

An example of simulated conditions is provided by a study conducted by Gast, Wellons, Young, Vail, and Clees (1992), in which students with mental retardation were taught to discriminate spoiled and fresh foods using their visual and olfactory senses. Because of the unnecessary risks involved with using real spoiled foods, simulations of spoilage were devised, with particular attention given to the most salient cue. Dairy products (e.g., milk, yogurt) and foods made with dairy products (e.g., potato salad) were made to smell spoiled by rubbing limburger cheese (a *very* potent smelling cheese) on the containers. Bread and canned vegetables and fruits were made to look moldy by adding clothes dryer lint. In this way, students were able to learn the fresh versus spoiled discrimination, without risk.

The ecological inventory may reveal an exceedingly large number of natural cues that could signal a dangerous situation. In such cases, it is typically not feasible to teach a student to respond to every cue. To address this problem, a general case approach is recommended. This strategy facilitates behavior generalization to nontrained conditions (Albin & Horner, 1988). The general case programming strategy, as it relates to safety skill instruction, involves the following steps:

1. Identify the range of stimulus conditions or cues that may signal the need for a particular safe response.
2. Determine safe response variations for each dangerous situation being trained.
3. Select a set of cues to be used during instruction that will sample the range of natural cues that signal an unsafe condition. Teaching examples should include the most common and obvious cues, as well as the least common and more subtle cues.
4. Develop a set of test situations for the assessment of response generalization to novel unsafe conditions.
5. Teach the appropriate safe response to each of the dangerous situation cues being trained.
6. Test for safe response generalization by using a sample of nontrained dangerous situation cues.

Following this strategy for identifying the conditions to which an individual should respond increases the likelihood that the targeted skill will be functional. If the learner fails to exhibit generalized safe responses to nontrained test conditions, it is necessary to train him or her to respond to these new conditions, as well as to those already learned. Adherence to the general case strategy, in conjunction with teaching within the context of natural routines, teaches students to respond to those natural cues that signal the possibility of danger and the need for appropriate action.

How to Teach

Because there are few studies in the special education and applied behavior analysis literatures that have focused on teaching safety skills to children or adults with disabilities, recommendations on how to teach safety skills should be viewed as tentative and subject to formative evaluation. Nevertheless, Gast and Wolery (1988) have forwarded the following guidelines:

> First, the procedure should minimize errors during acquisition as well as promote proficient responding. Errors potentially will expose students to unnecessary risk or harm; thus, should be avoided. Second, the procedure must be applicable for teaching chained tasks in the context of an activity model (e.g., total task presentation format). Third, the procedure must be appropriate for use in the natural environment with naturally occurring material and stimuli. Thus, the procedure must not appear intrusive, restrictive, or harmful to students. Fourth, the procedure must be able to be used with high procedural reliability by a variety of teaching staff (e.g., teachers, teacher assistants). To be implemented with high reliability, the procedure should be relatively simple and easy to implement with few "on-the-spot" decisions. Fifth, the procedure must be generalizable across skills, situations, and students. Sixth, the prompts provided to ensure correct responding should be easily faded and should require minimal teacher preparation time. Seventh, the procedure should be amenable to small group, dyad, and one-to-one instructional arrangements. (p. 3)

These criteria for selecting instructional procedures are consistent with previously recommended guidelines for teaching individuals with mental retardation other functional, community-referenced skills (Wolery, Ault, & Doyle, 1992). Several instructional methods have been identified as being "errorless" or near errorless in teaching this population. These procedures include progressive and constant time delay (Handen & Zane, 1987), system of least prompts (Doyle, Wolery, Ault, & Gast, 1988), most-to-least prompting (Demchak, 1990), stimulus shaping, stimulus fading, and stimulus shaping or fading with superimposition (Etzel & LeBlanc, 1979). The latter methods are discussed in Chapter 1 of this volume.

Although errorless or near errorless learning is associated with each of these strategies, stimulus shaping and stimulus fading do not lend themselves to teaching response chain skills in a total task presentation format. These stimulus modification procedures, however, may be appropriate for teaching students to direct their attention to the critical characteristics of an unsafe condition through the use of stimulus prompts. The remaining procedures, all of which are response prompting strategies, have been found effective in teaching individuals a variety of community-referenced skills (Snell, 1993).

Two procedures that have an extensive history of effectiveness, but require on-the-spot decisions that tend to lengthen the time of instructional trials, are the most-to-least prompting procedure and the system of least prompts. These two procedures are recommended for students who are not imitative or who require a physical prompt to perform the skill. If a student is imitative and can respond appropriately to a teacher's model or gestural or verbal prompt, a progressive or constant time delay procedure is recommended. Both these procedures meet all the criteria previously stated. Constant time delay (CTD) and progressive time delay (PTD) have been used successfully to teach a variety of discrete (object naming, sight word reading) and chain (food preparation, bed making) response skills. Typically, response chain skills have been learned with less than 10% errors using CTD or PTD. For a comprehensive description of progressive and constant time delay procedures, see Wolery et al. (1992).

Figure 1 presents a sample lesson plan that utilizes a time delay prompting procedure for teaching correct responding when confronted with dangerous objects. A 4-second constant time delay procedure is used to teach a student to verbalize the correct response to the sighting of a dangerous object. This is accomplished through the presentation of a sequence of photographs that show different people coming in contact with various dangerous objects. The learner is then asked what the pictured person should do. In the initial session, the teacher asks the question and immediately provides the controlling prompt (a verbal model of safety rules). In all subsequent sessions, a 4-second delay is inserted between the presentation of the question and the delivery of the controlling prompt.

After reaching the criterion level, demonstration of the correct safety responses are assessed outside of the training setting. Should the student fail to exhibit the motor behavior that corresponds to the verbal safety rule, direct instruction on the motor responses will occur. Assessment will take place in a variety of natural settings with a variety of "dangerous" objects. Maintenance of the behaviors will be tested at a minimum of once every 2 weeks.

PREPARATION OF THE TRAINING ENVIRONMENT AND MATERIALS

Instruction of safety skills should always be conducted in an environment where the learner is not exposed to unnecessary risks or dangers. Until the individual is able to perform certain safety behaviors independently, it is the responsibility of the educator to ensure that precautionary measures are taken specific to the skill being taught. For example, during a food preparation activity that requires the use of an electrical appliance (e.g., toaster oven), basic precautions should be taken, such as ensuring the presence of a fire extinguisher, baking soda, and first-aid kit within the kitchen area; examining the placement of the electrical cord on a regular basis; maintaining heat-resistant surfaces; placing all flammable materials at a safe distance from the appliance; and seeing that the learner is not wearing loose fitting or highly flammable clothing. Such precautionary measures may be identified through an examination of similar instructional programs, role playing in the instructional setting, visual inspection of the area, adherence to general appliance manufacturers' guidelines, and review of established safety regulations specific to the skill in training.

Part of preparing the environment for instruction includes adapting potentially danger-

Instructional objectives: When confronted with a dangerous object on the school grounds, the learner will not touch the object and will tell an adult what was found along with its location within 3 minutes of approaching the object (within 5 feet) with 100% accuracy in three sessions over a 3-day period.

Precautions: All dangerous objects will have been made safe or simulations will be used (e.g., plastic bottle pieces to simulate broken glass).

Setting/materials/equipment: Initial instruction will be carried out in a small group instructional setting in the classroom. Verbal responses to the question, "What should he or she do?" will be taught in response to photographic sequences in which individuals come in contact with various unsafe objects. Representations will vary within classes with multiple examples of items used and rotated throughout the training sessions. Untrained items from these classes will be used in assessing generalization. Demonstration of the skills in the natural environment will take place in various locations on school grounds.

Response components: Demonstration or verbalization of the three responses will be recorded in each session. During training, the learner will verbalize the following responses:

1. "Don't touch."
2. "Tell an adult what was found."
3. "Tell an adult where it is."

Demonstration requires the learner to perform the three responses outside of the instructional setting.

Instructional procedures: A 4-second constant time delay procedure will be used during group training. In the initial session, the teacher will present the picture sequence and ask the student what the individual in the picture should do. The teacher will immediately provide the learner with the correct verbal responses. Correct responding requires verbal imitation of the three rules. In all subsequent sessions, a 4-second delay will be inserted between the presentation of the teacher's question and delivery of the controlling prompt. Multiple examples of training items within the class of objects will be systematically rotated throughout sessions. Each student in the group will receive five trials per session. Descriptive verbal praise will be delivered for correct responding, with learners selecting a back-up reinforcer from a reinforcement "menu" at the conclusion of each session if no errors were made.

Evaluation: Individual assessment of the generalization of corresponding motor responses to areas outside of the training setting will be conducted, following achievement of the 100% unprompted correct level of responding in group training. Should individual data reveal that the learner is not performing to criterion level, a return to training will occur, which will require the learner to demonstrate both verbal and motor responses under role-play conditions. Following assessment in the natural environment, maintenance of the learned behaviors will be assessed at a minimum of once every 2 weeks.

Figure 1. Lesson plan: Responding to dangerous objects.

ous materials and equipment (e.g., kitchen knives, guns, lighters) to make them safer for use by the learner. Examples of material adaptations include filing down sharp blades, removing firing pins from firearms, draining butane from disposable lighters, covering sharp points with clear plastic shelving material, and removing tips from matches. Whenever possible, it is preferable to use real materials that have been adapted and made safe rather than to use simulated materials (e.g., a cardboard knife, toy gun). While the primary concern in the preparation of materials and equipment must be the learner's safety, the need to maintain realism is critical if target safety behaviors are to be functional in the natural environment. The following steps will assist in identifying adaptations and safety precautions that may be necessary during instruction:

1. List all identifying features of the object or situation based upon an examination of sensory areas.
2. List and prioritize safety-related features based upon the most salient cue(s) identifying the object as unsafe or dangerous (e.g., hot steam—visual; spoiled milk—olfactory).
3. Determine which (if any) of the features may be adapted to make the object safe while retaining a realistic appearance (e.g., steam—dry ice; spoiled milk—limburger cheese).

4. After adapting the materials, secure the opinions of others regarding the object's degree of safety and realism.
5. Determine whether to use the actual object, make further changes, or prepare to use a simulated version of the real material (e.g., rubber knife).

When real objects cannot be made safe through adaptations, or when adaptations are impractical, the effects of simulation may be achieved through substitution. Examples of simulation through substitution include the use of miniature breath mints as medication and cut plastic bottle pieces as broken glass. The realistic effect required for instruction may also be achieved through altering an imitation of an unsafe object (e.g., removing logos from toy guns, using powder to lessen gloss of plastic snakes). Features that detract from the substituted object's realistic appearance must be examined to determine whether alterations could eliminate its unrealistic image. If possible, the object may then be adapted to produce a realistic version of the training item.

In many cases, the use of simulations allows for realistic presentation; however, simulated objects, features, or sensations may not always be appropriate for instructional use. The most obvious reason why some simulations are inappropriate is the cost of duplication. Although there is a technology for simulating explosions or producing robotic animals that appear rabid, the expense of such simulations is beyond the means of most school districts. In such cases, it may be necessary to use a photograph or video format to set the occasion for the target safety response.

A second concern relates to creating excessive fear in students. As previously mentioned, the educator may use a role playing or story telling approach. The problem with these teaching formats can be the lack of generalization to the natural environment. Only through direct testing of the target behavior under natural conditions can instructors be assured that the safety skill taught is functional.

Finally, the use of simulations involves the difficulty of safely duplicating an object or sensation. Some sensations, such as heat from a hot appliance, require regulation by the instructor. In order to provide the sensation of heat realistically, while ensuring the safety of the learner, precautions must be incorporated into the instructional program. These precautions may include the adjustment of heat regulators or the substitution of warm items for hot items through "sleight of hand." True temperatures should not be permitted until the learner has reached a predetermined level of safe responding.

TEACHING SAFE RESPONSES TO SKILL-RELATED ACCIDENTS

During the performance of many skills, incorrect responding could result in an immediate danger to the learner. In order to reduce the number of risks associated with teaching many functional skills, potentially dangerous steps of a task analysis must be pinpointed during the development of the instructional program. In particular, those programs that require a student's direct contact with an object that has the capacity to inflict some form of discomfort or injury (e.g., cut, poison, burn) need to address this concern.

Through careful examination, the teacher can designate the specific steps of a task analysis that will require training of a safety response to prevent injury if the steps are performed incorrectly. For example, if during a cooking activity an individual were to spill soup on a hot burner while stirring, he could burn himself if he tried to clean up the spill without proper instruction. Similarly, if a learner were to cut herself while slicing vegetables, she may not know what to do. It is recommended that the teacher identify and break down the *task performance skill* (e.g., making microwave popcorn) and all associated *accident response skills* (e.g., responding to a steam burn due to improper opening of the popcorn bag). In this way, the teacher will be alerted to possible dangers associated with various tasks and will identify needed precautions prior to the initial instruction.

Following acquisition of the task performance skill, the individual should be taught each of the identified accident response skills. If an actual accident should occur during initial instruction, the teacher may use this naturally occurring opportunity to teach the appropriate accident response skill. Figure 2 presents a lesson plan for teaching coffee maker useage and related accident response skills. Precautionary measures are taken to ensure the learner's safety.

Figure 3 provides a breakdown of the task analyses for both skills in the lesson plan, the discriminative stimulus and the response the learner should perform for each step. The system of least prompts procedure is used to teach both of these chained tasks. Following probe sessions to determine the learner's present performance levels, training of the new performance skill begins with a presentation of the materials and the task request. The three types of prompts to be used are the verbal prompt, material prompt, and gestural prompt. Each prompt level provides an increasing amount of assistance to the learner.

Correct responding results in the delivery of descriptive verbal praise and consumption of the prepared item at the conclusion of each session. Following training of the task performance skill using multiple exemplars of the materials, training of the accident response skill begins, using the same type of prompts,

Instructional objectives: When presented with a coffee maker, materials necessary to prepare a warm drink, and the task direction to make a drink, the student will prepare the drink following the designated steps, initiating each step within 3 seconds of the discriminative stimulus from the previous step with 100% accuracy in three sessions over a 3-day period.

When presented with a hot liquid spill and asked to clean the spill from the surface, the student will clean the spill following the designated steps, initiating each step within 3 seconds of the discriminative stimulus from the previous step with 100% accuracy in three sessions over a 3-day period.

Precautions: Availability of fire extinguisher and first aid kit in area, inspection of electrical cords, removal of flammable materials from area, inspection and correction of student's clothing to ensure that no contact with heat occurs.

Setting/materials/equipment: Initial instruction will be carried out in the sink area of the classroom. Generalization of the skill will also be assessed in the teacher's lounge of the school and in the learner's home. Materials required for instruction at the sink area include coffee makers, preferred drinks, plastic mugs, spoons, and sponges. These materials will vary in size, color, and/or form in order to provide multiple examples of training materials.

Instructional procedures: A least to most prompting procedure will be used to teach these skills. Prior to initiation of training sessions, assessment of the learner's current level of performance in both chained tasks will take place over a minimum of three sessions. Training of the appliance skill will begin with the teacher providing the training materials and delivering the task direction to make a drink. The learner will then be given 3 seconds to initiate the first step of the task analysis. Correct responding will be reinforced with verbal praise. If the student responds incorrectly or not at all, a verbal prompt is delivered and the student is given another opportunity to respond. If necessary, two additional prompts will be provided, thereby increasing the level of assistance (i.e., a material prompt, showing a picture card of the correct response, and a gestural prompt, pointing to materials required to perform the response). These procedures will be followed for each step of the task analysis. The student will perform each step in response to the discriminative stimulus of the previous step and with assistance provided by the prompts when necessary.

Sessions will continue until the learner meets the 100% level of correct responding in three sessions over a 3-day period. Consumption of the drink will be permitted at the end of each session during training of both tasks to reinforce the behavior. Upon reaching criterion with the appliance skill, training of the related accident response skill will begin. Procedures, prompt levels, and reinforcement delivery identical to those used in teaching the appliance skill will be used. Training sessions for the safety skill will continue until the student reaches the 100% level of correct responding in three sessions over a 3-day period.

Evaluation: Assessment of the skill will occur in the school's teachers' lounge and in the learner's home. Should data reveal that the individual is not performing to criterion level in the different settings, additional training sessions in those settings will be conducted. Following achievement of the 100% level of accuracy, maintenance of the learned skills will be assessed at a minimum of once every 2 weeks.

Figure 2. Lesson plan: Using a coffee maker and related accident response skills.

Appliance skill: Coffee maker usage

Discriminative Stimulus	Response
1. Materials on counter, coffee maker unplugged, switch in "off" position. Teacher provides general task request.	1. Learner plugs coffee maker into outlet.
2. Coffee maker plugged into outlet.	2. Learner removes pot by handle.
3. Empty pot with pouring lid in place.	3. Learner removes pouring lid.
4. Empty pot with pouring lid removed.	4. Learner fills pot halfway with cold tap water.
5. Pot is half filled with cold water, no pouring lid.	5. Learner replaces pouring lid.
6. Pot is half filled with cold water, pouring lid in place.	6. Learner opens reservoir lid.
7. Pot is half filled with cold water, pouring lid on, reservoir lid open.	7. Learner pours cold water into reservoir.
8. Water poured into reservoir.	8. Learner closes reservoir lid.
9. Water in reservoir, lid closed, pot empty.	9. Learner places pot on burner.
10. Water in reservoir, lid closed, empty pot on burner.	10. Learner pushes switch into "on" position.
11. Coffee maker makes final surge and becomes silent, no water dripping.	11. Learner removes pot by handle and pours hot water into cup until cup is three-quarters full.
12. Cup is three-quarters full of hot water.	12. Learner replaces pot on burner.
13. Partially emptied hot pot on burner.	13. Learner pushes switch to "off" position.
14. Coffee maker turned off with remaining hot water in pot.	14. Student unplugs coffee maker.

Accident response skill: Hot liquid spill clean-up

Discriminative Stimulus	Response
1. Hot liquid spilled, teacher tells student to clean up spill.	1. Student replaces pot on burner.
2. Hot liquid on countertop.	2. Student gets sponge from sink.
3. Hot liquid on countertop, student holding sponge.	3. Student places sponge over hot liquid.
4. Sponge placed over hot liquid spill.	4. Student allows minimum 5 seconds for liquid to absorb and cool.
5. Liquid absorbed into sponge on spill.	5. Student lifts sponge, places it in sink.
6. Sponge with hot spill in sink.	6. Student turns on cold water, rinses sponge.
7. Sponge saturated with cold water in sink.	7. Student turns off cold water, wrings out sponge.
8. Spilled liquid cleaned from countertop, student with sponge.	8. Student places sponge to dry at sink following final rinse.

Figure 3. Task analyses: Task performance and accident response skills.

variety of materials and settings, and delivery of reinforcement. After meeting the criterion performance level, maintenance of the learned skills is assessed a minimum of once every 2 weeks.

TEACHING SAFE RESPONSES TO SOCIAL DANGERS

Although Chapter 11 of this volume focuses specifically on crime prevention and personal safety, we feel this issue to be such an integral part of home and community safety that it warrants mention here. In addressing this important issue, we will discuss teaching safe responses to social dangers by utilizing the same behavioral-instructional strategies we have presented thus far. Those wishing further information on this topic should refer to Chapter 10.

The potential for encountering social dangers, such as abduction and abuse, exists both in the home and community and has become an undeniable reality. The National Center for Missing and Exploited Children (1990) reported 24,655 cases of missing children during their first 5 years of operation. Of these, 920 were classified as nonfamily abductions (e.g., strangers, acquaintances, babysitters), with 199 children located alive, and 119 found deceased. Although figures are unavailable as to the number of individuals with disabilities who have been abducted, the abduction and murder of a woman with intellectual disabilities reported by the *Lexington Herald-Leader* (1990) provides one example of how an individual with disabilities may be an "easy mark" for strangers.

National information compiled by the Lexington Child Abuse Council (1991) revealed that 2.4 million children were reported as child abuse cases (physical, emotional, or sexual) to child protective service agencies in 1989. Among the reported cases were 1,237 abuse-related deaths. There are data to indicate a correlation between child abuse and parental stress associated with having a child with disabilities (Gallagher, Beckman, & Cross, 1983). In addition, the growing number of "latchkey" children who must fend for themselves while parents work (Heller & Spooner, 1991) and the increased emphasis on providing instruction for individuals with developmental disabilities and mental retardation within the context of the community (Sailor et al., 1986) indicate that the potential for individuals with disabilities to encounter social dangers is increasing. However, the authors believe that with the proper precautions, teaching within the community is well worth the risk.

Several procedures have been documented as effective in teaching responses to social dangers with persons without disabilities. These include discussion of hypothetical scenarios (Stevens & Long, 1982); use of picture cards (Peterson, 1984); role playing within the home (Miltenberger & Thiesse-Duffy, 1988), classroom (Wurtele, 1990), and on school grounds (Poche, Brouwer, & Swearingen, 1981); and videotaped instruction with behavioral rehearsal (Poche, Yoder, & Miltenberger, 1988). Some of the studies that have specifically documented teaching responses to social dangers to individuals with developmental disabilities include a focus on responding to the lures of strangers (Collins, Schuster, & Nelson, 1992; Gast, Collins, Wolery, & Jones, 1993), teaching appropriate social/sexual skills (Foxx, McMorrow, Storey, & Rogers, 1984) and teaching self-protection skills (Haseltine & Miltenberger, 1990; Watson, Bain, & Houghton, 1992).

What Social Safety Skills Should Be Taught

Social safety skills may be grouped into three types:

1. Avoidance or preventive measures
2. Safe practices within potentially dangerous activities or settings
3. Reaction skills when a dangerous situation arises

Like all individuals, it is important that individuals with disabilities be able to respond to strangers at home, on the telephone, or in the community; to give personal information only to the appropriate persons when lost; to recognize the difference between "good" and "bad" touches; and to have an appropriate escape response when confronted with acts of physical aggression. A list of safety concerns compiled from a national survey of special education teachers across disabilities (Collins, Wolery, & Gast, 1992) and from a local survey that included the safety concerns of parents of students with disabilities (Collins et al., 1991) indicated that several social safety skills are considered important for designated age groups. A compilation of these skills is presented in Table 2.

As indicated by the table, the total number of skills considered important for a student appears to increase as the student matures. This may correspond to an increasing level of independence and amount of time spent in the community. Although there is some overlap between skills selected by professionals and by parents, there are also differences as to which skills are considered important, indicating the value of parental input as a measure of social validity in the selection of the skills that will be taught.

Table 2. A compilation of social safety concerns for students with special needs[a]

	Preschool		Elementary		Adolescent	
Skill	Professional	Parent	Professional	Parent	Professional	Parent
Responding to strangers	x	x	x		x	x
Recognizing strangers	x	x	x	x		x
Attracting attention if attacked		x			x	x
Saying "no" to approaches			x		x	x
Getting adult help			x		x	
Using caution in public restrooms				x	x	x
Knowing private body parts				x	x	x
Saying "no" to drugs				x	x	x
Avoiding dangerous sites					x	x
Responding to doorbell/telephone					x	
Avoiding stranger's conversation						x
Refusing stranger's gifts						x
Avoiding empty elevators						x

Source: Collins, Wolery, & Gast (1991).

[a]Note: Xs indicate that 75% of the respondent group identified the skill as important to teach.

Coleman and Apts (1991) identified a number of specific skills that should be taught to children with developmental disabilities whose intellectual ability and level of social maturity make them acceptable candidates for going home from school without supervision. The skills related to social dangers are presented in Table 3; although these were identified by the authors as important for children to know, they would certainly be applicable to adults with developmental disabilities as well. Because these skills pertain to using a house key, crossing streets, identifying routes, and answering the telephone, they may easily be taught within their naturally occurring context. While these skills provide a starting point for identifying social safety skills that should be included in a functional curriculum, an ecological inventory is the most useful tool for individualizing and prioritizing what skills to teach.

Once appropriate skills have been selected, it is imperative that they are analyzed for critical components that will render them functional in an actual situation. A measure of social validity is necessary and can be attained in several ways. First, information from law enforcement experts can be used to validate a response selected for instruction. For example, the police department can be contacted to provide data as to the type of response that has enabled potential victims to escape dangerous situations in the past (e.g., running from a stranger, calling for help). Second, the teacher can practice (or observe others practicing) the target response within the natural setting, in order to identify important variables. For example, the distance a person should remove himself or herself from a dangerous stranger and the amount of time in which a response to a lure from a stranger should be initiated and completed are critical variables that should be predetermined. Third, once a response has been learned, experts can again be contacted to validate whether the response acquired by the learner is functional (e.g., a policeman could pose as a stranger and approach the learner to observe his or her response).

Table 3. Social safety skills of importance for "latchkey" children

Protecting the house key
- Keep house key in pocket, wallet, or purse.
- Keep house key a secret.
- Do not let others play with house key.

Getting home from school
- Take safest route, avoiding intersections, alleys, construction areas.
- Walk with friends when possible.
- Go straight home without stopping.
- Go straight home without talking to strangers.
- Go straight home without accepting gifts or rides from strangers.
- Check doors and windows of house for forced entry before going inside.
- Call parents from neighbor's house if house shows signs of entry by others.
- Lock door when inside house.
- When alone, do not allow strangers to enter house.

Using the telephone
- Do not tell caller you are alone.
- Tell caller parents cannot come to the phone and take message.

Source: Coleman & Apts (1991).

Where Social Safety Skills Should Be Taught

As previously stated, the best way to teach a functional response is to teach that response within its natural context (see section on Teaching in Natural Contexts, this chapter). For example, Gast et al. (1993) found that preschool children with developmental disabilities who were taught to respond to lures within the classroom setting using a constant time delay procedure of prompts did not exhibit generalized responding to community settings until training was actually conducted at community sites. If daily training within the community setting is not possible, training should be conducted using a combination of good classroom simulation and in vivo instruction or, at the very least, periodic testing for generalization within the community setting. In addition, it is important that multiple exemplars of stimuli (e.g., strangers, lure types) be used to facilitate generalization across all potential situations and that testing be conducted using novel exemplars to validate the usefulness or functionality of the response. Training should not be discontinued until the learner has demonstrated the ability to perform the target response across a variety of novel situations.

How Social Safety Skills Should Be Taught

While the potential is always present, dangerous social situations are not daily occurrences. It is not likely that strangers will call or present themselves at the front door on a regular basis. Thus, it is necessary, when possible, to contrive realistic situations in which to practice social safety skills. Role playing is a viable alternative (Gast et al., 1993; Haseltine & Miltenberger, 1990). Teaching procedures are available that can be employed within the context of role playing to prompt the learner through the correct response, while minimizing the likelihood that the learner will perform incorrectly. This increases the opportunity for the learner to experience success, while decreasing the opportunity for the learner to practice an incorrect response.

The time delay prompting procedure (see chap. 1, this volume, section on Fading) is an example of a teaching procedure that has been effective in teaching a response to social dangers within the context of realistic role play (Gast et al., 1993). The delay procedure employs a single controlling prompt (e.g., verbal direction, model, or physical guidance) to guide the learner through the correct response. The type of prompt chosen will depend on the degree of assistance necessary to control the behavior of the learner. During initial instruction, the learner is immediately prompted through the response (0-second delay) upon presentation of the danger (e.g., stranger's lure). In other words, time is not allowed for an error to occur because the learner is immediately prompted through the correct response. During subsequent sessions, a predetermined delay interval (e.g., 3 seconds) is inserted between the presentation of the danger and the prompt, allowing the learner to perform the response independently or to wait for a prompt if assistance is needed. Once criterion performance is reached, the learner has acquired a response that is performed with the desired degree of fluency.

Another near errorless procedure that is recommended is the system of least prompts (Doyle et al., 1988; see also chap. 1, this volume, section on Fading). This procedure allows the teacher to use a hierarchy of prompts from the least to most assistance necessary to guide the learner through the correct response. Once the stimulus that signals danger is presented, the teacher waits a set interval (e.g., 3 seconds) for the learner to respond independently. If the student fails to respond, each level of prompting from least to most intrusive is presented with a delay interval inserted between each level to allow the learner to respond. In the event the student attempts an incorrect response, the response is interrupted by the teacher and the next level of assistance is presented. The trial ends when the student is presented with a level of prompting that produces the desired response. The type and number of prompts selected may vary to include verbal direction, gesture, modeling, and physical guidance.

While systematic teaching procedures, such as progressive and constant time delay and the system of least prompts, increase the likelihood that students will behave in a prudent and safe manner, the power of natural aversive consequences for unsafe behavior cannot be ignored. Although it would be unethical to allow students to experience such consequences intentionally due to the possibility of undesirable side effects (e.g., excessive fear, personal harm), it is important that they learn the potential dire consequences of their unsafe behavior. One approach to this instructional dilemma is to provide learners with "vicarious instruction," that is, to expose them to the natural consequences experienced by others who have failed to behave in a safe manner. Such experiences may be conveyed through the use of newspaper or magazine articles and television programs. The teacher should proceed with caution, however, being alert to each student's reaction to this type of presentation so as not to frighten students unnecessarily.

Some social safety skills are of a nature that prohibits instruction in simulation (e.g., discriminating appropriate and inappropriate touching). In teaching such discriminatory skills, a verbal format supplemented with pictures may be the only acceptable practice. However, once students are taught the discrimination, they should be given the opportunity to practice, through modeling and role play, how they would avoid or escape these situations. To be prudent, particularly with regard to sex-related safety behaviors, teachers should consult with their sex education curriculum coordinator and their school district or agency's policies. It is important to keep in mind that the more discrepant an instructional arrangement is from the conditions under which the safety skills are likely to be needed, the less likely the skills will generalize to a real situation.

Lesson Plans

Figures 4 and 5 illustrate how safe responses to social dangers can be taught to students with mental retardation. Figure 4 presents a lesson plan for teaching a response to the lures of strangers based on a study conducted by Gast et al. (1993) with preschool children with developmental disabilities. This lesson plan uses a constant time delay procedure in combination with multiple exemplars of lure types, strangers, and settings. After the initial 0-second delay trial in which the learner is guided through the correct response, a 3-second delay interval

Instructional objectives: When presented with a lure from a stranger within the community setting, the student will say "no" within 3 seconds of the lure and walk away from the stranger in the direction of an appropriate adult for a minimum of 5 feet within 3 seconds of the verbal response with 100% accuracy over three consecutive opportunities and days.

Precautions: During the sessions, an adult will be stationed between the learner and the street as a safeguard should the student run toward the street or to intervene in the event that the person is actually approached by a real stranger. The student will be monitored across settings for undesirable side effects stemming from the instruction (e.g., nightmares, excessive fear of strangers).

Settings/materials/equipment: Initial instruction will take place in the classroom setting. Once the learner demonstrates criterion performance in classroom simulation, instruction will take place across a minimum of three community settings. A minimum of three "strangers" with varying physical characteristics (e.g., gender, age, hair color, physical build) will be recruited to approach the student. No setting or stranger will be used across 2 days in succession.

Response components: During testing, one point will be given for each of the following response components:

1. Saying "no"
2. Saying "no" within 3 seconds of the lure delivery
3. Moving away from stranger toward an appropriate adult
4. Walking away for a minimum of 5 feet
5. Walking away within 3 seconds of the verbal "no" response.

Instructional procedures: Instruction will consist of a constant time delay procedure within the context of a simulated dangerous approach by a stranger. During the first session, the instructor will immediately (0-second delay) provide the student with verbal prompts for completing the target response (i.e., "say 'no,' " "go get help"). During all subsequent sessions, the instructor will wait 3 seconds before prompting the verbal response and 3 additional seconds before prompting the motor response. Sessions will consist of three trials, one for each of the following lure types:

- Incentive ("Would you like to go get some candy?")
- Authoritarian ("Your mother wants you to go with me.")
- Generalized ("Would you like to go for a walk?")

The order in which the lure types are presented will vary daily. The instructor will provide descriptive praise for correct responses.

Evaluation: The instructor will test for generalization of the response at least once per week by conducting a realistic session using a novel lure, stranger, and setting. Although the student may be performing at criterion level during instructional sessions, training will continue until the student has demonstrated a generalized response to novel exemplars over three sessions.

Figure 4. Lesson plan: Responding to lures of strangers.

Instructional objectives: When alone in the community, the learner will call home from a public pay telephone and give his or her name and location to the person who answers with 100% accuracy across three consecutive sessions.

Precautions: An adult will be positioned near the student to ensure safety during instruction and testing. The student will have the prerequisite skills to safely cross the street, if necessary, in order to get to a public telephone.

Settings/materials/equipment: Instruction will take place on a public pay telephone on the school grounds. The learner will have a variety of coins available, including the quarter needed to place the call. If the target skill fails to generalize to a novel setting once instructional criterion is met, instruction will take place in that setting.

Response components: The following steps will constitute the correct response. An asterisk (*) indicates those responses that signal the correct terminal step of the chain, depending on whether the call results in a busy signal, no answer, or someone answers.

1. Learner approaches telephone.
2. Learner selects quarter from variety of coins.
3. Learner lifts receiver.
4. Learner inserts quarter in coin slot.
5. Learner dials entire home telephone number (7 digits).
6. Learner waits for up to 5 rings (20 seconds) for answer if number is ringing or hangs up receiver if number is busy.*
7. Learner states both name and location if someone answers or hangs up receiver if no one answers.*
8. Learner hangs up receiver when other person terminates call.*

Instructional procedures: Prior to instruction, the instructor will ask the student to state his or her location to ensure the student's awareness of this before the call is placed. Instruction will consist of a progressive time delay procedure within a total task presentation, allowing the student the opportunity to perform each step of the task during each trial. During the first session, the instructor will immediately (0-second delay) provide the student with physical guidance on each step of the task, with the exception of step 7 where the instructor will provide a verbal model for stating the caller's name and location. The delay interval before the corresponding prompt is presented will increase by 1-second increments per session, until a ceiling of 5 seconds is reached. There will be three trials per session. The instructor will provide descriptive praise for each correct response.

Evaluation: The instructor will test for generalization of the response at least once per week by testing the student in the community using novel exemplars of sites and telephones. Failure to generalize to a novel setting will indicate the need to train in that setting. Training and testing will continue in this manner until the student has demonstrated a generalized response across three untrained settings.

Figure 5. Lesson plan: Calling home from a pay telephone and giving necessary information when lost.

is inserted between the stimulus (i.e., the presentation of the lure by the stranger) and the prompt (i.e., verbal direction). This interval allows the learner to perform the correct response if it is known or to wait for help if it is not known. Multiple exemplars of lure types are presented during each session, while the "strangers" vary daily. Once the learner demonstrates acquisition of the correct response within the classroom setting, instruction continues in the community until the learner demonstrates generalized responding to untrained situations during weekly tests, using novel lure types, strangers, and settings.

Figure 5 presents a lesson plan for teaching students to call home and give necessary information from a pay telephone when lost. This example is based on a study by Collins, Stinson, and Land (1992). This lesson plan combines a progressive time delay procedure with in vivo instruction. After the initial 0-second delay trial in which the learner is guided through the correct response, the delay interval between the stimulus (e.g., "call home") and the prompt (i.e., physical guidance or verbal direction) is increased by a 1-second increment per session until a ceiling of 5 seconds is reached. All instruction is conducted on a public pay telephone on the school grounds. Instruction continues until the learner demonstrates generalized responding during weekly tests, using novel settings and telephones. Failure to generalize to an untrained site indicates the need for specific training in that site.

SUMMARY GUIDELINES

The following guidelines should be considered when planning instruction to teach safe responses to physical and social dangers within the home and the community:

1. Use a combination of techniques to determine safety skills that will be useful to the learner. These can include consulting published lists of safety concerns, conducting an ecological inventory to ascertain the learner's present and future environments and activities and to become aware of caregivers' concerns, and interviewing safety experts.
2. Validate the skills that will be taught by having others practice their performance within the natural context to set training criterion. Ask the opinion of professionals when evaluating skills once they are acquired.
3. Take the necessary precautions and be consistent in preparation of the teaching environment and materials prior to each instructional and testing session in order to reduce any unnecessary risks.
4. Whenever possible, conduct and assess training in the natural environment. If instruction must be conducted solely in simulation, be sure to test for generalization in the natural setting.
5. Teach and assess skill generalization using multiple exemplars of stimuli.
6. Consider the use of errorless teaching procedures (e.g., constant time delay) to increase the learner's opportunities to experience success and to decrease practice of unsafe responses.
7. Take advantage of opportunities for vicarious instruction that demonstrate the natural aversive consequences of unsafe responding.
8. For skills that do not lend themselves to realistic simulations, consider discussions that employ hypothetical scenarios. Training materials should be made as realistic as possible in order to facilitate generalization.
9. Conduct periodic testing to ensure that acquired skills are being maintained at criterion levels.

CONCLUSIONS

Preliminary research (Gast et al., 1993; Vail, Gast, Manley, Butts, & Clees, 1992; Wellons, Gast, Young, Clees, & Vail, 1992) indicates that the traditional approach of simply teaching students to recite safety rules (e.g., "don't touch, move away, tell an adult") does not result in behavioral correspondence. This has been shown to be true with preschool and elementary-age children with mental retardation. Whenever possible, natural instructional conditions, such as role playing and realistic simulations, may be the most appropriate formats for teaching safety skills. Certainly, "doing" rather than "saying" is necessary for students to respond appropriately to the lures of a stranger or the presence of a dangerous object.

It is hoped that in the years ahead, applied researchers will investigate the effectiveness of other instructional formats, including videodisc and computer technologies. "Errorless" teaching procedures (e.g., constant time delay), specific strategies, and combinations of strategies (e.g., progressive time delay and stimulus shaping) are in need of further investigation. For researchers interested in methodological issues, research designs that can be implemented in classroom settings and that do not waste valuable instruction time by requiring extended baseline phases (e.g., multiple probe design) merit attention. Only through increased interest in this research area will service providers and caregivers be given the guidelines needed to prepare their students to respond independently to the dangers associated with life in the community. Although such dangers may be infrequent in occurrence, individuals with developmental disabilities must be prepared to respond in an appropriate and effective manner.

REFERENCES

Albin, R.W., & Horner, R.H. (1988). Generalization with precision. In R.H. Horner, G. Dunlap, & R.L. Koegel (Eds.), *Generalization and maintenance: Life-style changes in applied settings* (pp. 99–120). Baltimore: Paul H. Brookes Publishing Co.

Bambara, L., & Warren, S. (1993). Massed trials revisited: Appropriate applications in functional skills training. In R.A. Gable & S.F. Warren (Eds.), *Strategies for teaching students with mild to severe mental retardation* (pp. 165–190). Baltimore: Paul H. Brookes Publishing Co.

Browder, D., & Snell, M. (1993). Daily living and community skills. In M. Snell (Ed.), *Instruction of students with severe disabilities* (pp. 480–525). Columbus, OH: Merrill.

Coleman, M., & Apts, S. (1991). Home-alone risk factors. *Teaching Exceptional Children, 23,* 36–39.

Collins, B.C., Schuster, J.W., & Nelson, C.M. (1992). Teaching a generalized response to the lures of strangers to adults with severe handicaps. *Exceptionality, 3,* 67–80.

Collins, B.C., Stinson, D.M., & Land, L. (1993). A comparison of in vivo and simulation prior to in vivo instruction in teaching and generalized safety skills. *Education and Training in Mental Retardation, 28,* 128–142.

Collins, B.C., Wolery, M., & Gast, D.L. (1991). A survey of safety concerns for students with special needs. *Education and Training in Mental Retardation, 26,* 305-318.

Collins, B.C., Wolery, M., & Gast, D.L. (1992). A national survey of safety concerns for students with special needs. *Journal of Developmental and Physical Disabilities, 4,* 263–276.

Demchak, M.A. (1990). Response prompting and fading methods: A review. *American Journal on Mental Retardation, 94,* 603–615.

Donnellan, A.M. (1984). The criterion of least dangerous assumption. *Behavior Disorders, 7,* 531–556.

Doyle, P.M., Wolery, M., Ault, M.J., & Gast, D.L. (1988). System of least prompts: A review of procedural parameters. *Journal of The Association for Persons with Severe Handicaps, 13,* 28–40.

Etzel, B.C., & LeBlanc, J. (1979). The simplest treatment alternative: Appropriate instructional control and errorless learning procedure for the difficult-to-teach child. *Journal of Autism and Developmental Disorders, 9,* 361–382.

Falvey, M.A. (1989). *Community-based curriculum: Instructional strategies for students with severe handicaps.* Baltimore: Paul H. Brookes Publishing Co.

Foxx, R.M., McMorrow, M.J., Storey, K., & Rogers, B.M. (1984). Teaching social/sexual skills to mentally retarded adults. *American Journal of Mental Deficiency, 89,* 9–15.

Gallagher, J.J., Beckman, P., & Cross, A.H. (1983). Families of handicapped children: Sources of stress and its amelioration. *Exceptional Children, 50,* 10–18.

Gast, D.L., Collins, B.C., Wolery, M., & Jones, R. (1993). Teaching preschool children with developmental disabilities to respond to the lure of strangers. *Exceptional Children, 59,* 301–311.

Gast, D.L., Wellons, J., Young, J., Vail, C., & Clees, T. (1992). *Teaching students with moderate intellectual disabilities to discriminate fresh and spoiled foods.* Unpublished manuscript. The University of Georgia, Safe Activities in Future Environments Project, Athens.

Gast, D.L., Winterling, V., Wolery, M., & Farmer, J.A. (1992). Teaching first aid skills to students with moderate handicaps in small group instruction. *Education and Treatment of Children, 15,* 101–124.

Gast, D.L., & Wolery, M. (1988). *Safe activities for future environments (Project SAFE)* (Grant No. H023C90128). Washington, DC: U.S. Department of Education, Office of Special Education Programs.

Handen, B.L., & Zane, T. (1987). Delayed prompting: A review of procedural variations and results. *Research in Developmental Disabilities, 8,* 307–330.

Haseltine, B., & Miltenberger, R.G. (1990). Teaching self-protection skills to persons with mental retardation. *American Journal on Mental Retardation, 95,* 188–197.

Heller, H.W., & Spooner, F. (Eds.). (1991). Special focus: Latchkey kids. *Teaching Exceptional Children, 23,* 34–51.

Hillman, H.S., Jones, R.T., & Farmer, L. (1986). The acquisition and maintenance of fire emergency skills: Effects of rationale and behavioral practice. *Journal of Pediatric Psychology, 11,* 247–258.

Holvoet, J., Guess, D., Mulligan, M., & Brown, F. (1980). The Individualized Curriculum Sequencing Model (II): A teaching strategy for severely handicapped students. *Journal of The Association of the Severely Handicapped, 5,* 337–351.

Horner, R.H., Jones, D.N., & Williams, J.A. (1985). A functional approach to teaching generalized street crossing. *Journal of The Association for Persons with Severe Handicaps, 10,* 71–78.

Janicki, M.P., Krauss, M.W., & Seltzer, M.M. (Eds.). (1988). *Community residences for persons with developmental disabilities: Here to stay.* Baltimore: Paul H. Brookes Publishing Co.

Jones, R.T., & McDonald, D. (1986). Childhood injury: A prevention model for intervention. *Education and Treatment of Children, 9,* 307–319.

Jones, R.T., Ollendick, T.H., McLaughlin, L.J., & Williams, C. (1989). Elaborative and behavioral rehearsal in the acquisition of fire emergency skills and the reduction of fear of fire. *Behavior Therapy, 20,* 93–101.

Lehman, G.R., & Geller, E.S. (1990). Participative education for children: An effective approach to increase safety belt use. *Journal of Applied Behavior Analysis, 23,* 219–225.

Lexington Child Abuse Council. (1991, October). Lexington, KY.

Lexington Herald-Leader. (1990, July). Lexington, KY.

Meyer, L.H., Peck, C.A., & Brown, L. (Eds.). (1991). *Critical issues in the lives of people with severe disabilities.* Baltimore: Paul H. Brookes Publishing Co.

Miltenberger, R.G., & Thiesse-Duffy, E. (1988). Evaluation of home-based programs for teaching personal safety skills to children. *Journal of Applied Behavior Analysis, 21,* 81–87.

National Center for Missing & Exploited Children. (1990, April). Arlington, VA: Author.

Neel, R.S., & Billingsley, F. (1989). *IMPACT: A functional curriculum handbook for students with moderate to severe disabilities.* Baltimore: Paul H. Brookes Publishing Co.

Nietupski, J., Hamre-Nietupski, S., Clancy, P., & Veerhusen, K. (1986). Guidelines for making simulation an effective adjunct to in vivo community instruction. *Journal of The Association for Persons with Severe Handicaps, 11,* 12–18.

Peterson, L. (1984). The "safe at home" game: Training comprehensive prevention skills in latchkey children. *Behavior Modification, 8,* 474–494.

Peterson, L., & Mori, L. (1985). Prevention of child injury: An overview of targets, methods, and tactics for psychologists. *Journal of Consulting and Clinical Psychology, 53,* 586–595.

Poche, C., Brouwer, R., & Swearingen, M. (1981). Teaching self-protection to young children. *Journal of Applied Behavior Analysis, 14,* 169–176.

Poche, C., Yoder, R., & Miltenberger, R. (1988). Teaching self-protection to children using television techniques. *Journal of Applied Behavior Analysis, 21,* 253–261.

Rivera-Tovar, L.A., & Jones, R.T. (1988). An extension and refinement of telephone emergency skill training: A comparison of training methods. *Behavior Modification, 12,* 445–465.

Sailor, W., Halvorsen, A., Anderson, V., Goetz, L., Gee, K., Doering, K., & Hunt, P. (1986). Community intensive instruction. In R. Horner, L. Meyer, & H. Fredericks (Eds.), *Education of learners with severe handicaps: Exemplary learning strategies* (pp. 251–288). Baltimore: Paul H. Brookes Publishing Co.

Schleien, S.J., & Ray, M.T. (1988). *Community recreation and persons with disabilities: Strategies for integration.* Baltimore: Paul H. Brookes Publishing Co.

Snell, M. (Ed.). (1993). *Instruction of persons with severe handicaps.* Columbus, OH: Merrill.

Snell, M.E., & Grigg, N.C. (1987). Instructional assessment and curriculum development. In M.E. Snell (Ed.), *Systematic instruction of persons with severe handicaps* (pp. 64–109). Columbus, OH: Charles E. Merrill.

Sowers-Hoag, K.M., Thyer, B.A., & Bailey, J. (1987). Promoting automobile safety belt use by young children. *Journal of Applied Behavior Analysis, 20,* 133–138.

Stevens, M.L., & Long, L. (1982). Individual and group training of social and health-related behaviors in young children. *Education and Treatment of Children, 5,* 233–248.

Vail, C., Gast, D.L., Manley, N., Butts, J.J., & Clees, T. (1992). *An assessment of stimulus conditions for teaching safety responses to dangerous items.* Unpublished manuscript, The University of Georgia, Safe Activities for Future Environments Project, Athens.

Watson, M., Bain, A., & Houghton, S. (1992). A preliminary study in teaching self-protective skills to children with moderate and severe mental retardation. *Journal of Special Education, 26,* 181–194.

Wehman, P., & Moon, M.S. (Eds.). (1988). *Vocational rehabilitation and supported employment.* Baltimore: Paul H. Brookes Publishing Co.

Wellons, J., Gast, D.L., Young, J., Clees, T., & Vail, C. (1992). *Teaching students with severe disabilities to respond to dangerous objects.* Unpublished manuscript, The University of Georgia, Safe Activities in Future Environments Project, Athens.

Winterling, V., Gast, D.L., Wolery, M., & Farmer, J.A. (1992). Teaching safe handling of broken materials to students with moderate disabilities during domestic skill instruction. *Journal of Applied Behavior Analysis, 25,* 217–227.

Wolery, M., Ault, M.V., & Doyle, P.M. (1992). *Teaching students with moderate to severe disabilities.* New York: Longman.

Wurtele, S.K. (1990). Teaching personal safety skills to four-year-old children: A behavioral approach. *Behavior Therapy, 21,* 25–32.

Chapter Three

Nutrition and Diet

Mary Ann Harvey Smith

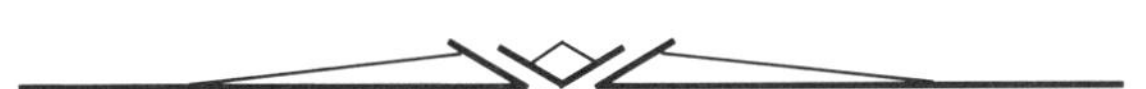

The nutritional needs and requirements for persons with developmental disabilities are not necessarily different from those of other persons of the same age and sex (Smith et al., 1982). As with people without disabilities, every person has unique and individual needs based upon his or her height, weight, metabolism, and, if applicable, physical and psychosocial circumstances. The purpose of this chapter is to report on the nutrient needs of persons with disabilities in terms of daily dietary intake, illustrate the problems that may prevent persons with disabilities from obtaining optimal nutrition, review the current literature on approaches that have been used to assist those with disabilities in nutrition education and food preparation with the goal of enhancing independence, and explore the issues that impinge upon this goal. The importance of nutrition to the health and well-being of persons with disabilities and/or special health care needs cannot be minimized. These individuals must learn the skills that will enable them to cope with the activities of life in the community, including knowledge of nutrition, food selection, preparation, and service.

NUTRITION AND HEALTH

Nutrition is the science of nourishing the body—it involves selecting, preparing, serving, eating, metabolizing, transporting, utilizing, and excreting food (Nieman, Butterworth, & Nieman, 1992). All living organisms have specific nutritional requirements that vary within each stage of growth and development. Recommendations to satisfy these specific nutritional requirements have undergone changes in the past few years as research in nutrition and health has more clearly demonstrated the effects of diet on a number of chronic degenerative diseases.

The United States Department of Agriculture (USDA) and the United States Department of Health and Human Services (DHHS) took the lead in introducing this recent information to the public through *Nutrition and Your Health: Dietary Guidelines for Americans* (USDA & DHHS, 1990). These guidelines were established for healthy individuals, and therefore they do not always apply to those with special dietary needs or specific diseases. However, the publication does offer general principles that may be followed by people with disabilities for the promotion of health and the prevention of disease. Included among thcsc principles are the following recommendations:

1. Eat a variety of foods.
2. Maintain a healthy weight.
3. Choose a diet low in fat, saturated fat, and cholesterol.
4. Eat foods with adequate starch and fiber.

5. Consume sugars, salt, sodium, and alcoholic beverages, only in moderation.

Nutrition scientists are unable to define an "ideal" diet for every individual because food needs vary substantially depending on one's age, sex, body size, physical activity, presence or absence of disease, and special conditions (e.g., pregnancy, some types of disabilities). When asked what constitutes a good diet, nutritionists often hedge the question. The USDA and DHHS dietary guidelines suggest that if people include a variety of foods in their total diet, all nutrients will be included, and if moderation in the intake of fat, saturated fat, cholesterol, sugar, sodium, salt, and alcohol are practiced, normal levels of blood cholesterol will be assured.

These guidelines, however, cannot guarantee perfect health. Individuals are subject to genetic and environmental stressors that may negate the value of nutritional intervention. For most people, these guidelines will ensure a balanced food plan, as well as provide a variety of needed vitamins and minerals.

Figure 1 illustrates the Food Guide Pyramid released by the USDA (1992) to provide guidance to the public about how to use the information included in the national dietary guidelines (Burros, 1992; Ingersoll, 1992). The pyramid is the first graphic to clearly illustrate the importance of moderation in consuming certain groups of food, namely meat, dairy food, fats, and sugars. Its simple, straightforward design well lends itself as a user-friendly menu planning tool for persons with developmental disabilities and mental retardation. Its base is made up of complex carbohydrates, including bread, cereal, rice, and pasta, all of which should provide the most calories in a diet. The next largest portion of the pyramid is made up of two food groups: vegetables and fruits. The third layer of the pyramid includes milk, yogurt, and cheese as one group in an equal portion to another food group representing meat, poultry, fish, dry beans, eggs, and nuts. The tip of the pyramid includes fats, oils, and sweets with a cautionary note to "USE SPARINGLY." At a glance, this graphic conveys that fruits, vegetables, and grains should make up the bulk of a person's diet, with other foods to be eaten less often.

NUTRITION EDUCATION FOR PEOPLE WITH DEVELOPMENTAL DISABILITIES

Teaching nutrition skills to individuals with developmental disabilities involves several related, yet different, areas:

- Meal planning
- Food purchasing
- Meal preparation
- Meal service

It is hoped that, when given the responsibility for determining his or her own eating plan, an individual with developmental disabilities will be able to comprehend the misleading and often controversial information regarding good nutrition, and learn which foods to eat for maintenance of optimal nutrition and health, how to plan menus on limited budgets, and how to prepare and serve meals. Teaching, as well as learning, these skills can be overwhelming. It is not surprising that studies conducted on the dietary intakes of individuals with developmental disabilities have revealed significant nutritional deficits (Green & McIntosh, 1985; Kalisz & Ekvall, 1984; Springer, 1987).

Menu Planning and Grocery Shopping

If individuals with developmental disabilities are to learn basic menu planning using a budget, attention must be paid to the development of teaching materials and references that are appropriate to the learner's level of understanding. Basic menu planning involves preparing lists of foods from every food group, including the approximate cost of each item per serving. Good menus take into consideration many different factors other than cost. These factors include ensuring that a variety of colors, shapes, textures, and types of foods are consumed throughout the day and the week. Also considered are the ease of preparation, length of cooking time, blending of flavors, daily consumption of foods from all levels and groups of

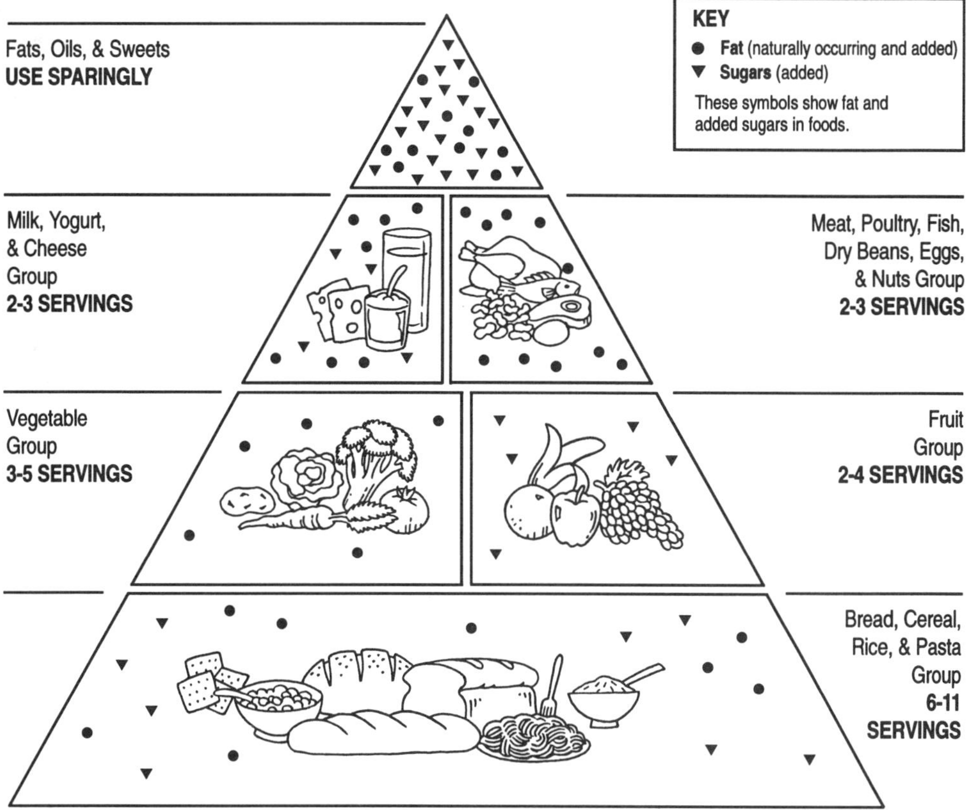

Figure 1. The food guide pyramid. (From United States Department of Agriculture, Human Nutrition Service. [1992]. *The Food Guide Pyramid* [Home and Garden Bulletin, No. 252]. Hyattsville, MD: Author.)

the pyramid, and, of course, the preferences of the consumer.

Suggested instructional activities for teaching menu planning might include using models or shapes representing various food types or constructing written menus. For example, colored pictures of items from each food group can be cut out. Learners can then be directed to plan a meal using various food cutouts in a variety of colors. The activity can be repeated until the learner is able to plan the menu with at least three to four different colors. Finally, the learners may practice writing or drawing menus for 1 day, then 2 days, and so on until a week's plan can be developed.

Frequent practice in the preparation of menus and grocery lists, along with continued reinforcement, are crucial to the maintenance of the behavior when persons with developmental disabilities live independently. Teachers and counselors in group homes or other independent living situations should check residents' menus and grocery lists for accuracy and evaluate them for wholesomeness. A few attempts at developing a comprehensive curriculum for meal planning have been reported; however, these reports do not include experiential and evaluative components (Drieth, 1979; Matson, 1981).

Trips to the supermarket can be intimidating to those who have never been oriented to the thousands of food items available. In teaching grocery shopping, it may be helpful to introduce the learner to a simulated store in the classroom before taking him or her on a field trip to the actual market. Maps illustrating the location of each type of food on the various aisles can assist with this field experience. Guided practice is a recommended method for teaching this skill.

For example, individuals may be guided through the simulated store experience in the classroom, with specific assignments to purchase the items necessary to prepare preplanned meals with a designated shopping list on a preset budget. They could be given food baskets to fill with pictures or other replicas of the food items to be purchased within a given time limit. At the end of the time period, each person would be asked to total the cost of the food items and compare the cost with the preset budget, check the foods chosen to be certain that all necessary items were selected for preparing the meals as planned, and determine if the meals planned for that day were nutritionally complete using the pyramid food guide. Each person would be instructed to repeat these tasks until they are able to master shopping at a preset level of 80%–90% proficiency before being taken to the actual store to shop.

Field trips and study sessions within the store should be scheduled to follow meals. If the learner is not hungry, he or she is less likely to select foods not included on the prepared shopping list. If possible, it is best to begin the shopping experience in a smaller market rather than in a "superstore."

Unique approaches to teaching grocery shopping skills have been reported with varying degrees of success (Gaule, Nietupski, & Certo, 1985; Nietupski, Welch, & Wacker, 1983; Sarber, Halasz, Messmer, Bickett, & Lutzker, 1983; Wheeler, Ford, Nietupski, Loomis, & Brown, 1980). Sarber et al. (1983) used the following methods for teaching these skills to a mother with mental retardation. Pictures of food items were glued to color-coded index cards. Four different colors were used to represent the different food groups, including grains, milk, fruits and vegetables, and meat. A menu-planning chart was used, consisting of pockets arranged in four columns, one for each group of foods, and three double rows, one for each meal. At the bottom of each column was a

Gaule et al. (1985) taught supermarket skills to three males with mental retardation, ranging in age from 17 to 20 years old. The young men were helped in preparing shopping lists by using a *Pictorial Meal Preparation Manual* developed by Bates and Pancsofar (1979). The manual contained picture recipes that were used to devise shopping lists for supermarket items. Recipes were selected based on meal complexity and individual preference. The first page of the recipe contained pictures of the food items and utensils needed to prepare the meal.

Food purchasing was taught to the men with an adaptive shopping aid described by Sarber et al. (1983). This aid was placed in a three-ring binder in the bottom of their shopping carts. The shopping aid contained the food pictures of all of the items in the preselected recipes. Adjacent to each pictured item were squares that denoted the item's approximate cost. A system was established that used Velcro stickers in square shapes to depict the costs: one sticker equaled 1¢–50¢ and two stickers = 51¢–$1.00. Thus, for example, a picture of a quart of milk with a cost of $1.45 had three stickers next to it, whereas a single yogurt costing 45¢ had one sticker next to it.

Another feature of the shopping aid was a numbered money line made up of squares used to determine the total approximate cost for all the items selected. The participants counted the number of dollars available for shopping and used a marking pen to show the amount of available funds on the money line. After each food item was placed in the cart, the number of squares representing the cost of that item were checked off the money line from left to right. If the total number of slashed squares did not exceed the total number of squares representing the full amount of money on hand, a participant knew he had enough money to purchase all items. In addition, each participant could determine the correct number of dollars to give the cashier by reading the number directly below or one square to the right of the last crossed off square.

Data from this study indicated initial skill acquisition by all participants. Partial skill maintenance was reported as much as 4 weeks following training. The authors reported that the costs for such simulations were minimal because food preparation was not a part of the teaching–learning process.

color-coded index card with the number of servings needed per day from that food group and a space for tallying the number of servings planned for the day. The charts were sized to fit onto an 8½ × 11 inch sheet of paper that could be placed in a looseleaf notebook. One chart was used for each day's menus.

The procedure for training included breaking down the learning tasks into small segments. These segments included identifying picture and food group relationships; sorting food cards by groups; choosing the correct number of foods from each group and dividing them into complete meals; and, finally, devising sample menus for breakfast, lunch, and dinner.

Grocery list preparation followed mastery of the meal planning instruction and used the stack of food picture cards, deleting the cards that represented items already on hand from inventory. Each step of the training was repeated until it was mastered successfully. For grocery shopping, the food cards in the binder were used to locate and place foods in the shopping cart. Rather than initially teaching food shopping for all food groups, selection of items from one food group at a time was taught. Once proficiency (90% performance) was achieved, training proceeded to the next food group.

Food Selection and Preparation

Educators who teach food selection and preparation skills to individuals with developmental disabilities should ensure that recommended food products are edible, do not violate any dietary restrictions, are liked by the individuals, and are nutritious (Snell & Browder, 1987). Important ethical considerations arise when educators opt to include foods that are easy to prepare, regardless of their nutritional value, because the program participants are likely to continue to prepare the foods in which they received training (Marchand-Martella, Windham, Wyse, & Martella, 1991). Therefore, lean cuts and types of meats should be used, preparation techniques such as broiling versus frying should be taught, and foods without hidden sources of fat (e.g., palm kernel or coconut oils) should be selected (Marchand-Martella et al., 1991). Training should include appropriate and inappropriate examples of nutritious and healthful foods so that participants will be encouraged to develop discrimination abilities and to plan meals according to the foods they have selected. The case example below illustrates a possible approach to teaching food discrimination to learners with special needs.

Several studies have been conducted in the

Mrs. Jones, the resource room teacher at Schooner High School, decided to teach nutrition skills to students in her class. She sought the help of a dietitian and, with her guidance, developed a program for teaching students to select nutritious and healthful foods. Students in the class were responsible for helping Mrs. Jones cut out pictures of food from popular magazines; additional pictures were obtained from grocery store ads or hand-drawn if necessary. These foods were placed on index cards. Mrs. Jones prepared a lesson (again with the dietitian's help) on the importance of good nutrition and on foods that fit into the USDA Food Guide Pyramid. The pyramid graphic was exhibited and discussed in class, and a model of the pyramid was provided for each student. Following the discussion, Mrs. Jones placed the foods into the different groups and levels of the pyramid; she further divided the index cards into foods that were nutritious and healthful or foods that were high in sugar, sodium, fat, or cholesterol. Based on these two piles of appropriate and inappropriate examples of nutritious and healthful foods, Mrs. Jones had students point to and verbalize which foods they would choose for snacks or meals. Based on every choice, the students had to provide a rationale. Positive or constructive feedback was provided for each selection. For example, if skim milk and whole milk were the choices, the student (unless he or she was underweight) needed to choose skim milk and say, "I would choose skim milk because it is lower in fat." For the next session, Mrs. Jones will bring in packages and containers from real food items (e.g., whole and skim milk gallon jugs) to determine if generalized responding has occurred.

area of food selection and preparation. The teaching techniques used in these studies were quite successful, and those developing their own training programs may wish to follow them. Modifications, in terms of the nutritional values of the foods prepared in these studies, may be appropriate.

Johnson and Cuvo (1981) taught four adults with mental retardation to boil eggs and vegetables, bake cornbread and biscuits, and broil hot dogs and English muffins. Each cooking task was analyzed, and its content validity established by nutrition experts. These task analyses were written on recipe cards used by participants. Training involved a system of least-to-most prompts, ranging from no assistance at all to verbal instruction and physical guidance. Positive and constructive feedback, both graphic and verbal, were provided on the participants' performance. Results showed relatively rapid acquisition of each of the three cooking skills.

Robinson-Wilson (1977) utilized picture recipe cards to teach preparation of gelatin dessert, hot dogs, and hot chocolate to three adults with mental retardation. The pictures were drawn on 5 × 8 inch index cards that provided a task-analyzed approach to preparing each item. One-on-one instruction using the cards was given, including positive or constructive feedback after each step of the recipe was completed. Results indicated that the participants acquired the necessary skills to prepare the three items.

Understanding Nutrition Labels Food labels in the United States are being reformed to make them more user-friendly and accessible to consumers in choosing a healthy diet. The new labelling will be on most foods and will provide specific information on the amount of saturated fat, cholesterol, dietary fiber, and other nutrients per serving. Nutrient reference values will be listed to help shoppers determine how a particular food fits into their meal plans. Uniform definitions for such misunderstood or meaningless terms as "light," "low fat," and "high fiber" will be spelled out. These descriptors are helpful to consumers whose intent is to modify their diets with respect to calories, fat, fiber, or other nutrients. Claims about the relationship between a nutrient and a disease (e.g., calcium and osteoporosis) will be consistent with specified guidelines. Standardized serving sizes will simplify nutritional comparisons. The actual percentage of juice in juice drinks must be specified. Voluntary nutrition information will be provided for many raw foods. The new labels are available as of May 1994, and regulations with regard to health claims are now in effect.

The new food label is titled "Nutrition Facts." A preview of the label as designed by the Food and Drug Administration (1992) is shown in Figure 2. The "Daily Value" comprises two new sets of dietary standards: *Daily Reference Values* and *Reference Daily Intakes.* Only the daily value will appear on the label. Daily values are being introduced for micronutrients that are sources of energy (i.e., fat, carbohydrate [including fiber], and protein) and for cholesterol, sodium, and potassium that do not provide calories. The Daily Reference Values for the energy-producing nutrients are based on the number of calories consumed per day. A daily intake of 2,000 calories is used as a reference.

Reading and Following Recipes Recipe books are available that have been designed using pictographs for those who have difficulties reading (Robinson-Wilson, 1977). Practice in reading recipes is one of the best methods for teaching this skill. After learners have mastered mock-reading and direction-following activities, actual cooking lessons are quite effective because learners are reinforced by tasting the prepared products. Teachers can guide learners to prepare simple recipes with a limited number of ingredients and a few preparation steps.

For example, one simple recipe involves the preparation of a sandwich using two slices of bread, meat or cheese filling, and a spread. Multiple variations can be made. Usually it is best to initiate new cooks with recipes that do not have to be heated. Examples include sandwiches, salads, raw fruits and vegetables, and beverages. As students advance in their cooking skills, more complex recipes can be intro-

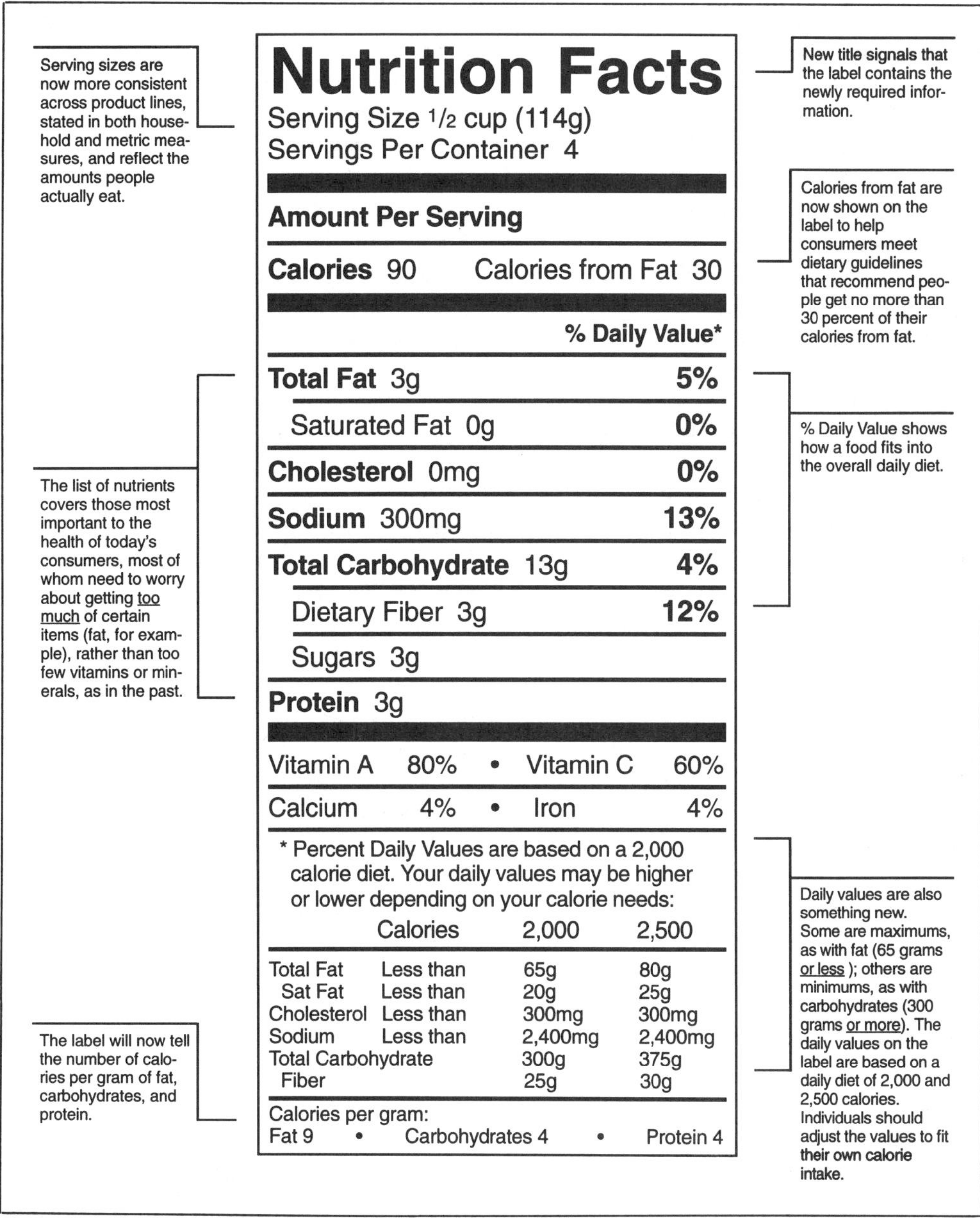

Figure 2. The new food label with easier-to-use nutrition information guide is required on almost all packaged foods. This figure is only a sample. Exact specifications are in the final rules. (From United States Food and Drug Administration. [1992]. *The new food label.* Washington, DC: FDA Backgrounder.)

duced. At this stage, cooking lessons often begin with instruction on how to boil water.

Recipes are already broken down into steps or tasks that simplify the process of learning. These steps may need to be further modified (e.g., break step 2 into three separate steps) to accommodate learners who require greater levels of assistance. Name recognition of various cooking utensils, such as pans, pots, casserole dishes, measuring cups and spoons, spatulas, knives, and cutting boards is an important concept to include in the curriculum for teaching recipe use. In the teaching kitchen or food laboratory, individuals should be taught to identify and assemble all equipment and food items to be used in the recipe prior to beginning the food preparation activity.

Selecting Appropriate Cooking Methods Cooking methods include baking, broiling, boiling, steaming, frying, grilling, and microwaving. Students need to know how to perform each of these as well as the kinds of foods that are usually prepared with each method. Cooking with conventional methods includes using both moist and dry heat. Moist heat methods, such as boiling, cooking in the oven or on the range top with a covered pan, or using a "slow cooker," are used to cook foods that require tenderizing. Baking large cuts of meat in a covered pan or wrapped with aluminum foil is an example of moist heat cooking. Dry heat methods require less time, but are reserved for foods that are already tender. Dry heat methods include broiling, frying, baking without a top or aluminum foil cover, grilling, and microwaving.

Individuals with developmental disabilities who are learning how to prepare food need to understand not only the various methods of cooking, but also how to choose the appropriate length of cooking time and the correct temperatures for each type of food that they wish to prepare. For example, large roasts or hams, even when tender, require longer cooking times and lower oven temperatures. Dried beans and peas require extensive cooking times using slow boiling (simmering); however, the level of the heat must be monitored with additional water added during the cooking period to prevent these legumes from boiling dry and burning.

Convenience foods also play a part in the total menu. Selection of nutritious foods from the vast array of mixes and packaged premade items, such as main dish entrees, pasta salads, pizzas, tacos, and frozen entrees, add even greater diversity to menu planning. These prepared items have directions for heating or cooking directly on the packages. Although aimed at an elementary reading level, the directions may still be too complex for use with persons with developmental disabilities, unless additional, more specific directions are provided.

In selecting these types of foods, students must be taught to read the labels first. Premade items are usually combinations of the different pyramid food groups. Individuals must be taught to separate mixtures by the components within them. For example, lessons could be provided on what is in lasagna (i.e., tomato sauce from the vegetable group, meat from the meat group, ricotta cheese and mozzarella cheese from the dairy group, pasta from the bread and cereal group). By analyzing the preprepared food, individuals can learn to recognize food groups and understand more about nutritional value. Learners should also be made aware that most premade dishes are higher in sodium and other additives and typically cost more than home-prepared versions.

Modifying Recipes for Healthy Food Preparation Favorite recipes can often be modified to reduce their fat, sodium, or sugar content. Through experimentation, the same kind of taste and quality of the original recipe can be achieved. A ready reference to assist individuals with developmental disabilities on how to modify recipes is not available. However, several simple rules from the American Dietetic Association (Hermann, 1991) can be applied to an educational program. These rules include the following:

1. Reduce fat in cooking meats and vegetables by baking, broiling, microwaving, or stewing foods, as opposed to frying them.
2. Decrease the salt content of most recipes by half, or, in the instance of baked products, simply leave out the salt entirely.
3. The amount of sugar can be reduced in cooked items or a sugar substitute may be used in recipes that do not require cooking (e.g., beverages, ice cream, fruit salads). (Aspartame [Equal®] is heat labile and should not be used in cooked dishes.)

Recently, a number of cookbooks have been published that provide low fat, calorie-specific recipes. Although most of these are not directed toward persons with developmental disabilities and the reading levels of these cookbooks have not been determined, many books are relatively easy to read and understand. The

American Dietetic Association has a consumer information hotline (1-800-877-1600) for obtaining information on menu modification and other ideas for improving diets for healthy lifestyles.

Meal Service

Setting the table is a task that can be presented in segments to learners with developmental disabilities. Drawings of items required for correct table settings can be easily made. Students can learn first to recognize and verbalize the names of each utensil and type of dinnerware. Paper or cardboard cut-outs of table appointments may be obtained from department or gift store displays. Repetitive teaching strategies can be used to help each learner become proficient with the cardboard settings before progressing to real dinnerware, flatware, and napkin placement.

Actual eating/serving can also be taught using repetition or practice. Different styles of meal service can be introduced. To keep it simple, the family style service is probably best to teach. The foods are served in bowls or platters and placed on the set table for the group to pass and serve themselves. Another service, the "plate" service, may be applicable, as well. Here, the food is pre-served on each plate and set on the table at mealtime. The "plate" service adapts well to small or large groups. The buffet service is another style that those with disabilities might find useful and one they may already be accustomed to using in large residential cafeterias.

NUTRITIONAL ASSESSMENT OF INDIVIDUALS WITH DEVELOPMENTAL DISABILITIES

Before determining what foods an individual with developmental disabilities might be taught to prepare for himself or herself, or what foods the person should learn to include in his or her own meal planning, it is important that service providers assess the individual's current nutritional status. Unfortunately, the nutritional status of people with developmental disabilities is often less than desirable. Specifically, persons with developmental disabilities may experience problems relating to any of the following:

- Weight problems, including being overweight, obese, underweight, or emaciated
- Specific feeding difficulties, including lack of feeding skills and difficulties in chewing, swallowing, or sucking
- Anemia
- Poor or bizarre eating habits
- Inborn errors of metabolism or other genetic disorders
- Nutritional deficiencies caused by medications
- Growth retardation (Green & McIntosh, 1985; Smith, 1976; Smith et al., 1982)

Specific nutritional deficits often reported include iron, vitamin A, and calcium, with over 40% of some groups of adults with mental retardation receiving less than 50% of the RDAs for one or more nutrients (Green & McIntosh, 1985). Obesity has been shown to occur in almost half of the adults with mental retardation in several studies (Green & McIntosh, 1985). Table 1 shows various syndromes or disabilities and how they impact nutritional status.

In 1976, Smith published guidelines for the nutritional assessment of children with disabilities. These guidelines have not been widely disseminated, and are therefore often inaccessible to caregivers. They are reprinted by permission in Table 2. The suggested standards for comparison mentioned in the table are included in the references. Although Smith focuses specifically on children in these guidelines, Chernoff (1991) identifies the same areas of assessment as Smith as being crucial in the assessment of adults and elderly persons both with and without disabilities.

Improper development, malnutrition, and/or undernutrition have been linked to stunted growth, developmental lags, changes in psychological functioning, difficulties with learning, and even mental retardation (Blyler & Lucas, 1987). Signs of malnutrition may include listlessness, apathy, limited attention span, fatigue, and even improper labeling at a lower degree of intellectual ability than is actually correct (Blyler & Lucas, 1987). Even in individuals with typical development, nutritional

Table 1. Nutrition problems and causes for nutritional risk in persons with developmental disabilities

Syndrome or disability	Altered growth rate/growth retardation	Altered energy needs/intake	Altered nutrient needs, nutrient deficiencies	Constipation, diarrhea	Feeding problems	Others
Cerebral palsy	X	X	X	X	X	Poor appetite, orthopedic problems
Epilepsy			X	X		Dilantin-induced hyperplasia of gums, drug-nutrient interaction
Muscular dystrophy		X		X	X	
Myelomeningocele	X	X	X	X	X	
Cleft lip/palate	X (during infancy)	X	X		X	Orthodontic problems
Down syndrome	X	X		X	X	Gum disease
Prader-Willi syndrome	X	X		X	X	
PKU and other inherited metabolic disorders		X	X		X	May need specialized nutrients/medication
Mental retardation of unknown etiology	X	X		X	X	Drug-nutrient interaction, pica
Autism					X	Drug-nutrient interaction, pica

From Blyler, E., & Lucas, B. (1987). Nutrition in comprehensive program planning for persons with developmental disabilities. *Journal of the American Dietetic Association, 87,* 1070; reprinted by permission.

deficits can impinge upon learning (Smith, 1976). For those who already have developmental disabilities, this additional burden on learning should certainly be avoided.

Individuals with genetic disorders may require nutritional intervention as the key to their survival. For others, sound nutrition plays a preventive role in helping to achieve maximal performance. The diagnosis of malnutrition should be made at as early an age as possible, and its etiology should be determined before devising the plan of care with the help of a physician or registered dietitian (Blyler & Lucas, 1987; Smith, 1976). The following sections address various areas of assessment.

Anthropometric Assessment

Anthropometric assessment is the measurement of the body by weight, height, circumferences, and fat folds (Smith, 1976). Accurate

Table 2. Guidelines for nutritional assessment of persons with developmental disabilities

I. Anthropometric
    A. Purpose: To collect data related to growth and body composition
    B. Levels of assessment
        1. Minimal
            a. Weight*
                (1) Conditions: no shoes, light clothing[a]
                (2) Suggested standard: reference data assembled by National Center for Health Statistics[b]
            b. Height*
                (1) Conditions[a]: recumbent length○
                (2) Suggested standard: reference data assembled by National Center for Health Statistics
            c. Head circumference*
                (1) Conditions: up to age 6 years
                (2) Suggested standard: reference data assembled by National Center for Health Statistics[b]
        2. In-depth
            a. Skin fold: triceps and subscapular desirable[a] *
                (1) Conditions: obtain duplicate readings[a]
                (2) Suggested standard: reference data assembled by Fomon[a] and National Center for Health Statistics[b]
            b. Arm circumference*
                (1) Conditions[a]: desirable, if possible
                (2) Suggested standard: Gurney and Jelliffe nomogram[c]
    C. Equipment specification and maintenance[a]
        1. Calibrated weight scale (balance-type)
        2. Measuring board (stadiometer) for measuring recumbent length or vertical surface with leveler for measuring standing height
        3. Narrow flexible steel or plastic coated tape measure for measuring circumference of head and arm
        4. Calibrated calipers
II. Clinical
    A. Purpose: To observe clinical signs of chronic or subacute disease
    B. Levels of assessment
        1. Minimal review of past and present records of medical and dental examinations for signs suggestive of poor nutritional status
        2. In-depth
            a. Collection of health history with special attention to areas of nutritional risk, e.g.
                (1) Prenatal: pattern and total amount of maternal weight gain, complications of pregnancy, etc.
                (2) Postnatal: client or family history of diabetes, coronary heart disease, infections, anemia, constipation, diarrhea, hyperactivity, food intolerances, pica, inborn errors of metabolism, malabsorption syndromes, etc.
            b. Observation
                (1) General appearance
                (2) Speech
                (3) Oral hygiene
    C. Suggested standards
        1. Fomon[a,d]
        2. Christakis[e]
        3. Goldsmith[f]

(continued)

Table 2. (*continued*)

III. Biochemical
  A. Purpose: To obtain objective data related to present nutrition status or recent dietary intake
  B. Levels of assessment
    1. Minimal
      a. Complete blood count
      b. Routine urinalysis including microscopic
      c. Semi-quantitative amino acid screening▪
    2. In-depth
      a. Serum total protein and albumin
      b. Fasting blood glucose
      c. Serum urea nitrogen
      d. Transferrin saturation
      e. Organic acids as primary screening for metabolic disorders
      f. Quantitative urinary and plasma amino acid screening
    3. Other tests to respond to special conditions or problems (examples only)

Condition/problem	Tests+
a. anticonvulsants	Folic acid, ascorbic acid, calcium, vitamin D, alkaline phosphatase, B_6
b. Prader-Willi syndrome	Glucose tolerance test
c. Pica	Lead, hemoglobin

  C. Suggested standards
    1. Fomon[a,d]
    2. Christakis[e]

IV. Dietary
  A. Purpose: To determine a usual dietary pattern and/or nutrient intake
  B. Criteria for dietary assessment
    1. Family income
    2. Mechanical feeding problems
    3. Growth deviations
    4. Age
    5. Specific nutritional disorders or inborn errors of metabolism
    6. Feeding behavior problems
    7. Response to parents' or other professionals' concerns
  C. Levels of assessment
    1. Minimal
      a. Twenty-four hour recall using food models and/or measures and food frequency with verbal questioning
      b. Feeding history questionnaire to include parents' concerns regarding nutrition status
    2. In-depth
      a. Three-day dietary intake kept by parent
        (1) Verbal instruction in dietary record keeping
        (2) Kept during 2 weekdays and 1 weekend day
        (3) Dietary supplements and/or medications included
        (4) Occurrences affecting validity recorded, i.e., illness or holidays
        (5) Quantity, preparation, and brand names of food included
        (6) Where, when, and with whom client eats included
      b. Activity record (as needed)
      c. Pertinent historical information related to feeding
      d. Present influences on dietary intake
    3. Other
      Certain conditions (i.e., inborn errors of metabolism or syndromes) may require further dietary investigation necessitating more detailed data collection)
  D. Suggested standards
    1. Recommended Dietary Allowances[g]
    2. Fomon[a,d]
    3. FAO[b]

V. Behavioral and Feeding Skill Development
  A. Purpose: To determine the influence of level of feeding development and behavior on nutritional status
  B. Levels of assessment
    1. Minimal
      a. Parental perception of feeding skills and behavior
      b. Professional perception of feeding skills and behavior

(*continued*)

Table 2. (*continued*)

2. In-depth
   a. Review of past history and interview to determine feeding skill development and present level of functioning
   b. Observations ♦
      (1) Physical
         (a) Oral structure and function including primitive reflexes, sucking, swallowing, biting, chewing, occlusion, and caries
         (b) Neuromuscular development including gross and fine motor skills, head and trunk control, eye-hand coordination, and position for feeding
      (2) Behavioral
         (a) Parent (caregiver)-child-interaction
         (b) Reinforcement patterns (positive and negative)
         (c) Environmental influences

C. Suggested standards
   1. Gesell and Amatruda[i]
   2. Vineland Social Maturity Scale[j]

From Smith, M.A.H. (Ed.). (1976). *Guides for nutritional assessment of the mentally retarded and developmentally disabled.* Memphis: University of Tennessee, Child Development Center; reprinted by permission.

[a]Fomon (1976).

[b]National Center for Health Statistics (1976).

[c]Gurney and Jelliffe (1973).

[d]Fomon (1974).

[e]Christakis (1973).

[f]Goldsmith (1959).

[g]Food and Nutrition Board (1974).

[h]Passmore, Nicol, and Rao (1974).

[i]Knobloch and Pasamanick (1975).

[j]Doll (1965).

* Measurement to be made by well-trained, motivated personnel.

○ Standards for recumbent length for normal children are available only up to 2 years of age; however, this method yields more accurate measurement of children with physical disabilities over 2 years, especially when they are unable to stand without support.

▪ Screening with multiple Guthrie tests and/or thin layer chromatography or chromatography alone.

\+ Professional judgment is warranted and a current search of literature should be done to determine appropriateness of tests before they are used.

♦ Observations both at home and outside home with and without primary caregiver and/or conjoint professional assessments are valuable.

scales for measuring weight and height and boards for measuring standing height are fairly inexpensive and should be standard equipment in all classrooms that serve children and young adults with disabilities. For students unable to stand, measuring boards to assess recumbent body length can be constructed. For those individuals with contractures, segmental measurements can be made beginning with the foot, then the lower leg, upper leg, trunk, neck, and head (Kalisz & Ekvall, 1984; Smith, 1976). Height measures are needed for calculating basal energy needs. Determination of weight for height, height age (age at which a person's height falls at the 50th percentile for height on standard growth charts), Z-scores, and body mass index are objective ways to assess height and describe growth (Blyler & Lucas, 1987). Determination of arm muscle and arm fat areas may be made with an understanding of the degree of musculature in those individuals with special problems such as *myelomeningocele* (a congenital defect of the spine). Arm length has been suggested as an alternative measure to length and height in children with myelomeningocele and others who are nonambulatory (Blyler & Lucas, 1987). Knee height measurements have recently been suggested as appropriate measurements to estimate the height of nonambulatory individuals.

Growth charts (including height, weight, and height/weight ratio) include comparisons of a child or adolescent's height and weight with national standards, provide a percentile indication of growth, and show discrepancies in the growth proportions of children and adolescents (Kalisz & Ekvall, 1984). Growth charts were developed on groups of children without disabilities; however, they have been shown to be effective as tools for monitoring the growth of children with developmental disabilities and special health care needs (Smith, 1976). In growing children, the importance of longitudinal growth is a significant consideration in their overall development. By measuring heights as frequently as every 3 months, any growth deviations can be detected as they occur and assistance can be sought. Because some children with genetic disorders have an altered metabolism that predisposes them to obesity, serial measures of weight and height can determine subtle changes in body fat and allow children to begin learning at an early age what they can do to prevent obesity.

Teachers and service providers need an awareness of their unique roles in the assessment of heights and weights in the classroom. The activities associated with body measurements can be integrated into math lesson plans. Body size can be monitored by actually tracing the size of the students on lengths of wrapping paper, cutting out the shapes, and using them for decorations within the classroom.

Clinical Assessment

Clinical assessment includes an appraisal of the general appearance and well-being of the individual. It includes observation of the hair, skin, nails, eyes, mouth and tongue, teeth, joints, lower extremities, skeleton, and general musculature. Signs of malnutrition include bowed legs, skin eruptions not related to insect bites, dental decay and missing teeth, tongue discoloration and mouth lesions, hair color changes, swollen ankles, and other physical anomalies. These signs are indicative of particular nutritional deficits and warrant discussion with the individual and his or her caregivers or service providers; a referral to the school nurse or a physician may be necessary. Such physical defects as craniofacial anomalies or abnormal tongue movements can result in severe feeding deficits and require specialized assessment with appropriate care plans by a team of health care professionals (Blyler & Lucas, 1987; Chernoff, 1991; Smith, 1976).

Biochemical Assessment

Biochemical parameters for nutritional assessment include blood and urine tests to determine body stores with respect to essential nutrients. Often physicians monitor blood counts using hemoglobin and hematocrit tests. These parameters give indications of the body's store of iron and protein. Another test particularly relevant for nutritional assessment is to check levels of *albumin* (a protein in the blood) as an indicator of body protein stores necessary for maintaining body repair. Interested readers can seek this type of information by consulting with a physician. If caregivers observe that an individual is experiencing excessive tiredness or sleepiness, the problem may be related to poor nutrition. A physician should be notified immediately so that the appropriate tests can be conducted (Blyler & Lucas, 1987; Smith, 1976; Smith et al., 1982).

Dietary Assessment

Dietary assessment is a general appraisal of food intake and habits over a specific period of time. Data can be collected by observing the individual at mealtimes, or food records may be sent to parents or group home service providers to complete for one to several days and then return to a nutritionist. A food frequency checklist has also been found to be an effective tool (Kalisz & Ekvall, 1984). This checklist reports the frequency with which individuals eat certain types of food on a daily, weekly, or monthly basis.

In addition to the collection of data pertinent to the daily intake of food, data must also be obtained on the medications or supplements being taken on a routine basis (Blyler & Lucas, 1987). An important element of the diet is fluid; therefore, some indication of the amount of water and other fluids consumed on a daily basis is also needed (Chernoff, 1991). After obtaining these data, comparisons of the daily number of servings of each type of food with those recommended by the USDA pyramid

Table 3. Sample diets for one day at three different calorie levels

Number of servings	Lower[a] 1,600	Moderate[b] 2,200	Higher[c] 2,800
Bread group	6	9	11
Vegetable group	3	4	5
Fruit group	2	3	4
Milk group	2–3[d]	2–3[d]	2–3[d]
Meat group (ounces)	5	6	7
Total fat (grams)	53	73	93
Total added sugars (teaspoons)	6	12	18

Adapted from United States Department of Agriculture, Human Nutrition Service (1992).

[a]1,600 calories is about right for many sedentary women and some older adults.

[b]2,200 calories is about right for most children, teenage girls, active women, and many sedentary men. Women who are pregnant or breastfeeding may need somewhat more.

[c]2,800 calories is about right for teenage boys, many active men, and some very active women.

[d]Women who are pregnant or breastfeeding, teenagers, and young adults to age 24 need three servings.

food guide are possible, although caregivers may wish to seek further guidance from a registered dietitian. Tables 3 and 4 provide further information on dietary recommendations from the USDA.

Behavioral Assessment Behavioral assessments during meals and snacktimes may provide insight about such behaviors as "acting out" (e.g., disrupting mealtime by throwing food, excessive noise-making), food rejection, food aversions, unusual eating habits, and how the feeding situation is approached by the individual in general. People with developmental disabilities are sometimes anorectic or bulimic. They may reject food because of its texture, color, odor, or flavor. Persons with autism may have unhealthy responses to the feeding situation or to any change in the feeding regime. Some of these responses may include *rumination,* a self-regurgitative behavior, which can result in esophagitis, aspiration, dehydration, or malnutrition (Blyler & Lucas, 1987). *Pica,* ingestion of nonfood items, is another unusual response, which may lead to intestinal blockage and could result in nutritional deficits. Gaining an understanding of food acceptance allows caregivers to make suggestions to the individual and his or her family or to make referrals to the appropriate health professionals. Behaviors that occur at mealtimes are often present in other activities of daily living, social, and learning situations; thus, mealtimes are a good time to detect these behaviors (Smith, 1976).

Table 4. What counts as a serving?

Food groups	One serving
Bread, cereal, rice, and pasta	1 slice of bread 1 ounce of ready-to-eat cereal ½ cup of cooked cereal, rice, or pasta
Vegetable	1 cup of raw leafy vegetables ½ cup of other vegetables, cooked or chopped raw ¾ cup of vegetable juice
Fruit	1 medium apple, banana, or orange ½ cup of chopped, cooked, or canned fruit ¾ cup of fruit juice
Milk, yogurt, and cheese	1 cup of milk or yogurt 1½ ounces of natural cheese 2 ounces of process cheese
Meat, poultry, fish, dry beans, eggs, and nuts	½ cup of cooked dry beans, 1 egg, or 2 tablespoons of peanut butter count as 1 ounce of lean meat

Adapted from United States Department of Agriculture, Human Nutrition Service (1992).

Economic and Environmental Assessment

The economics of the food and feeding of children and adults with disabilities is another important area of assessment. The income level of the individual and his or her family or the funding available to a group home or other residential facility can strongly affect the ability to purchase and provide adequate food. Some assistance for older persons may be available through "Meals on Wheels," which is sometimes funded by Title XIX programs via state offices on aging. School systems participating in the National School Lunch Program can provide children with free or reduced price breakfasts and lunches if the child's family income falls within specified criteria. However, some families are uncomfortable with providing this information to the school and will send food for the child that is of marginal quantity and quality. Teachers should try to become aware of the economic situation of their students so they can assist the family in meeting nutritional needs through the use of school and other community resources (Chernoff, 1991; Smith, 1976).

Equally important to economic assessment is an understanding of the environment in which the individual lives. Who is mainly responsible for food preparation and service, when and where the individual eats, and the general treatment of the individual in his or her social environment are some of the factors that directly impact nutritional status. Sometimes the meals consumed at school or in adult care programs are the only meals an individual might have all day (Chernoff, 1991; Smith, 1976).

Assessment of Feeding Skill and Ability

Feeding skill development is often extremely difficult for some individuals with disabilities, and delays in feeding skills can sometimes cause nutritional deficits. Some individuals are unable to finger feed, spoon feed, or drink from a cup. Others have mechanical feeding difficulties that preclude sucking, chewing, or swallowing; in these cases, the consistency of their food must always be modified. Others require tube feeding.

Feeding skill development parallels all other areas of development. Several feeding assessment tools are available that illustrate a person's progression across developmental areas and the interdependence of these areas with one another (Bagnato, Neisworth, & Munson, 1989; Smith et al., 1982). These feeding assessment scales can be used within the classroom in a prescriptive developmental assessment.

In order to establish an appropriate educational program, each person's feeding skill level must be determined. Occupational therapists, physical therapists, speech pathologists, and registered dietitians are health professionals who can assess these abilities and help plan appropriate modifications to facilitate independent feeding methods, if possible, and to improve the person's nutritional status. Coordination with these consultants can be time consuming; however, it can prove extremely valuable in promoting the individual's nutritional well-being and overall health.

WORKING WITH SPECIFIC NUTRITIONAL CONCERNS

If a gross deficit is suspected, the problem should be discussed with the individual and his or her caregivers; perhaps the individual will need to be referred to a registered dietitian and/or a physician. In larger school systems or care facilities, registered dietitians may be on staff to assist with the food service program. These dietitians may be available as consultants to assist with nutritional assessments and nutrition education programs. The Public Health Department also has nutrition consultants who are available to work with a variety of community agencies. Dietitians are usually employed in all major hospitals. These dietitians can be called upon as consultants to community programs as needed. The following sections address specific nutritional concerns, including difficulties with achieving a healthy weight, problematic drug–nutrient interactions, and mechanical feeding difficulties.

Achieving a Healthy Weight

A weight management program for either underweight or overweight conditions can be established following nutritional assessment. This enables caregivers to assist an individual in choosing foods that will meet their nutritional needs and help them to achieve balanced weight (Blyler & Lucas, 1987). Also, exercise programs can be designed with the individual's input to assist with energy balance. Following are suggestions for assisting individuals who are either overweight or obese or underweight or emaciated.

Overweight/Obesity

Overweight/obesity is often precipitated in persons with hypotonia, gross motor limitation, immobility, short stature, lack of nutrition knowledge, inappropriate eating habits, and obesity-related syndromes such as Prader-Willi, Lawrence-Moon Beidel, or Carpenter (Blyler & Lucas, 1987). Obese persons with limited ability for movement are more susceptible to the development of skin breakdown at pressure points, less able to transfer from a wheelchair, and require more care with activities of daily living (Blyler & Lucas, 1987).

For those who are extremely overweight, a behavior management system using nonfood rewards for weight loss (e.g., tokens for each pound lost that can be "cashed in" for prizes) has been effective (Neely & Smith, 1977). For growing children, severely restricted calorie regimes are not recommended; it is better to maintain weight, while monitoring growth in stature, until weight can be normalized (Neely & Smith, 1977). Choosing foods of high nutrient density, yet with a lower level of calories, and eliminating high fat, low nutrient foods, along with a reasonable exercise program, is the best method of weight control. Permanent change in life style holds the only promise to continued weight maintenance after ideal weight is achieved (National Research Council, 1989a).

Underweight/Emaciation For severely underweight people, the capacity for volume is often very small; thus, high caloric, nutrition-

Susie, a 15-year-old girl with mental retardation, presented at a diagnostic center at 130% of her ideal body weight. She lived with her parents and two older siblings in a rural area. The family raised a garden, had a history of cooking large quantities of high fat foods, and enjoyed eating as one of their main activities. Susie liked to eat and loved sweets and fried foods most of all. However, she was beginning to have pride in her appearance and had a desire to lose weight.

During the nutrition assessment session, Susie indicated her desire to be on a weight management program. Weight goals were established. The dietary pattern developed for Susie followed the pyramid food guide and allowed for 1,600 calories a day. At the onset, a picture of Susie was taken in her swimsuit and given to her to tape to her bedroom dresser mirror. Susie and her mother were instructed on the diet that was tailored to the family's available and usual foods. They were requested to keep a daily diary of foods eaten and return for follow-up visits with the dietitian every 2 weeks.

During the follow-up visits, Susie was weighed and her height was measured. The food diaries were reviewed, and any exceptions to the diet were discussed with both Susie and her mother. The visits with the dietitian were held monthly after the first 2 months, and the follow-up weight loss program continued for 6 months. At the end of that time, Susie was photographed again in a "new" swimsuit. The weight loss was quite apparent from the before and after pictures. The pictures were framed together and given to Susie to place in her room as a constant reminder of her original appearance. The pictures provided continued incentive for Susie to eat correctly and keep off the weight.

She had been encouraged to walk a mile at a brisk pace at least three times a week during the 6-month program. For maintenance, the exercise program was continued. Susie was able to maintain her weight at 110% ideal body weight for 2 years of follow-up assessments.

ally dense foods should be eaten frequently in small amounts. When initiating a weight gain program, severely underweight individuals should start by eating small amounts, then gradually begin increasing the number of their feedings as tolerated. Specialized foods are available commercially for this purpose; however, these supplements are costly. The use of "Instant Breakfast" with whole milk, ice cream shakes, whole grain cereals with milk, lean meat, fish, poultry, and fruits and vegetables are the best choices.

Often, severely underweight people have mechanical feeding difficulties that preclude adequate oral feedings. Or they may have neural deficits that cause unpurposeful movements or such accelerated activity levels that energy needs cannot be met (Blyler & Lucas, 1987). Thus, tube feeding with or without oral feeding may be the only answer to meeting their energy and nutrient needs. If possible, oral feeding should be the method used as long as the gut is intact. After persistent oral feeding programs have proven to no avail, a referral back to the physician for further consultation is necessary.

Methods of self-monitoring of either weight loss or gain might include the following:

1. Pictures could be taken of the individual at the onset of the weight management program and each month thereafter, and these pictures could be placed on a poster or on the person's refrigerator as a means of monitoring progress.
2. Food intake can be self-monitored by using shapes or colored tokens to represent servings from each food group; as food is consumed the markers could be placed in a jar. At the end of the day, the individual could count the number of servings of foods from each group. The person could then reward himself or herself with a nonfood treat (e.g., a shopping trip, movie) for eating the correct number of servings.
3. A self-chart for exercise could be kept by recording the number of blocks walked or other units of exercise completed, with rewards given for meeting preset goals.

Problematic Drug–Nutrient Interactions

Drug–nutrient interactions are often the causes of specific nutritional and medical problems, which sometimes go unnoticed until a crisis presents itself (Blyler & Lucas, 1987). Such interactions are fairly common with the drugs prescribed for attention-deficit/hyperactivity disorders, seizure control, epilepsy, behavioral disturbances, recurrent infections of the pulmonary or renal systems, and chronic constipation. Heavy usage of anticonvulsant medicines can cause problems with vitamin D, mineral, and bone metabolism. Particularly vulnerable are those individuals who are nonambulatory, as they may be more prone to bone loss due to lack of weight-bearing exercise. Others at risk are those who are house-bound without the benefit of vitamin D from the sunlight.

Folate deficiencies are another effect of prolonged use of anticonvulsant medications. Folate supplements render the anticonvulsant medications ineffective; the medications affect the utilization of folate. Thus, folic acid deficiencies result in anemia, unless blood tests are monitored.

Overuse of laxatives for constipation, often a chronic condition in individuals with developmental disabilities because of hypotonia and lack of physical activity, can result in protein-losing enteropathy and potassium depletion. Mineral oil, when used for its laxative effect, also results in decreased utilization of vitamin A, vitamin D, calcium, and phosphorus (Springer & Fricke, 1975).

Appetite depression has been reported in those with long-term use of such stimulant medications as dextroamphetamine and methylphenidate, which are often prescribed for attention-deficit/hyperactivity disorders (Blyler & Lucas, 1987). Such suppression of appetite can also retard growth. Thus, when assessing nutritional status, a review of medications should be completed (Smith, 1976). With drug usage, vitamin-mineral supplementation may be needed and continual monitoring is essential.

Mechanical Feeding Difficulties

As mentioned earlier, difficulties in feeding can cause nutritional deficits. Once a complete assessment of the level of the individual's feeding ability has been done by a team of professionals, a feeding training program can be developed tailored to the individual's needs. These programs have been shown to be effective when an interdisciplinary approach is used including the disciplines of medicine, nursing, nutrition, occupational therapy, physical therapy, and behavior analysis. Such plans include the proper placement or seating for eating, providing specialized feeding equipment, preparing foods of an appropriate consistency, and taking a behavioral approach to the training situation (Neely & Smith, 1977).

Training for mechanical feeding problems begins by proper placement of the individual in an upright position for eating. The feet must be flat on the floor, the body in an upright, midline position, and the arms and hands free for movement. Food is placed before the person at midline. For example, suppose the individual needed to learn to use a spoon for feeding semisolid food, the caregiver would place the spoon in the hand so that the person was using a palmar grasp; the caregiver would then stand behind the person and place his or her hand over the hand of the learner. The caregiver would guide the person's hand to the dish, dip the food, and guide the spoon into the learner's mouth. This activity would be repeated many times until the person being trained could actually hold the spoon, dip the food, bring the food to the mouth, and take the food from the spoon. Gradually fading hand-on-hand assistance in a sequential manner, replacing it with touch, and then with verbal cues, would allow the learner to become independent in spoon feeding.

Training for sucking and swallowing needs the expertise of those with special training and experience in techniques that minimize aspiration. An occupational therapist or speech pathologist can best assist and teach caregivers in this realm. Each person is unique; mechanical feeding training must be tailored to meet individual needs, and programs for training cannot be generalized.

CONCLUSIONS

Problems in promoting greater independence and nutritional well-being of persons with developmental disabilities include difficulties in following "prescribed dietary and medicinal practices, deliberate or inadvertent encouragement of overdependence on caregivers, and service providers' vulnerability to following nutrition fads and accepting misinformation" (Blyler & Lucas, 1987, p. 1070). Teachers, families, and service providers continue to decry the lack of appropriate resource materials available for training purposes and for daily use by individuals with disabilities. Every effort must be made to provide them with an up-to-date knowledge base.

Reviews of menu planning and food preparation programs for people with developmental disabilities have emphasized the shortcomings of current practice (e.g., Marchand-Martella, Smith, & Agran, 1992). Specifically, the following limitations have been identified: 1) lack of inclusion of nutrition information consistent with national dietary guidelines, and 2) the use of a "shotgun approach" to teaching by singling out one preparation technique, while neglecting the provision of comprehensive information relative to planning menus across time (Marchand-Martella et al., 1991). Varied methods for teaching these skills have been studied, including food buying via computer programs; task analyses approaches (Sarber & Cuvo, 1983); instruction on simple preparation techniques using constant time-delay procedure resulting in chained responses (Schuster, Gast, Wolery, & Guiltinan, 1988); teaching shopping skills in supermarkets via the use of pocket calculators, adaptive shopping lists, food slides, menu planning boards, and food serving keys (Nietupski et al., 1983; Sarber et al., 1983; Wheeler et al., 1980); and using skill transfer techniques to teach simple housekeeping tasks including food preparation (Livi & Ford, 1985).

Most of the above methods have merit. However, a thorough search of the literature revealed no studies directed toward nutrition monitoring in residential or home facilities for persons with mental retardation, evaluation of nutrition and food teaching methods and programs, or teaching of food safety and sanitation skills. Marchand-Martella et al. (1991) pointed to the need for more research with collaboration between special educators and nutritionists with the goal of designing more effective programs to teach adequate nutrition and health practices to those with special health care needs. Recognition of the lack of appropriate teaching curricula and resources provides incentives for those in the field of nutrition and special education to collaborate in the design and field testing of appropriate educational materials for persons with developmental disabilities.

To promote greater independence and well-being, a strong partnership among teachers, service providers, caregivers, families, health professionals, and individuals with developmental disabilities themselves is essential. Closer alliances between schools, home residential facilities, community programs, public health, and specialized health facilities must be formed. Teachers need to develop new skills in referral, consultation, and technical assistance both as the provider and the receiver of services (Kozlowski & Powell, 1989). Collaboration among dietitians, occupational and physical therapists, psychologists, speech pathologists, and dentists, who can provide assistance with special feeding and nutrition problems, will help these specialists to work with individuals with developmental disabilities and their caregivers to create functional nutrition curricula.

In the past, nutrition education has been unavailable to most people. Only recently has attention been given by the media and the government to the fact that what we eat can prevent or impact the chronic diseases of later life. Educators, registered dietitians, and other health professionals with specific expertise in nutrition and feeding must make every effort to ensure that people with disabilities acquire skills in these areas. These individuals must be assisted with taking an active role in their own nutritional health.

REFERENCES

Bagnato, S.J., Neisworth, J.T., & Munson, S.M. (1989). *Linking developmental assessment and early intervention: Curriculum-based prescriptions* (2nd ed.). Rockville, MD: Aspen.

Bates, P., & Pancsofar, E. (1980). *Pictorial preparation manual.* Des Moines: Iowa Department of Public Instruction.

Bates, P., Renzaglia, A., & Wehman, P. (1981). Characteristics of an appropriate education for severely and profoundly handicapped students. *Education and Training of the Mentally Retarded, 16,* 142–149.

Blyler, E., & Lucas, B. (1987). Nutrition in comprehensive program planning for persons with developmental disabilities: Technical support paper. *Journal of the American Dietetic Association, 87,* 1069–1074.

Burros, M. (1992, April 28). U.S. agrees to rank food with symbol of a pyramid. *New York Times,* p. B1.

Chernoff, R. (1991). *Geriatric nutrition.* Rockville, MD: Aspen.

Christakis, G. (Ed.). (1973). *Nutritional assessment in health programs.* Washington, DC: American Public Health Association, Inc.

Doll, E.A. (1965). *Vineland Social Maturity Scale.* Circles Pines, MN: American Guidance Service.

Drieth, R. (1979). Nutrition for the developmentally disabled. *Nutrition News, 42,* 9–10.

Fomon, S.J. (1974). *Infant nutrition* (2nd ed.). Philadelphia: W.B. Saunders.

Fomon, S.J. (1976). *Nutritional Disorders of Children: Screening, follow-up, prevention.* Rockville, MD: United States Department of Health and Human Services/Public Health Service/Office of Maternal and Child Health.

Food and Drug Administration. (1992). *The new food label.* Washington, DC: FDA Backgrounder.

Food and Nutrition Board. (1974). *Recommended dietary allowances* (8th ed.). Washington, DC: National Academy of Sciences.

Gaule, K., Nietupski, J., & Certo, N. (1985). Teaching supermarket shopping skills using an adaptive shopping list. *Education and Training of the Mentally Retarded, 20,* 53–59.

Goldsmith, G. (1959). *Nutritional diagnosis.* Springfield, IL: Charles C Thomas Publishers.

Green, E.M., & McIntosh, E.N. (1985). Food and nutrition skills of mentally retarded adults: Assessment and needs. *Journal of the American Dietetic Association, 85,* 611–612.

Gurney, M., & Jelliffe, E. (1973). Arm anthropometry in nutritional assessment: Nomogram for rapid calculation of muscle circumference and crosssectional muscle and fat areas. *American Journal of Clinical Nutrition, 26,* 912.

Hermann, M.G. (1991). The ABCs of children's nutrition. *Supplement to the Journal of the American Dietetic Association, 91.*

Ingersoll, B. (1992, April 28). U.S. picks pyramid to show how to eat. *The Wall Street Journal,* p. B1.

Johnson, B.F., & Cuvo, A.J. (1981). Teaching mentally retarded adults to cook. *Behavior Modification, 5,* 187–203.

Kalisz, K., & Ekvall, S. (1984). A nutritional interview for clients with developmental disorders. *Mental Retardation, 22,* 279–288.

Knobloch, H., & Pasamanick, B. (Ed.). (1975). *Gesell and Amatruda's developmental diagnosis* (3rd ed.). New York: Harper and Row.

Kozlowski, B.W., & Powell, J.A. (1989). Position of the

American Dietetic Association: Nutrition services for children with special health care needs. *Journal of the American Dietetic Association, 89,* 1133–1137.

Livi, J., & Ford, A. (1985). Skill transfer from a domestic training site to the actual homes of three moderately handicapped students. *Education and Training of the Mentally Retarded, 20,* 69–82.

Marchand-Martella, N.E., Smith, M.A.H., & Agran, M. (1992). Food preparation and meal planning for persons with disabilities: A review of the literature. *British Columbia Journal of Special Education, 16*(1), 13–28.

Marchand-Martella, N.E., Windham, C.T., Wyse, B.W., & Martella, R.C. (1991). Teaching food skills to individuals with mental retardation: A review and recommendations for incorporating nutritious and healthful foods. *Journal of Nutrition Education, 23,* 116–119.

Matson, J. (1981). Use of independence training to teach shopping skills to mildly mentally retarded adults. *American Journal of Mental Deficiency, 86,* 178–183.

National Center for Health Statistics. (1976). *Reference data.* Rockville, MD: United States Department of Health and Human Services/Public Health Service/Office of Maternal and Child Health.

National Research Council. (1989a). *Diet and health: Implications for reducing chronic disease risk.* Washington, DC: National Academy Press.

National Research Council. (1989b). *Recommended dietary allowances* (10th ed.). Washington, DC: National Academy Press.

Neely, R.A., & Smith, M.A. (1977). *Program for feeding training of developmentally delayed children.* Memphis: University of Tennessee, Child Development Center.

Nieman, D.C., Butterworth, D.E., & Nieman, C.N. (1992). *Nutrition.* Dubuque, IA: William C. Brown.

Nietupski, J., Welch, J., & Wacker, D. (1983). Acquisition, maintenance, and transfer of grocery item purchasing skills by moderately and severely handicapped students. *Education and Training of the Mentally Retarded, 18,* 279–286.

Passmore, R., Nicol, B.M., & Rao, M.N. *Handbook on human nutritional requirements.* (FAO nutritional studies, no. 28). New York: UNIPUB.

Robinson-Wilson, M.A. (1977). Habilitation. *Education and Training of the Mentally Retarded, 12,* 69–73.

Sarber, R.E., & Cuvo, A.J. (1983). Teaching nutritional meal planning to developmentally disabled clients. *Behavior Modification, 7,* 503–530.

Sarber, R.E., Halasz, M.M., Messmer, M.C., Bickett, A.D., & Lutzker, J.R. (1983). Teaching menu planning and grocery shopping skills to a mentally retarded mother. *Mental Retardation, 21,* 101–106.

Schuster, J.W., Gast, D.L., Wolery, M., & Guiltinan, S. (1988). The effectiveness of a constant time-delay procedure to teach chained responses to adolescents with mental retardation. *Journal of Applied Behavior Analysis, 21,* 169–178.

Smith, M.A.H. (Ed.). (1976). *Guides for nutritional assessment of the mentally retarded and developmentally disabled.* Memphis: University of Tennessee, Child Development Center.

Smith, M.A.H., Connolly, B., McFadden, S., Nicrosi, C.R., Nuckolls, L.J., Russell, F.F., & Wilson, W.M. (1982). *Feeding management of a child with a handicap: A guide for professionals.* Memphis: University of Tennessee, Child Development Center.

Snell, M.E., & Browder, D.M. (1987). Domestic and community skills. In M.E. Snell (Ed.), *Systematic instruction of persons with severe handicaps* (pp. 390–434). Columbus, OH: Charles E. Merrill.

Springer, N. (1987). From institution to foster care: Impact on nutritional status. *American Journal of Mental Deficiency, 91,* 324–327.

Springer, N.S., & Fricke, N.L. (1975). Nutrition and drug therapy for persons with developmental disabilities. *American Journal of Mental Deficiency, 80,* 317–322.

Thomas, P.R. (Ed.). (1991). *Improving America's diet and health.* Washington, DC: National Academic Press.

United States Department of Agriculture, Human Nutrition Information Service. (1992). *The food guide pyramid* (Home and Garden Bulletin, No. 252). Hyattsville, MD: Author.

United States Department of Agriculture, & United States Department of Health and Human Services. (1990). *Nutrition and your health: Dietary guidelines for Americans* (Home and Garden Bulletin, No. 232). Washington, DC: U.S. Government Printing Office.

Wheeler, J., Ford, A., Nietupski, J., Loomis, R., & Brown, L. (1980). Teaching moderately and severely handicapped adolescents to shop in supermarkets using pocket calculators. *Education and Training of the Mentally Retarded, 15,* 105–112.

Chapter Four

Self-Medication Skills

Alan E. Harchik

Taking medication is a routine part of the day for many people. Although medication can be properly prescribed, correct administration is required if optimal benefits are to occur. Unfortunately, many people do not correctly and consistently follow their prescriptions. Without proper instruction, monitoring, and feedback, people with developmental disabilities are at least as likely as the majority of the population to fail to follow their medication regimens. Due to the potential serious consequences of taking medication incorrectly, people with developmental disabilities are often never taught to participate in their own medication regimens, and it is the individual's teachers, parents, or service providers who take full responsibility for this task. Consequently, many people with developmental disabilities are prevented from having opportunities to live or work in community settings primarily due to their dependence on others for managing their own medications.

Nevertheless, current knowledge, practice, and research suggest that people with developmental disabilities can learn to participate to some degree in the administration of their own medications. Allowing independent opportunities for self-administration of medications, while maintaining high levels of safety, is the ultimate goal, as well as the ultimate challenge, for all self-medication programs. In addition to an increased sense of personal control, another advantage to teaching self-medication is that it can reduce the costs of paying special direct service or nursing staff to administer medications.

Still, the greatest risk of any self-medication process is that a serious error will be made that will jeopardize the health or even the life of the individual. Medication errors can include errors in amount (too much or too little), schedule (at the wrong times, too often, not enough, discontinuing before prescribed time), or type of medication (taking the wrong medication, taking medication for the wrong reasons) (Boczkowski & Zeichner, 1985). Any self-medication program needs to ensure proper safeguards and monitoring to alleviate any undue risk.

Because self-medication is clearly an important skill, some human services agencies have developed their own programs for providing people with developmental disabilities the opportunity to participate in their own medication regimens. The Medication Education and Self-Administration program (Coudreaut, Hinson, & McMorrow, 1990) is an example of a detailed, data-based self-medication training pro-

Frank Bird, John Clayton, and Tom Zwicker provided valuable assistance in the preparation of this chapter.

Components of the self-medication programs at the Choate Center in Anna, Illinois, Community Living Opportunities in Lawrence, Kansas, and the May Institute in Centerville, Massachusetts, have been incorporated throughout this chapter. Contributions from these agencies are greatly appreciated.

gram for people with developmental disabilities. Programs designed for people with other types of disabilities can also be used; however, extensive adaptation will be required (e.g., Wallace, Boone, Donahoe, & Foy, 1986).

The purpose of this chapter is to review procedures and discuss issues relevant to teaching individuals with a variety of developmental disabilities to administer their own medications safely. In general, the self-medication skills described in this chapter are most appropriate for adolescents and adults because younger children (with or without disabilities) are rarely given opportunities to be responsible for administering their own medication. Table 1 summarizes general guidelines and considerations addressed in this chapter for developing a self-medication program.

Table 1. General guidelines for developing a self-medication program

1. Ensure proper consents are obtained.
2. Examine current medication regimen, and consult with physician and pharmacist regarding modification of the regimen for ease of administration.
3. Determine the necessary skills for administering the medication by conducting a task analysis.
4. Assess the individual's current skill level.
5. Interview program participant and others who know the individual well regarding his or her skill level and abilities.
6. Determine the individual's preferences and goals.
7. Develop a teaching procedure and reinforcement system; make any special stimulus modifications.
8. Implement a monitoring system.
9. Specify criteria for discontinuation.
10. Upon repeated correct performance of self-medication skills, fade supervision, while maintaining frequent, unobtrusive monitoring to evaluate maintenance of skills.

PRELIMINARY STEPS TO IMPLEMENTING A SELF-MEDICATION PROGRAM

Prior to embarking on any self-medication program, some preliminary actions need to be taken. These steps are addressed in the following sections and they include:

1. Understanding caregiver liability
2. Obtaining informed consent
3. Understanding the participant's current medication regimen
4. Evaluating necessary prerequisite behaviors on the part of the individual learning the skills
5. Predetermining discontinuation criteria

Understanding Caregiver Liability

Parents, teachers, direct service staff, and health care professionals have typically been responsible for administering medications to people with developmental disabilities in order to reduce the likelihood of medication errors and consequent injury. When people with disabilities are given opportunities to self-administer, those caregivers who had previously administered the medication remain responsible for health outcomes over which they now have less control. Thus, issues surrounding liability when allowing someone with disabilities to self-administer medications must be addressed.

Each agency should have written policies and procedures that are always followed regarding informed consent, human rights committee approval, interdisciplinary team recommendations, prerequisite and discontinuation criteria, staff training procedures, and intense monitoring of the self-administration activities of each person with developmental disabilities. Further, state and federal regulations regarding medication storage, dispensing, and documentation must be followed. With the proper safeguards, liabilities can be reduced, while safety is maintained (Coudreaut et al., 1990; Yunker, Flint, & Carpenter, 1990).

Obtaining Informed Consent

Every self-medication program should include approval and informed consent from the person with disabilities, his or her parents, guardian, physician, interdisciplinary team, and the human rights committee that is involved with the person or agency teaching self-medication skills. Informed consent implies voluntary participation in the program following a thorough explanation of the skills to be taught, methods to be used, potential benefits, possible risks, any costs that might be incurred, and the expected length of training. Participants should also be assured that an acceptable monitoring system will be in place and that there will be ongoing, regularly occurring reviews of the person's progress.

Understanding the Participant's Current Medication Regimen

Data suggest that more than one-third of people with developmental disabilities living in the community regularly receive some sort of medication, such as anticonvulsants or psychotropics (Burd et al., 1991; Zaharia & Struxness, 1991). Oral medications (e.g., pills, tablets, capsules, liquids) and topical medications (e.g., ointments, creams) are most commonly prescribed. Medications may be administered long term to address chronic conditions (e.g., seizure disorders, psychiatric problems, hypertension, vitamin or dietary deficiencies) and short term for more temporary conditions (e.g., infections, pain). These medications are obtained by a prescription or bought over the counter.

The focus of this chapter is on oral and topical medications; however, there are a number of other types of medications and health-care procedures that might be taught to people with developmental disabilities (e.g., eye or ear drops, suppositories, insulin injections, bandaging wounds, self-catheterization). Instruction in these skills is likely to require a high level of involvement and supervision by licensed health care professionals. These types of health care procedures are addressed in Chapter 5 of this volume.

People with developmental disabilities and their parents, teachers, and service providers should work closely with physicians, psychiatrists, neurologists, and pharmacists to determine the best medication regimen for each individual based upon his or her medication needs, preferences, skills, and daily schedule. Once the medication regimen has been prescribed, it must be adhered to as closely as possible. Examples of some medications typically prescribed for people with developmental disabilities are listed in Table 2.

Evaluating Prerequisite Behaviors

People with developmental disabilities exhibit a wide range of abilities; thus, any self-medication program must be geared to each individual's strengths, needs, and preferences. Certainly, every person, regardless of his or her level of ability, can participate in a self-medication training program to some degree. For example, the immediate goal for some individuals may be to acquire some component skills of self-administration, such as setting up medications, using a self-recording chart, or closing a pill container. The concept of partial participation (Ferguson & Baumgart, 1991) suggests that every person should be taught as much of each skill as possible and should not be excluded from all participation simply because he or she is likely to continue to require support, supervision, and assistance.

Although the concept of partial participation strongly suggests that all people with developmental disabilities can participate in their own self-medication program to some extent, there are some prerequisite skills to embarking on a detailed self-medication training program that will include opportunities for unsupervised self-administration. These prerequisites can be targeted for direct training if not currently in the person's repertoire.

Prerequisite behaviors include the following:

1. Consistent acceptance of the medication (i.e., individual does not regularly refuse)
2. Current exhibition of the behaviors necessary to administer the medication (or can exhibit similar behaviors that suggest that the person can learn the specific behaviors needed)
3. Emotional stability
4. A stable medication regimen
5. Recommendations from the interdisciplinary team (Coudreaut et al., 1990; Yunker et al., 1990)

Table 2. Medications often prescribed for people with developmental disabilities

Brand	Generic	Purpose	Adult dose	Form	Side effects
Tegretol	Carbamazepine	Seizure control	800–1200 mg daily	Tablet	Dizziness, unsteadiness, nausea
BuSpar	Buspirone HCL	Anti-anxiety	20–30 mg daily	Tablet	Dizziness, nausea, headache, excitement
Keflex	Cephalexin	Antibiotic	1–4 g daily	Capsule	Diarrhea, rash
Hismanal	Astemizole	For allergies	10 mg daily	Tablet	—
Caltrate	Calcium	Dietary	600–1200 mg daily	Tablet	—
Tagamet	Cimetidine	Ulcer treatment	800 mg daily	Tablet, liquid	Diarrhea, dizziness, headache
Colace	Docusate sodium	Stool softener	50–200 mg daily	Capsule, liquid	—
Tylenol	Acetominophen	Pain relief	325–650 mg every 4 hours	Tablet, liquid	—

Predetermining Discontinuation Criteria

Once a person begins a self-medication program, a predetermined criterion for discontinuing the program, if necessary, should be made. Such criteria may include the occurrence of any intentional errors (e.g., intentional overdose, intentional destruction of medications) or frequent errors (e.g., forgetting to take medication 3 times within 24 hours) (Coudreaut et al., 1990). Once discontinued, a decision must be made whether to resume training with appropriate supervision or to delay a return to training altogether.

TOPICS FOR SELF-MEDICATION CURRICULA

Self-medication curriculum topics typically focus on instruction in the following areas:

- Recognizing and understanding one's medication
- Learning necessary skills for self-medication
- Handling problems or errors in self-medication

Table 3 presents some basic curriculum topics covered by two currently existing self-medication programs.

Recognizing and Understanding One's Medication

Many self-medication programs teach individuals to name their medications and state why they need to take them. Although sometimes of interest for the individual, there appears to be little correlation between knowledge of one's medication and successful adherence to a medication regimen (e.g., Boczkowski & Zeichner, 1985; Robinson, Gilbertson, & Litwack, 1987). Nevertheless, being informed about one's own medications and health status is an important aspect of informed consent and client rights (Dow, Verdi, & Sacco, 1991).

Self-Medication Skills

Skills taught in a self-medication program include being able to choose and locate the correct medication, manipulate and set up the medication (e.g., using a lock box, opening containers, matching words to labels, counting out the correct number), consume medications correctly (e.g., with water), apply medications correctly (e.g., correct amount of topical ointment applied to correct area of skin), initial and sign a self-medication record (see Figure 1, p. 64), and correctly handle and store the

Table 3. Sample self-medication curriculum topics

Example 1[a]

1. Basic skills: using a lock box, opening containers, matching words, counting, responding to time
2. Self-administration steps: get water, open box, identify medications, open containers, take out correct amount, take pills with water, put cap on containers, restore medication box
3. Conceptual skills: obtaining information, self-administering, understanding side effects and precautions, self-monitoring medication times and medication
4. Supervised self-administration
5. Unsupervised self-administration

Example 2[b]

1. Recognizing the time medications should be administered within 30 minutes of the correct time by approaching the appropriate area or staff
2. Seeking attention from appropriate personnel in the event that medication is needed and identifying the process
3. Selecting appropriate medications from a field of two
4. Obtaining additional material if needed (e.g., water, cloth, bandages)
5. Opening containers and removing the correct amount of medication
6. Consuming medication appropriately
7. Recording and documenting the process
8. Self-administering medications under staff supervision until independent for five consecutive opportunities
9. Maintaining correct self-administration of medication
10. Seeking attention and assistance in event of injury or illness
11. Identifying symptoms, only reporting those that are valid
12. Identifying appropriate medication interventions for personal needs (e.g., aspirin for headache)

[a]Adapted from Coudreaut, Hinson, and McMorrow (1990).
[b]Adapted from self-medication programs at the May Institute in Centerville, Massachusetts.

medication (Coudreaut et al., 1990; Wallace et al., 1986).

Table 4 shows two examples of task analyses for self-administering medication. Each skill can be further divided into even smaller component steps depending upon the medication, the person, and the setting. In addition to learning how to actually administer medication, some people may be taught how to identify symptoms, obtain additional information from physicians and pharmacists, discuss medication treatments with physicians and psychiatrists, and pick up medication from the pharmacy.

Learners should also be taught to verbalize the time that they are to take their medication and to initiate administration of their own medications at the appropriate times. Discriminating the correct time for administration is one of the most difficult skills to teach. Consequently, prompting systems are often used (see Teaching Methods, below). Knowing *how* to self-medicate and knowing *when* to self-medicate are two different skills, and it is not uncommon for a person to learn one skill and not the other.

Table 4. Sample task analyses for self-administration

Example 1[a]

1. Get water.
2. Open box.
3. Take out correct medication containers.
4. Open containers.
5. Take out correct number of pills.
6. Consume pills with water.
7. Put cap back on containers.
8. Restore medication box.

Example 2[b]

1. Say, "Time for my pills," when the nurse arrives.
2. Get a cup of water and go to the office.
3. Take keys from side of medication cabinet.
4. Remove medication box from cabinet using blue key.
5. Open medication box with red key.
6. Take pill box out of medication box and open correct lid.
7. Take out three pills and name the medication.
8. Take pill with water and throw cup away.
9. Take ledger out of medication box and sign sheet.
10. Put all items back into medication box.
11. Lock medication box in cabinet.
12. Hang keys back up on side of medication cabinet.

[a]Adapted from Coudreaut, Hinson, and McMorrow (1990).
[b]Adapted from self-medication programs at the May Institute in Centerville, Massachusetts.

Problem Solving

Learning to deal with problems that might arise is an important aspect of self-medication. Examples of problem solving include knowing what to do if there is not enough medication, if the medication is lost, or if a medication error is made (e.g., excess medication consumed, medication not taken at all). One typical response to this situation is for the individual to call his or her pharmacist, physician, family members, or service provider. Furthermore, learners should also be taught to discriminate between correct and incorrect medications and to obtain assistance when needed. Presenting incorrect examples of medication can contribute to successful self-administration, while reducing medication errors (Horner, Albin, & Ralph, 1986).

TEACHING METHODS

A number of researchers examining the teaching of self-medication skills to individuals with developmental disabilities have found that multiple-component teaching strategies are most effective. For example, Hinson, McMorrow, and Coudreaut (1990) and Lundervold and Enterman (1989) found that a combination of cues, direct teaching, and positive reinforcement for the exhibition of desired behaviors were required for success. Potential reinforcers include praise, special treats, and participation in preferred activities. Specific examples include returning small amounts of money that were initially deposited with the trainer (Epstein & Masek, 1978) or setting up special contingencies, such as social activities or special outings (Lundervold & Enterman, 1989). Individualized, contingent, and immediate positive reinforcement, paired with behavior-specific praise, is critical for learning any new skill, including self-medication skills. (See chap. 1, this volume, for a more detailed description of the use of reinforcement procedures.)

Overall, self-medication teaching programs include three broad phases. First, the skill is established within well-structured teaching sessions. Second, the person is allowed opportunities to self-administer under highly supervised conditions. Third, self-administration is allowed in unsupervised (but highly monitored) situations.

Teaching about Medications

Individuals may be taught about their medications and medication regimen through didactic instruction; discussion; and role playing, either individually or in small groups. Information can be presented verbally, with visual aids, and with sample medications and materials. During teaching sessions, participants should learn to respond to verbal questions (e.g., "How should medication be stored in your home?", "Why is it important to follow your doctor's instructions?"). Correct verbal responses should be reinforced, and prompts should be provided for incorrect responses.

Establishing a New Skill

To establish new skills, positive teaching procedures are used in much the same manner as when teaching other self-care, domestic, and leisure skills. (See chap. 1, this volume, for a full discussion of general behavioral-instructional strategies.) This includes repeated discrete trial training, positive reinforcement for correct responses, shaping by reinforcing successive approximations to the desired response, prompting responses (e.g., with verbal, modeled, or physical guidance), and fading of prompts following criterion levels of performance.

In discrete trial training, for example, each opportunity to practice self-administration (or a component of self-administration) is considered a trial. Instructions, prompts, and reinforcement are provided during each independently presented trial. Typically, multiple trials are presented during each teaching session. Thus, an individual might practice opening a medication container and counting out the correct number of pills for five trials. If praise was a known reinforcer for the person, behavior-specific praise would follow every correct trial. Each incorrect trial would be followed by a demonstration by the teacher and another opportunity for practice by the learner.

Teaching sessions should coincide with the times during the day that the person normally receives his or her medication, thereby assuring that all the relevant stimuli are present. In order to establish the skill, however, more frequent and intensive training opportunities will usually be needed. Thus, the person will participate in additional sessions with repeated trials during each session. Simulated medications are used during these additional sessions and trials (e.g., mints, candies, raisins, juice, water).

Component steps and their sequences are determined for each self-medication skill (see, for example, the task analyses described in Table 4). Then, backward chaining, forward chaining, or total task teaching can be done. Chapter 1 of this volume provides a detailed description of chaining strategies.

Special adaptations are often needed for people who do not have basic functional academic skills (e.g., reading, counting, writing). Adaptations might include the use of specially color-coded medication containers, counting templates for counting out a specified number of pills, prepackaged medications for each session, and medications placed in 3- or 7-day medication containers (Gehres, 1986; Lundervold & Enterman, 1989). These adaptations are most likely to have a positive impact on learning self-medication when used in conjunction with intensive teaching, reinforcement, prompting, and monitoring (i.e., these adaptations are likely to be ineffective when used alone).

Making the medication regimen simpler is another adaptation that has a positive effect on correct self-administration. Many people need to take several types of medication every day. The physician or pharmacist must look closely at the prescribed regimen and attempt to simplify it. Sometimes the number of medication administrations each day or the number of medications administered at each session can be reduced.

Implementing Prompting Systems

For many people with developmental disabilities, the environmental cues to take medication at prescribed times are not salient and, thus, are not discriminated. Consequently, medications are either administered at the incorrect time or not at all. This is one of the primary factors contributing to the failure of many self-medication programs. Many people without developmental disabilities respond to more subtle environmental cues throughout the day or develop their own set of prompting systems. A prompting system is required in almost every case.

Fortunately, a variety of prompting systems can be developed based upon each person's individual situation. Examples include timing devices such as alarms, watches, or cue lights (Lundervold & Enterman, 1989); picture schedules; tailoring times to daily activities (Boczkowski, Zeichner, & DeSanto, 1985); phone calls from an assigned person; or a medication-monitoring service (Gehres, 1986). Table 5 summarizes these examples. Again, implementation of a positive reinforcement system is critical to the success of these prompting systems.

Table 5. Examples of self-medication prompts

Timing devices

Wristwatches: Many watches can be set to ring 3–5 times each day without any need for resetting.

Alarms: Alarm clocks can be set in a manner similar to wristwatches.

Cue light: A special light can be set on a timer to go on at a particular time and to stay on until turned off.

Routine

Activity schedule: The individual's daily routine or schedule should include self-medication as an activity. The prompt to self-administer would be on the person's picture, audio, or written schedule.

Tailoring: Self-medication can occur with or immediately after the same activity every day (e.g., breakfast, evening TV news). In this manner, the naturally occurring activity becomes a prompt for self-administration.

Prompts from others

Telephone calls: A telephone service, family, or staff member can call and prompt the individual to take his or her medications.

Regular visits: A pharmacist or physician can visit regularly to observe and provide feedback.

Teaching Problem-Solving Strategies

How to respond correctly and safely when problems with medication arise is taught in much the same manner in which new skills are taught. Problem situations (e.g., wrong medications are present, medications are missing) are presented to the learner and positive reinforcement is used to shape and maintain correct response (e.g., calling a physician or staff member for assistance). Repeated discrete trials, prompting, and fading of prompts are used. Any presentation of incorrect medication set-ups, however, must be highly supervised to avoid possible injury. Once mastered, supervised and well-monitored probe situations should be presented periodically to allow staff to assess the maintenance of each person's skill at rejecting incorrect medications and calling for assistance. The case study on page 63 illustrates how the various teaching methods presented here might be applied.

MONITORING SELF-MEDICATION

Self-medication programs must be monitored in order to determine accurately and reliably whether the participant has correctly taken his or her medication. This will reduce the potential for medication errors, which can cause serious injury to the person's health. At first, self-administration should be completely and directly observed by another person. Once the individual can perform the component skills of self-administering the medication and an effective prompting system is in place, a systematic procedure for fading supervision, while maintaining intensive monitoring, can be implemented. After a predetermined criterion is met (e.g., 14 consecutive days with no errors), supervision may be reduced and monitoring should be less intrusive. During this transitional period, only small amounts of medication should be available to the individual at any one time (e.g., medication for 2–3 days only) (Coudreaut et al., 1990; Yunker et al., 1990). A number of monitoring procedures are presented in the following sections.

Laura is 35 years old and was recently living in a group home with seven other adults. She can express herself clearly, reads many simple words, and can tell time to the hour. She has a seizure disorder, and staff at the group home were giving her Tegretol and Depakote three times a day at 8:00 A.M., 4:00 P.M., and 8:00 P.M.

Laura was offered the opportunity to move into her own apartment; however, the situation required that she first learn to administer her own medications. Laura was very excited about the possibility of living on her own, and informed staff that she wanted to learn how to self-medicate. After consent was obtained from Laura, her guardian, her physician, and the human rights committee of the agency operating the group home, a self-medication teaching program was developed.

Laura was first taught to state the names of her medications, the dosages, and the prescribed times for administration. This was done 10–20 times throughout the day, with praise for each correct response. Laura's medication was color-coded, and she was taught to identify her medications when they were shown to her and to choose her medications when other medications were also present. This was accomplished by placing her medication on the table, along with medications of other residents of the group home (no more than three medications were put out at a time). Laura was asked to point to and name her medication, and again, specific praise was given for each correct response.

The next step was to teach Laura how to actually self-administer her medications. This was done by first creating a task analysis, and then teaching Laura the component skills through demonstration, opportunities for practice within her natural routine, verbal prompts, and behavior-specific praise. At medication times, Laura was taught to get a cup of water, remove her key for her lock box from the side of the table, open the box, take out the correct number of pills, close the box, consume the pills with water, replace the key, and put her initials in the appropriate box on her record sheet.

Once Laura was able to perform these skills correctly, it was time for her to learn to initiate self-administration of her medications at the correct times. To teach this, a prompt fading strategy was implemented. Initially, Laura was told 10 minutes prior to the scheduled time that it would be time to take her medication in 10 minutes. If she then took her medication at the correct time with no further assistance or prompts, she was given behavior-specific praise. Once she correctly performed self-medication in this manner for 10 consecutive administrations, the prompt was given 20 minutes prior, 30 minutes prior, and then 1 hour prior to the scheduled time. In addition to verbal praise, Laura received a special outing for coffee if she correctly took her medications for all three scheduled times that day. If Laura failed to take her medication, she was prompted by staff after 15 minutes. Finally, all prompts were removed.

During this time, a staff member was always present. Once Laura correctly performed self-medication with no prompts for 15 consecutive administrations, staff presence was faded. That is, over successive trials, staff stood further and further away from her.

Next, Laura was taught to administer her medications with little supervision from staff. Staff checked her record and did a pill count within 30 minutes after each scheduled administration time. A number of times errors occurred (e.g., medication was missed, pill count off by one pill). After each error, staff directly observed her self-administration until no errors occurred for 10 consecutive administrations (e.g., 3–4 days).

On two occasions during this teaching sequence, Laura became toxic to her medication. These opportunities were used to teach her to identify feelings of dizziness, upset stomach, and "tingling" sensations in her fingers. Subsequently, on a regular weekly basis, staff had Laura describe what she would do if she again felt these sensations (e.g., call a staff member, call her physician). Fortunately, perhaps due to slight changes in dosage prescribed by her physician, Laura has not become toxic again.

By the time Laura was able to move into her apartment, she had been correctly self-administering her medications for over 30 consecutive days. Once in her apartment, Laura's self-medication was monitored every 2 days by staff members (a pill count and a check of her self-recording were done). Because she now lives by herself, a locked box for the medication is no longer required. Laura continues to self-record after each administration, and she has not had any serious medication errors. Laura tells staff members that she is really enjoying her new-found independence.

Interviews

Many people have difficulty accurately reporting their own compliance when following a medication regimen. During interviews, people often tend to overestimate their compliance. In addition, low correlations between self-reports and actual pill counts have been demonstrated (Boczkowski et al., 1985). Interviews with people with developmental disabilities are at least as likely to be an inaccurate measure of medication regimen compliance as they are with the general population and should not be considered as a sole means of monitoring self-medication skills.

In some cases, interviews with other people (e.g., parents, direct service staff, physicians) have been used to obtain information about the person's compliance with the regimen. These types of interviews should also be considered inaccurate for monitoring the person's self-administration activities. However, interviews with other people may prove helpful in ascertaining information about the person's skills, typical habits, and potential problem areas.

Self-Recording

Self-administration logs or charts are often used to record whether or not one has taken his or her medication. Figure 1 illustrates a typical self-monitoring chart. The person using this chart self-administered medications four times each day. He recorded his initials after his medication was taken. Staff initials at the bottom of each column indicate that a pill count was done at the end of the day. In addition to self-recording, other monitoring procedures (e.g., pill count) will also be required because self-recordings are frequently overestimated. Self-recording, when used in conjunction with other monitoring procedures, can contribute to long-term independence and an increased sense of personal control.

Direct Observation

Service providers, teachers, and parents can directly observe the person self-administering medication. This type of monitoring provides an accurate, potentially reliable, and valid measure of whether the person has followed his or her self-medication regimen. Direct observation at each medication time is particularly recommended during the early stages of skill acquisition and supervised self-administration.

However, direct observation poses many problems for long-term monitoring. First, it defeats the purpose of self-medication training, that is, learning to perform a skill indepen-

DAYS

TIME	20 MONDAY	21 TUESDAY	22 WEDNESDAY	23 THURSDAY	24 FRIDAY	25 SATURDAY	26 SUNDAY
8 A.M. # OF PILLS 6	4-20-92 Take 6 DD	4-21-92 Take 6 DD	4-22-92 Take 6 DD	4-23-92 Take 6 DD	4-24-92 Take 6 DD	4-25-92 Take 6 DD	4-26-92 Take 6 DD
12 NOON # OF PILLS 2	4-20-92 Take 2 DD	4-21-92 Take 2 DD	4-22-92 Take 2 DD	4-23-92 Take 2 DD	4-24-92 Take 2 DD	4-25-92 Take 2 DD	4-26-92 Take 2 DD
4 P.M. # OF PILLS 3	4-20-92 Take 3 DD	4-21-92 Take 3 DD	4-22-92 Take 3 DD	4-23-92 Take 3 DD	4-24-92 Take 3 DD	4-25-92 Take 3 DD	4-26-92 Take 3 DD
8 P.M. # OF PILLS 5	4-20-92 Take 5 DD	4-21-92 Take 5 DD	4-22-92 Take 5 DD	4-23-92 Take 5 DD	4-24-92 Take 5 DD	4-25-92 Take 5 DD	4-26-92 Take 5 DD
	AR	AR	AR	JC	JC	GH	GH

Figure 1. Self-recording chart for monitoring self-medication.

dently without the presence of another person. Second, direct observation can lead to false assumptions; the presence of an observer may, in fact, prompt the individual to engage in self-administration, although he or she may not be correctly following the regimen when alone. For example, if an individual who is self-medicating lives in a residential home where medications are administered by nursing staff to other residents at the same time that the person is self-medicating, it is unclear as to whether the person may simply have been unintentionally "cued" by the presence of the nursing staff.

Despite these potential problems, observation by others is a useful technique when done unobtrusively, intermittently, and when used in conjunction with other monitoring procedures. Occasional direct observation under naturally occurring conditions also allows for evaluation of the maintenance of the person's skill level at administering the medication (e.g., set up, drinking water) and can help to pinpoint any specific problems in the performance of the skill. In many settings, it is helpful to set up a predetermined schedule for unobtrusive observation.

Physiological Measures

It might seem that the best way to monitor compliance with a medication regimen would be to obtain physiological measures of the presence of the medication in the person's body (e.g., blood, urine) or to obtain a measure of a tracer (e.g., riboflavin) attached to the medication, if the medication itself does not produce an observable change in blood or urine. These types of procedures, however, are fraught with difficulties. First, there are wide differences in the way that each person's body metabolizes medications. For example, differences in the speed with which medications are absorbed will yield a variety of results across people and across time (e.g., 1 hour vs. 3 hours post administration). Furthermore, there are cumulative effects of long-term compounds that reduce the validity of any physiological measurement.

An even greater problem with physiological measures is that they are often too complex or too expensive to implement on a regular basis in typical community settings. Obtaining frequent (e.g., daily) blood samples can be impossible for a family or a community program to accomplish. Specialized and expensive technology is usually required, as well as specific training in how to read the results of these tests correctly.

For example, Babiker, Cooke, and Gillett (1989) and Dubbert et al. (1985) found that a single 50 mg dose of riboflavin could be accurately discriminated by observers based on urine tests. They also found that the best time to assess was 4–5 hours postingestion and that levels returned to normal after about 15 hours. However, this procedure required use of a spectrofluoromoter, described by the authors as a relatively complex and expensive instrument, thus making this process impractical for most budgets.

Observing the Outcome of Medication

Measuring the desired outcome of medication is not an accurate method for monitoring self-administration. For example, the absence of epileptic seizures or psychotic symptoms or the improvement of an illness may or may not indicate that the person correctly self-medicated. Other nonmedicinal factors (e.g., normal course of illness, diet, behavior therapy) can contribute to an improvement in desired outcomes; therefore, reliance upon outcomes as the sole measure of correct self-administration may be incorrect and too delayed to prevent injury.

Pill Counts

The most frequently used monitoring method is to count the number of pills remaining in the container to determine whether this is the number that should be present had the person self-administered correctly (Eisen, Hanpeter, Kreuger, & Gard, 1987; Hinson et al., 1990). For example, if a person was prescribed two pills a day, one at 8 A.M. and one at 8 P.M., and given a 3-day supply to begin on Monday morning, a pill count on Tuesday morning should indicate four pills remaining. Frequent, unobtrusive pill counts can be very useful (e.g., counting pills between every administration when the person is not present, such as counting pills at 10 A.M. and 10 P.M. for medication prescribed for 8 A.M. and 8 P.M.). The primary problem with pill counts is that they do not indicate exactly what the person did with the pill. For example, a pill count cannot determine whether the person actually consumed the medication or, perhaps, flushed the pill down the toilet.

Coding

Another potential method for monitoring is coding oral medication so that each pill, capsule, or tablet produces a specified flavor, colors the tongue, or colors the urine. This coloring could be directly observed by another person, or the self-administering individual could independently record the flavor or color that was produced. The self-recordings could be examined at a later time to determine if they corresponded with the missing pills (Epstein & Masek, 1978).

This type of monitoring system could be useful because the outcome observed would be a direct result of consuming the medication. This method, however, has not yet received extensive application or evaluation. Issues surrounding altering of medication, appropriate and acceptable pharmaceutical practices, FDA approvals and regulations, and potential side effects need to be addressed.

Pill Counts Along with Direct Observation

Based on the literature and practices presented in this chapter, the best methods for monitoring appear to be a combination of unobtrusive and frequent pill counts along with unobtrusive and infrequent direct observation. For example, along with verbal feedback, behavior-specific praise, and other reinforcements, service providers should count the number of pills remaining at the end of each day. In addition, during ongoing activities when the person routinely takes his or her medication, and during which time service providers are present (e.g., dinner time), the individual's skill performance could be unobtrusively observed. In this way, the pill counts provide some indication of amount and time medication was taken, whereas direct observation indicates the process used by the person self-administering.

ASSESSMENTS AND EVALUATIONS

The trainee's performance should be assessed prior to beginning a self-medication program, during the course of training, following completion of training, and on a regular basis thereafter. The monitoring systems previously discussed can provide valuable information about the individual's performance. Structured role-play assessments may allow the observer to determine which component steps the individual already has in his or her repertoire. In addition, the following assessments are recommended.

Assessment of Participant Satisfaction

Every program can benefit from ensuring that the person is satisfied with his or her current medication regimen, with the support he or she receives for correct implementation, and with his or her own ability to self-administer. Similarly, listening to the opinions of parents, teachers, and direct service staff may help to determine the overall success of the program and the likelihood for continued participation once formal teaching has been completed. Satisfaction with the goals, procedures, and results of training can play a critical role in the successful maintenance of skills.

Assessment of Individual Preferences and Abilities

Individual assessments of each trainee's preferences and abilities are integral to ensuring program success. Once this assessment has been done, modifications or adaptations of the materials can be carried out to help the individual to perform self-medication procedures more successfully. To make this kind of assessment, the learner might be presented with different types of containers and packaging (e.g., bottles, bubble packs, plastic cases) to determine which is easiest for him or her to open and close, different labels (e.g., size of lettering, wording used, color-coding) to determine which are the easiest to read, and different types of instructions to determine those most easily understood (Morrow, Leirer, & Sheikh, 1988).

Assessment of Nonadherence

There are many reasons why a person may not adhere to a medication regimen; determining the reason can be critical. For example, noncompliance may be intentional or unintentional; that is, a person may not follow his or her regimen because he or she does not have the proper skills to follow the regimen, or the reinforcement schedule may not be effective. A skill deficit implies a need for skills training, whereas active noncompliance may be related to other factors, such as:

- An adverse reaction to the taste or side effects of the medication
- Issues of control and countercontrol
- Positive contingencies operating to maintain the noncompliance (e.g., attention from parents or staff)

Obtaining this type of information may recommend such actions as modifying the taste of the medication, aggressively combating side effects, providing new opportunities for choice making and personal control, and implementing new contingencies.

Studies of people without developmental disabilities have found noncompliance to be directly related to the complexity of the regimen (i.e., the more complex the regimen, the greater the nonadherence) (Boczkowski & Zeichner, 1985; Richardson, 1986). Regimens are more complex when a person is required to take several kinds of medication each day and when different medications or dosages are required at different times of the day. These researchers found that compliance was not related to gender, socioeconomic status, education, income, type of medication, cost of the medication, knowledge about the medications, or relationship between the patient and physician. Special reinforcement systems, such as requiring medications to be accepted before engaging in other desirable activities or including an instruction to take medications within a series of easy-to-follow requests, have been successful in encouraging individuals to follow instructions to take their medications (e.g., Harchik & Putzier, 1990).

MAINTAINING SELF-MEDICATION SKILLS

Once an individual has successfully completed a self-medication training program, several supports must be put in place to ensure correct maintenance of skills. As mentioned earlier, the individual's sense of satisfaction with his or her self-medication program is critical to maintenance. In addition, any changes to a medication regimen must be trained, and unobtrusive prompting and monitoring, as well as support and assistance when needed from the individual's family, agency, and friends, should be ongoing.

Ongoing Prompting and Monitoring

The two most difficult components of any self-medication program are ensuring that the person administers the medications correctly and at the prescribed times. Many people have chronic conditions that require medications to be taken for many years, often in the absence of any apparent symptoms. It should be expected, therefore, that ongoing systems for prompting and monitoring will remain as permanent parts of any self-medication program. A well-designed prompting system and an intermittent and unobtrusive monitoring system will allow the person to benefit from self-administration, while ensuring his or her safety.

Handling Changes to Established Medication Regimens

Changes in medication regimens frequently occur. For example, anticonvulsants may be changed depending upon the effectiveness of seizure control; psychotropic medications may be changed as the person's behavior improves or comes under control of environmental stimuli; and medications may be prescribed on a short-term basis to treat temporary conditions, such as illnesses or infections (e.g., Hancock, Weber, Kaza, & Her, 1991; Spirrison & Grosskopf, 1991). Any change to the medication regimen will require additional training and monitoring until the change has been incorporated safely and correctly into the individual's regular self-medication routine.

Making Use of Social Support Networks

The help and support of family, friends, and service providers can be very important for successful maintenance of a self-medication program. As more people with developmental disabilities are living and working in the community, social support networks have become crucial. Parents, siblings, staff members, roommates, and friends can play an important role in teaching, modeling, prompting, providing positive reinforcement, controlling consequences and rewards, providing assistance and support, ensuring that medications are taken correctly and at the appropriate times, and helping to solve any problems that may arise (Bentley, Rosenson, & Zito, 1990; Diamond, 1986). In addition, positive relationships between the individual who is self-medicating and his or her health care providers (e.g., physicians, pharmacists) can also have a beneficial impact on maintenance of self-medication skills.

CONCLUSIONS

Based upon the available literature and examples from existing self-medication programs, it is clear that self-medication skills can be taught to people with developmental disabilities. Interested parents, teachers, and direct service staff can use the suggestions provided in this chapter to develop a self-medication training program based upon characteristics unique to each individual (e.g., current skills, settings, regimen complexity, specific medications). Positive teaching procedures must be used, especially a detailed reinforcement system, and appropriate prompting and monitoring systems need to be implemented.

A number of issues in this area remain to be clarified by future research. First, as much of the published work that is available focuses upon research with people with psychiatric disabilities and the elderly, more work is needed to determine what can be generalized from this research for teaching self-medication skills to people with developmental disabilities. Second, further analysis is necessary to determine which skills are the easiest to teach and maintain and what skills are of the greatest benefit to all people concerned (e.g., program participant, parents, service providers, funding source).

Third, the conditions under which people are most likely to administer medications successfully without supervision need to be analyzed. Fourth, more research needs to be done on self-administering other nonoral medications (e.g., topical ointments, eye and ear drops) and other health care procedures. Fifth, attention must be given to the long-term maintenance of skills and to the continued development of safe, but unobtrusive, monitoring procedures. Finally, future application may address developing procedures that are specifically individualized to each person's unique needs, preferences, and abilities.

REFERENCES

Babiker, I.E., Cooke, P.R., & Gillett, M.G. (1989). How useful is riboflavin as a tracer of medication compliance? *Journal of Behavioral Medicine, 12,* 25–38.

Bentley, K.J., Rosenson, M.K., & Zito, J.M. (1990). Promoting medication compliance: Strategies for working with families of mentally ill people. *Social Work, 35,* 274–277.

Boczkowski, J.A., & Zeichner, A. (1985). Medication compliance and the elderly. *Clinical Gerontologist, 4,* 3–15.

Boczkowski, J.A., Zeichner, A., & DeSanto, N. (1985). Neuroleptic compliance among chronic schizophrenic outpatients: An intervention outcome report. *Journal of Consulting and Clinical Psychology, 53,* 666–671.

Burd, L., Fisher, W., Vesely, B.N., Williams, M., Kerbeshian, J., & Leech, C. (1991). Prevalence of psychoactive drug use among North Dakota group home residents. *American Journal on Mental Retardation, 96,* 119–126.

Coudreaut, E.A., Hinson, R., & McMorrow, M.J. (1990). *Medication education and self-administration for people with developmental disabilities: A teacher's guide.* Anna, IL: IDMH/DD Choate Mental Health and Developmental Center.

Diamond, R.J. (1986). Strategies for medication compliance with resistant patients. *Psychiatric Annals, 16,* 664–666.

Dow, M.G., Verdi, M.B., & Sacco, W.P. (1991). Training psychiatric patients to discuss medication issues. *Behavior Modification, 15,* 3–21.

Dubbert, P.M., King, A., Rapp, S.R., Brief, D., Martin, J.E., & Lake, M. (1985). Riboflavin as a tracer of medication compliance. *Journal of Behavioral Medicine, 8,* 287–299.

Eisen, S.A., Hanpeter, J.A., Kreuger, L.W., & Gard, M. (1987). Monitoring medication compliance: Description of a new device. *Journal of Compliance in Health Care, 2,* 131–142.

Epstein, L.H., & Masek, B.J. (1978). Behavioral control of medicine compliance. *Journal of Applied Behavior Analysis, 11,* 1–9.

Ferguson, D.L., & Baumgart, D. (1991). Partial participation revisited. *Journal of The Association for Persons with Severe Handicaps, 16,* 218–227.

Gehres, R.W. (1986). A medication monitoring service for elderly patients offered by the pharmacist on a fee-for-service basis. *Journal of Geriatric Drug Therapy, 1,* 81–89.

Hancock, R.D., Weber, S.L., Kaza, R., & Her, K.S. (1991). Changes in psychotropic drug use in long-term residents of an ICF/MR facility. *American Journal on Mental Retardation, 96,* 137–141.

Harchik, A.E., & Putzier, V.S. (1990). The use of high-probability requests to increase compliance with instructions to take medication. *Journal of The Association for Persons with Severe Handicaps, 15,* 40–43.

Hinson, R.L., McMorrow, M.J., & Coudreaut, E.A. (1990). *The effect of medication education and self-medication opportunities on knowledge of medication and self-medication accuracy in adults with developmental disabilities.* Anna, IL: IDMH/DD Choate Mental Health and Developmental Center.

Horner, R.H., Albin, R.W., & Ralph, G. (1986). Generalization with precision: The role of negative teaching examples in the instruction of generalized grocery item selection. *Journal of The Association for Persons with Severe Handicaps, 9,* 287–296.

Lundervold, D., & Enterman, M. (1989). Antecedent and consequent control of medical regimen adherence skills of an adult with developmental disabilities. *Education and Training in Mental Retardation, 24,* 126–132.

Morrow, D., Leirer, V., & Sheikh, J. (1988). Adherence and medication instructions: Review and recommendations. *Journal of the American Geriatrics Society, 36,* 1147–1160.

Richardson, J.L. (1986). Perspectives on compliance with drug regimens among the elderly. *Journal of Compliance in Health Care, 1,* 33–45.

Robinson, G.L., Gilbertson, A.D., & Litwack, L. (1987). The effects of a psychiatric patient education to medication program on post-discharge compliance. *Psychiatric Quarterly, 58,* 113–118.

Spirrison, C.L., & Grosskopf, L.G. (1991). Psychotropic medication efficacy graphs: An application of applied behavior analysis. *Mental Retardation, 29,* 1399–1470.

Wallace, C.J., Boone, S.E., Donahoe, C.P., & Foy, D.W. (1986). The chronically mentally disabled: Independent living skills training. In D.H. Barlow (Ed.), *Clinical handbook of psychological disorders* (pp. 462–501). New York: Guilford Press.

Yunker, N.S., Flint, N.B., & Carpenter, E.D. (1990). Patient self-medication on a rehabilitation unit. *Patient Education and Counseling, 15,* 261–268.

Zaharia, E.S., & Struxness, L. (1991). Comparative survey of drug use in a community service system. *Mental Retardation, 29,* 191–194.

Chapter Five

Meeting Special Health Care Needs of Students

Donna H. Lehr and Sally Macurdy

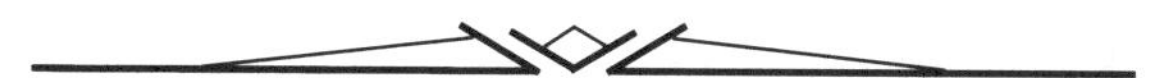

Some children require specialized health care that is beyond the routine for most school-age children. Very careful attention must be paid to the execution of that care. Inadequate implementation of procedures may often be life-threatening.

Many students with special health care needs who have developmental disabilities are dependent on others for their basic care, which places them in greater intimate contact with service providers. Because contact with others is the most frequent source of illness (Taylor & Taylor, 1989), high frequency of careproviding contact will increase the opportunity to contract diseases. The dependent care position also puts individuals with special health care needs at greater risk for abuse (Orelove & Sobsey, 1991; Sobsey, 1994; Sobsey & Varnhagen, 1989) and, consequently, at greater risk for being exposed to sexually transmitted diseases, including HIV (Jacobs, Samowitz, Levy, Levy, & Cabrera, 1992).

Becoming ill may be an added health risk for individuals with special health care needs. Some children have less resistance to communicable diseases due to genetic and metabolic anomalies, poorer nutrition, or lower activity levels (Orelove & Sobsey, 1991). For example, a cold, although uncomfortable, is not of grave concern for most children. However, for some children with compromised respiratory systems, colds can more readily turn into a serious upper respiratory illness. Additionally, children dependent on technology are at greater risk of being affected by such things as equipment breakdowns or clogged or dislodged tubes that could have serious repercussions.

Little emphasis has been placed on quality health care in schools. While childcare programs are licensed on the basis of their health and safety procedures, no similar standards are applied to schools that are educating groups of students who, due to developmental disabilities and/or special health care needs, often demonstrate a lack of control of body secretions that could lead to the spread of disease if not properly handled. The lack of strict standards can result in unsafe practices that compromise the health and safety of students and the adults with whom they interact.

The skill development of many children with developmental disabilities who have special health care needs can affect their susceptibility to infection. The lack of self-care skills (e.g., nasal hygiene and toileting skills) increases the risk for transmission of diseases and infections. An overwillingness to "share" mouthed toys and partially eaten snacks also increases disease transmission risks. Finally, difficulties in communicating aches and pains can sometimes result in undetected illnesses or diseases (Taylor & Taylor, 1989).

The implications of these concerns are clear. In educational programs for students with special health care needs, we must pay careful attention to care-providing practices, both those provided by staff and those performed by the students themselves. If we fail to provide hygienic care or to implement health care procedures correctly, we put students at risk. If we fail to model appropriate practices, instruction that leads to increased self-management of care becomes more difficult. If we fail to instruct students in their own care, we increase their dependency on others and put them at risk. Educators must be both knowledgeable and skillful in implementing procedures and in incorporating instruction on self-administration of procedures and practices into educational programs.

The overall focus of this book is on practical guidelines for teaching relevant health and safety skills to individuals with disabilities in order to increase their independence. However, this chapter deviates somewhat. Less emphasis is given to instruction of students with special health care needs in their own care, and more emphasis is given to informing practitioners about what comprises a healthy and safe environment for these individuals.

There are a few reasons why this focus has been chosen. The authors believe that information regarding special health care needs is not common knowledge among educators and other community-based service providers. The presence of individuals with complex special health care needs in schools and community settings is new. In the past, such individuals, if they survived, resided in hospitals and institutions, not within the community. As these individuals have moved to less restrictive settings, researchers and program developers have, as a first step, addressed how to provide a safe and healthy environment for them. This begins with the development of an understanding by practitioners of the nature of the needs of individuals requiring special health care procedures, as well as knowledge of the issues and practices surrounding their care. The next step, which is just beginning to occur, is to develop strategies for increasing the independence of individuals with special health care needs through instruction on methods for management and/or implementation of their own care.

At the present time, however, little information exists concerning specialized self-health care practices. What could be located is included later in this chapter, as are general recommendations by the authors based on their experience in the field. Although the focus of this chapter is on school-age children and school settings, much of the information is generalizable to individuals of all ages in all community settings.

SPECIAL HEALTH CARE NEEDS

Health care needs that have caused the greatest concern to school personnel, primarily due to their newness in schools, can be grouped into two categories: 1) special health care needs requiring use of technology and 2) infectious diseases. Even the typical diseases that occur in all children (e.g., measles, chickenpox, colds) may have greater impact on some students with special health care needs due to their increased susceptibility to contracting the diseases. Other diseases, such as the human immunodeficiency virus (HIV), cytomegalovirus, or hepatitis, require greater attention due to their unique relationship to children and youth with developmental disabilities (e.g., potential increased prevalence and/or risk of transmission). This section provides a brief description of specialized health care procedures for each of these categories and is designed to provide a basis of general understanding regarding why these procedures may be needed and how they are implemented.

Needs Requiring Technology-Based Procedures

Some students will be able to perform some of these procedures independently contingent on their motivation, fine motor control, and support from involved adults. As with any learning task, students will require varying degrees of prompting and supervision before becoming independent in performing a procedure (Graff, Ault, Guess, Taylor, & Thompson, 1990). Educators or others wishing to instruct individuals in implementing self-health care may wish to use the information presented here to develop task analyses. For a more detailed description of implementation procedures, readers are referred to Graff et al. (1990); Haynie, Porter, and Palfrey (1989); and Larson (1988).

Clean Intermittent Catheterization (CIC) Individuals with such conditions as spina bifida or other defects of the spinal cord often have no ability to control bladder emptying, no awareness of when the bladder is full, or no consistent sensation of wetness. The muscles required for urination function inconsistently. CIC is administered to empty the bladder to prevent urinary tract infection and kidney dysfunction (Graff et al., 1990). This procedure involves inserting a plastic or rubber tube (catheter) through the urethra into the bladder, thus bypassing the abnormal functioning area to allow the bladder to empty. This procedure can be scheduled at recess times to minimize school disruptions. Materials needed include:

- Catheter
- Cotton balls
- Soap
- Towelettes
- Syringe
- Urine collection container
- Antibacterial solution
- Water soluble lubricant for males (Graff et al., 1990)

Catheterization is a clean procedure, as contrasted with a sterile procedure, and requires only washing of equipment with soap and water after each use.

Tracheostomy Care A tracheostomy is a surgical opening through the neck and into the windpipe to aid in breathing. This procedure may be needed as a result of an injury; a condition requiring a bypass of the nose or mouth; or neurological, muscular, or other conditions that make it difficult for the individual to clear passages and cough up secretions. Within this opening, there may be a tracheostomy tube. Well-executed tracheostomy care is critical to ensure unobstructed breathing, prevent infection around the trachea or in the lungs, and prevent irritation around the opening into the trachea (stoma) (Graff et al., 1990).

Tracheostomy care procedures include suctioning, cleaning the inner tube known as the cannula, care of the skin around the stoma, changing the tracheostomy tapes, and changing the tracheostomy tube under clean, but not sterile, conditions. The most likely procedures needed during school hours include suctioning and cleaning of the inner cannula. Supplies necessary for removing secretions include:

- Catheters
- Gloves
- Sterile water
- Sterile saline
- Suction machine (Smith & Duell, 1989)

When suctioning, the catheter (attached to the suction machine) is inserted into the trachea. Force is created by placing a finger over an opening in the catheter and terminated by removing the finger. The inner cannula is cleaned by soaking it in a solution of hydrogen peroxide and water; cleaning with a small pipe cleaner brush; and rinsing in sterile water or saline, followed by tap water. It is then placed in a clean container to air dry. All cleaning activities should occur in a separate area in a sink not used for other purposes (Graff et al., 1990).

Nasogastrostomy and Gastrostomy Care Some children will be unable to take food by mouth because of inadequate suck, extreme difficulty chewing and swallowing, or episodes of pneumonia resulting from stomach contents being drawn into the lungs (Graff et al., 1990). To meet the nutritional needs of these students, a nasogastric tube is inserted into the nose, or a gastrostomy tube is inserted into the stomach through a surgical hole in the abdomen. There are several strategies for passing the liquid through the tube: the bolus method (formula flows through the tube in a few minutes), the intermittent gravity drip method (formula drips over a 20- to 30-minute period), the continuous gravity method (formula drips at a carefully controlled rate for 16–24 hours), and the continuous infusion by pump method (formula is given at a rate regulated by the infusion pump over 16–24 hours).

Ventilator/Respirator Care A ventilator (respirator) is used to aid breathing when conditions exist such as neurological damage, muscle weakness, or severe pulmonary disease. There are several different types of ventilators. Among them are positive pressure machines that are small and portable and help the individual to breathe by delivering air into the lungs, usually through a tracheostomy tube. Negative pressure ventilators pull air into the lungs by pulling the chest wall outward as the person lies inside a vacuum chamber. There are a variety of negative pressure machines such as the iron lung, the raincoat, and other portable home devices (Haynie et al., 1989).

Contagious and Infectious Diseases

The diseases that seem to generate the greatest amount of concern among school personnel responsible for educating groups of students with developmental disabilities and special health care needs are the human immunodeficiency virus (HIV), cytomegalovirus infection, and hepatitis. (For a more comprehensive discussion of infection and contagious diseases, readers are referred to Anderson, Bale, Blackman, & Murph, 1986.) Table 1 presents sample infection control regulations that schools may follow to prevent the spread of contagious diseases among their students.

In addition to the guidelines presented in Table 1, comprehensive school health care policies might include the following components taken from the *Day Care Regulations* of the Massachusetts Office For Children (1990):

1. Post emergency telephone numbers by each telephone.
2. Develop procedures for emergencies and illnesses.
3. Post procedures for using and maintaining first-aid equipment.
4. Develop policies for each of the following: emergency evacuation, injury prevention, infection control, and management of infectious diseases.
5. Formulate a plan to meet the needs of children with mild illnesses and distribute this plan to parents.
6. Develop guidelines for administration of medicine and distribute to parents.
7. Develop recommendations for meeting specific health care needs.
8. Formulate guidelines for identifying and responding to suspected cases of child abuse or neglect.

Human Immunodeficiency Virus (HIV) As HIV is the focus of Chapter 8, information concerning it will not be repeated here. However, no chapter on students with special health care needs is complete without reference to this increasing group of students present in today's schools. Many professionals, particularly those working in suburban and rural areas, feel a false sense of security regarding the likelihood of contact with individuals infected with the HIV virus. The rapid rate of increased incidence should cause all professionals, regardless of where they work, to be aware of the potential for contact and of the procedures necessary for cautious careproviding discussed in subsequent sections of this chapter.

Cytomegalovirus Infection (CMV) Cytomegalovirus infection (CMV) is usually a harmless virus. It is estimated that 40%–60% of children under the age of six have active cases of the virus and 75% of adults in the United States have had CMV at one time or another. In children and adults, CMV is manifested as either asymptomatic or mild flu-like symptoms.

CMV is transmitted through contact with feces, urine, and saliva, as well as prenatally from the placenta to the fetus. It is through placental transmission that the virus can be dangerous, causing abnormalities in fetal development. While the disease is prevalent and highly contagious, the potential for causing birth defects is very low. It is estimated that only 1% of all infants born in the United States will be infected; of that number, only 10%–15% will develop a disability that might include central nervous system damage and result in mild to

Table 1. Sample infection control regulations

(a) The licensee shall ensure that staff and children wash their hands with liquid soap and running water using friction. Hands shall be dried with individual or disposable towels. Staff and children shall wash their hands at least at the following times:

1. Before eating or handling food;
2. After toileting or diapering;
3. After coming into contact with body fluids and discharges;
4. After handling center animals or their equipment; and
5. After cleaning.

(b) The licensee shall ensure that the specified equipment, items, or surfaces are washed with soap and water and disinfectant using the following schedule:

1. After each use:
   a. Toilet training chairs which have first been emptied into a toilet;
   b. Sinks and faucets used for handwashing after the sink is used for rinsing a toilet training chair;
   c. Diapering surfaces;
   d. Toys mouthed by infants and toddlers;
   e. Mops used for cleaning body fluids;
   f. Bibs; and
   g. Thermometers.
2. At least daily:
   a. Toilets and toilet seats;
   b. Containers, including lids, used to hold soiled diapers;
   c. Sinks and sink faucets;
   d. Drinking fountains;
   e. Water table and water play equipment;
   f. Play tables;
   g. Smooth-surfaced nonporous floors;
   h. Mops used for cleaning; and
   i. Cloth washcloths and towels.
3. At least monthly or frequently as needed to maintain cleanliness, when wet or soiled, and before use by another child:
   a. Cribs, cots, mats, or other approved sleeping equipment;
   b. Sheets, blankets, or other coverings; and
   c. Machine washable fabric toys.

(c) The disinfectant solution shall be either a self-made solution consisting of ¼ cup of household bleach to each gallon of water (1 tablespoon per quart) which shall be prepared daily, labeled, and placed in a bottle that is sealed with a cap, or a commercially prepared disinfectant which indicates it kills bacteria, viruses, and parasites and which shall be used in accordance with label instructions. All such disinfectants shall be stored in a secure place and out of the reach of children.

From Massachusetts Office for Children. (1990). *Day care regulations* (103 CMR 7.07 [16] [a–k]). Commonwealth of Massachusetts: Author.

severe hearing loss, mental retardation, or motor abnormalities (Taylor & Taylor, 1989).

A child who has a disability due to CMV may have the etiology of the disability noted in his or her school records. Knowledge that a child has CMV may sometimes result in discrimination and avoidance. Because most adults who are responsible for careproviding have acquired immunities to the disease, avoidance is unnecessary. Furthermore, many other children with whom the adults typically have contact may also have active cases of the disease, but are not labeled as having it. Consequently, exclusion or avoidance of the child with CMV, who is labeled as such, will not protect the careprovider from the risks of transmission from other children in the class. A preferred procedure is careful adherence to hygienic care for all children and instruction of children in providing their own hygienic care.

Hepatitis A Hepatitis A refers to a viral disease of the liver caused by infectious organisms found in fecal matter. This disease has been common in childcare settings. In young children, about 25% will show no signs of illness; of the remaining 75%, 5%–10% will develop jaundice. In contrast, 75% of adults infected will develop jaundice (Hadler & McFarland, 1986). The symptoms will persist from 2 weeks to 2 months, with 99% of infected individuals recovering completely (Hadler & McFarland, 1986).

Hepatitis A is spread through fecal-oral contact. Studies on transmission in childcare centers indicate the risks of transmission are increased in facilities that include children who are in diapers and in centers that include large numbers of children (Hadler & McFarland, 1986). These are the same conditions that exist in many residential programs for individuals with developmental disabilities. Consequently, similar problems exist with individuals in these settings. Again, the solution is careful care provision and instruction of hygienic careproviding practices.

CRITICAL ISSUES

Until the 1970s, most students with special health care needs either did not survive the critical care period or were placed in restrictive hospital or home settings automatically (Lehr & Noonan, 1989). Changes in this trend have occurred due to the full inclusion movement, improvements in technology that have increased survival rates, increases in programs for younger children, and increases in the number of children with ongoing special health care needs who are surviving long enough to become students in regular schools and classrooms (Lehr & Noonan, 1989). Because the practice of including students with special health care needs in regular education settings is new, numerous questions arise regarding how to best provide services. Policy decisions related to program placement, procedure implementation, educational plan development, and training of school personnel and individual students are needed for all school districts.

Although arguments have been made that there are some children whose disabilities are so severe that they would not be able to benefit from an educational program, the focus of debate regarding students with special health care needs has instead been on whether these students should be attending school-based programs (as opposed to being educated at home or in a hospital) and who should be responsible for implementing and/or paying for the implementation of complex health care procedures. Few guidelines exist to recommend educational practices for students with special health care needs. Although some issues have been discussed in the courts, most have been local decisions that have not set firm standards for practice. Consequently, considerable variability exists in the ways in which issues are resolved. The following sections address some of these issues and practices, including inclusion, fiscal responsibility, and implementation.

Inclusion

One of the first challenges in regard to where education of students with special health care needs should take place occurred in *Department of Education, State of Hawaii v. Dorr* (1983). In this case, the school department refused to provide school-based services for Katherine, a child who required tracheostomy tube suctioning, reinsertion, and periodic medication. The State Department of Education determined that the child had health care needs that were more complex than could be provided by school personnel. They offered a home program of therapy and counseling. Appeals led to a ruling that a home placement did not meet the intent of the least restrictive provision of the Education for All Handicapped Children Act of 1975 (PL 94-142).

The question of inclusion of a student with developmental disabilities and AIDS was raised in *Martinez v. School Board of Hillsborough County, Florida* (1988). In this case, a child with developmental disabilities who contracted AIDS through transfusions at birth was offered home-bound instructional services. Upon appeal of that decision, the district court determined the child could be provided school-based services, but in a separate booth in a corner of a special educational classroom which would have a glass window and a sound system to enable contact with the rest of the class. The district offered the justification that her lack of continence, drooling, and thumb sucking increased the chances of her transmitting the HIV virus to others with whom she may have contact. The United States Court of Appeals remanded the decision, specifying that testimony indicated only theoretical risks of transmission and therefore was not sufficient cause for exclusion.

These two court decisions resulted in the inclusion of these students with special health care needs in their local school programs. Many other decisions regarding inclusion of students with special health care needs have been discussed through the individualized education program (IEP) process and have resulted in decisions to educate students with complex health care needs in schools, as in the cases of Dorr and Martinez. In other cases, decisions have been made that students should not attend school. Variability in school program placement continues because laws and regulations concerning inclusion of students with special health care needs are subject to interpretation, and administrative policies differ across programs.

Fiscal Responsibility

The question of who should pay for a student's health care services is being discussed extensively throughout the country. Central to the issue is interpretation of what is meant by medical and related services under the Education for All Handicapped Children Act of 1975 (PL 94-142) (Lehr & Haubrich, 1986; Lehr & Noonan, 1989; Martin, 1991). In PL 94-142, medical services are described as that which is necessary for diagnostic purposes to determine eligibility for special education. Related services are described as those supports necessary to enable a student to benefit from special education.

In the case of *Detsel v. Board of Education of the Auburn Enlarged City School District* (1987), the disagreement related to who should bear the financial responsibility for attending to the health care needs of Melissa Detsel, a school-age child born with severe physical disabilities. Due to her disabilities, she required the use of a ventilator with oxygen to assist with her breathing and was fed and received medications through a gastrostomy tube. When Melissa reached kindergarten age, her parents requested that the school district assume the cost for her nursing care during her attendance at school. The district denied the services based on their interpretation that the services were more complex than the typical school nursing services and more "medical" than required on the basis of the related services provision of PL 94-142. Their interpretation was upheld in the Second Circuit Court of Appeals in June of 1987 (*Detsel v. Board of Education of the Auburn Enlarged City School District,* 1987) on the basis of the complexity of the services, constancy of the care, level of skill of the staff necessary to implement the procedures, and cost of the care (Martin, 1991).

During the period of disagreement, the school district continued to pay the costs of Melissa's nursing services when she attended school. Due to the complexities of her health care needs, she was also authorized to receive 24 hours a day of private duty nursing services funded by Medicaid. Currently existing Medicaid regulations, however, did not permit Melissa's private duty nurse to provide her with nursing care in any location other than in the confines of her home, hospital, or skilled nursing facility (Omnibus Budget Reconciliation Act, 1981). Although the funding was available for her to receive nursing care throughout the entire day, those services could not be provided at her school.

After being denied funding for the provision of Melissa's health care services at school, her parents filed suit against the United States Department of Health and Human Services, challenging their regulations restricting the use of private duty nurses outside their home. Although this motion was originally denied in district court, it was upheld in the Second Circuit Court of Appeals (*Detsel v. Sullivan,* 1990); private duty nursing service for Melissa could be provided at her school. In time, the ruling was nationalized and was extended to all children receiving Medicaid private duty nursing services (*Pullen v. Cuomo,* 1991).

While this decision may appear to provide an answer to the question of who pays for health care services in the schools, it is far from a comprehensive solution. Only 27 states have private duty nursing services available through Medicaid (Golinker, 1991). The precedent set by Detsel only covered private duty nursing services; home health nursing services, which are available in all states, were not included. In addition, not all children with special health care needs are approved for Medicaid funding, and of those approved, many do not receive enough hours of coverage to include both needed school-time service and home services.

Responsibility for Implementation of Procedures

Of particular relevance to this chapter is the question of who should be responsible for implementing health care procedures in the schools. In the only case regarding the provision of health care services for students to be heard by the United States Supreme Court as of 1994, it was decided that clean intermittent catheterization (CIC) of a young girl with spina bifida was the school district's responsibility under the related services provision of PL 94-142, despite the district's arguments to the contrary (*Tatro v. Irving Independent School District,* 1984). The district argued that the procedure of catheterization was medically complex and beyond the responsibility of a school district. The courts upheld that CIC was not complex and was not medical in nature.

The Tatro case determined that it was the school district's responsibility for provision of the related service of CIC, and as this was a Supreme Court decision, the decision was extended to all children in this country. It did not address, however, the question of exactly who in the school district should be responsible for implementing CIC. In the Tatro case, the simplicity of the CIC procedure was emphasized. For other procedures that have not received similar scrutiny, much discussion continues regarding whose job it is to implement the procedures.

Issues regarding roles and responsibilities revolve around questions of how the role of a teacher should be defined, who can develop the necessary competence to implement the procedures, and how "medical" the procedures are in nature. In an attempt to clarify these questions, representatives from a number of associations, including the American Federation of Teachers, the Council for Exceptional Children, the National Association of School Nurses, and the National Education Association, formed a task force to develop guidelines for the delineation of roles and responsibilities relative to implementing health care procedures for children in the schools (Joint Task Force for the Management of Children with Special Health Care Needs, 1990). The resulting guidelines were published as a matrix which indicated who should have responsibility for implementing which health care procedures.

Concern has been expressed among some professionals, however, regarding strict adherence to these guidelines (Sobsey & Cox, 1991; TASH Critical Issues Committee on Individuals with Special Health Care Needs, 1990). Among these concerns are that the role, not the competence, of personnel implementing the procedures is what is stressed in the guidelines. Although nurses may appear to be the logical individuals to implement procedures, their designation as nurses alone cannot be used to imply competence. School nurses have indicated their lack of confidence in their skills in performing certain health care procedures that have not been routinely performed in school settings (Hester, Goodwin, & Igoe, 1980).

A second concern stems from the Joint Task Force's assumptions regarding the level of complexity of procedures based on the names of the procedures. As Sobsey and Cox (1991) indicated, according to the guidelines, teachers can assume responsibility for oral feeding of students, but not for tube feeding. The assumption is that tube feeding is more complex than oral feeding; however, "for some students . . . oral feeding requires extremely sophisticated training and skill while for others tube feedings are relatively trouble free" (Sobsey & Cox, 1991, p. 159). Determination based on the names of the procedures and not on the specifics of implementing the procedures with individual children is troublesome.

Because the guidelines recommend that most of the health care procedures be implemented by health care professionals, it is likely that students in need of those services will be located in centers where the personnel are located; thus, they will be placed in more restrictive educational settings. Additionally, these guidelines reinforce clear distinctions between roles and responsibilities among professionals providing educational services to students. These distinctions are in contradiction to the recent emphases on transdisciplinary service delivery to students with special health care needs (Sobsey & Cox, 1991).

However, this entire issue can be viewed from a different perspective: helping students to themselves become responsible for the management and/or implementation of their own care. The issue thus becomes not who will *implement* the procedure, but who will *teach* the student to implement the procedure. This places the focus on the area of teaching, not just on health care provision.

MEETING STUDENTS' SPECIAL HEALTH CARE NEEDS

This section focuses on how to meet students' special health care needs in the schools. Included in the discussion are suggestions for developing an individualized health care plan, training personnel to implement procedures, teaching self-care skills and encouraging greater independence, and normalizing education settings to assist students with special health care needs to feel more at ease in the classroom.

Developing a Comprehensive Health Care Plan

Well-implemented procedures are critical to the care of individuals with special health care needs. This begins with the development of a comprehensive health care plan that some have described as being analogous to an IEP (Palfrey et al., 1992). These plans should be developed by a team of professionals, including school nurses, educators, therapists, administrators, and parents, and should include descriptions of the child's health condition; his or her specific health care requirements, including nutrition, medication, and oxygen or other respiratory requirements; and specific emergency care procedures. Palfrey et al. (1992) further recommend that such a plan be reviewed and signed by the student's parents, physician, school administrator, and health care coordinator and be included as part of a student's IEP. A sample plan is shown in Figure 1. Haynie et al. (1989) have developed excellent materials to facilitate the development of such plans for individual children. These materials are a series of forms, which are included in the manual *Children Assisted by Medical Technology in Educational Settings: Guidelines for Care.*

Training Personnel to Implement Health Care Procedures

This section focuses on training personnel to implement special health care procedures; however, it is important to remember that the goal of this book is ultimately to encourage greater independence of individuals with disabilities. This section is included here because some procedures, due to their complexity or physical positioning, cannot be performed entirely by the individual himself or herself; however, the individual might be able to participate by letting others know when to begin or end a procedure, how to perform a procedure, or how to prepare or clean the necessary materials.

Numerous resources have emerged in the last 10 years that can serve as guides for personnel responsible for implementing specific health care procedures in schools (e.g., see Graff et al., 1990; Haynie et al., 1989). However, such resources alone cannot develop competence (Lehr, 1990b). They may be sufficient for development of a general awareness by other personnel in the school, such as building administrators and school secretaries, but they are not sufficient to prepare staff to actually implement such procedures.

Specialized training by individuals who have had considerable experience with the specific health care procedures required and the teaching of these procedures to significant others is critical. To assure that the needs of individual students are met, general procedures or protocols must be viewed merely as guides. Specific instructions for implementation of health care procedures must be received from each individual student's physician. Furthermore, parental input is essential. Parents can often identify methods that work best for their children. It is possible to be technically correct in execution of a procedure but not be effective. For example, positioning a child in a manner that does not allow for maximal relaxation can compromise the effectiveness of a particular procedure such as tube feeding.

Training must be provided at multiple knowledge and skill levels and to many different groups of individuals. Students in school settings interact with a wide range of school personnel and pupils. Some school staff likely to interact with students with special care needs may need only general awareness or desensitization training, while others must become competent in implementing specialized health care services. For example, the school cafeteria staff may only need to be aware that a child requires tube feeding and that his or her food must be kept in the kitchen's refrigerator, while the school nurse must be trained in implementing the feeding. The bus driver should

Name Kristin Smith Date 9/5/92

Health Care Needed gastrostomy tube feeding

Protocol attached

Plan Developed by mother, teacher, school nurse, in consultation with physician

Frequency daily, during scheduled lunch

Responsible staff teacher, teacher aide, school nurse as backup

Training

Date 8/25 Trainer public health nurse

Trainees teacher, aide, school nurse

Topics general first aid

Date 8/26 Trainer public health nurse

Trainees teacher, aide, school nurse

Topics CPR

Date 8/27 Trainer public health nurse

Trainees teacher, aide, school nurse

Topics tube feeding

Monitoring

Date 9/4 Trainer public health nurse

Trainees teacher, aide, school nurse

Date 10/2 Trainer public health nurse

Trainees teacher, aide, school nurse

Date 1/8 Trainer public health nurse

Trainees teacher, aide, school nurse

Emergency Indicators: color changes
breathing difficulties
g-tube comes out

Emergency Procedures: see emergency form

Figure 1. Sample health care plan.

be trained in regard to safe transport of a suction machine, while the aide accompanying the student with suctioning needs must know how to implement the procedure and how to instruct the student to participate in his or her own care.

The Council for Exceptional Children (1988) recommends that school personnel training programs include the following:

1. awareness and understanding of students' health care, emotional, and educational needs;
2. knowledge of common medical and health terms;
3. knowledge of medical characteristics including etiology and implications;
4. knowledge of physical, developmental, and emotional characteristics;

5. knowledge of appropriate curricular and environmental modifications;
6. knowledge of roles and responsibilities of the health care professional in the classroom;
7. knowledge of the importance and necessity for establishing support systems for personnel, students, and families; and
8. knowledge of resources for families. (pp. 5–6)

Lehr (1990b) recommends that personnel training programs be multifaceted and include the following characteristics:

1. Training should be designed to address the learning needs of the wide range of people with whom students with special health care needs are likely to have contact. This includes not only health care professionals and teachers, but also ancillary staff, such as cafeteria and school maintenance personnel.
2. Training should be individualized to meet the needs of personnel in differing roles; however, all should be aware of emergency procedures.
3. Training should use a variety of methods appropriate to the needs of the learners and their assigned roles relative to the delivery of health care services.
4. Training must be timely, systematic, and comprehensive.
5. Training must be sensitive to the needs of each individual student and family, respecting the child's right to be included in deciding what to tell peers about their health care conditions and needs.

The timing of training is critical. Training staff in implementation of procedures must occur prior to the student attending school. To do otherwise would put the student's health and safety at risk. Training must also be ongoing. That is, periodic review of implementation and refresher courses are necessary to assure that procedures continue to be implemented correctly.

Teaching Self-Care Skills

Once a health care plan has been developed and is being correctly implemented by well-trained personnel, an emphasis should be placed on the development of IEPs that include special goals and objectives related to each child's management of his or her own needs for care. It is typical to see numerous objectives on IEPs related to the partial participation of students with developmental disabilities in toileting and feeding; however, rarely do similar objectives appear in the IEPs of students with special health care needs. Typically, procedures are *done to* students, rather than *with* or *taught to* students.

Objectives for students with special health care needs and other students in their programs should include an emphasis on hygiene. Instruction in toileting, hand washing, and oral and nasal hygiene is critical. Fortunately, it is relatively commonplace to find such instruction occurring in programs for students with disabilities. The inclusion of students with special health care needs in school programs necessitates review of the emphasis placed on instruction in this area to assure that it is appropriate and sufficient to ensure their safety. Considerable literature exists on methods for instructing students in these areas, so it will not be replicated here. Readers are referred to Snell (1993) for a review of these methods.

Appropriate objectives for students with special health care needs might include teaching a student tolerance of, initiation of, partial participation in, implementation of, or termination of a health care procedure. Additional health care emphases that may be addressed in IEPs include increasing a student's understanding of the reasons for or implications of his or her health care needs or the indicators of problems related to the procedures. Sample objectives designed to generate ideas regarding possible IEP objectives are included in Table 2.

The lists in Table 2 are not comprehensive nor are the objectives written sequentially; they are merely proposed as examples. As for all children, the goal should be independence without a compromise of health and safety. In instances of self-implementation of procedures, 80% accuracy may not do!

The newness of our experiences in providing school-based education for students with special health care needs may account for the lack of research on the instruction of students in

Table 2. Sample IEP objectives related to special health care procedures

Tube feeding:
Student will explain (orally, in writing, or through other means) reasons for alternative eating method.
Student will describe steps necessary in implementing the procedure.
Student will indicate desire to eat.
Student will measure feeding liquid to be placed in feeding bag or syringe.
Student will pour food in feeding bag or syringe.
Student will direct cleaning of feeding equipment.
Student will clean equipment.
Student will feed self.

Tracheostomy suctioning:
Student will indicate need to be suctioned.
Student will turn on suction machine.
Student will hold suction tube while procedure is being implemented.
Student will describe steps necessary to suction.
Student will explain to others the indicators of need for suctioning.

Catheterization:
Student will indicate time to be catheterized.
Student will self-catheterize.
Student will describe steps in implementing the process.
Student will wash materials necessary.
Student will assemble materials necessary.
Student will hold catheter steady during procedure.
Student will describe indicators of problems related to catheterization.

self-health care. The exception is in the area of catheterization, about which several articles were located. Hannigan (1979) taught four 5-year-old children to self-catheterize using a combination of simulation with the use of a doll, verbal rehearsal, and supervised practice with use of a mirror. All four learned to self-catheterize, although no data were presented. In another study, which was conducted with two children with mental retardation, a detailed task analysis and praise for successful performance of each step of the task analysis were employed (Tarnowski & Drabman, 1987). Data showed that both students met criterion performance of all steps performed successfully for 4 consecutive days after 29 and 40 days of training, respectively.

In a multiple baseline design study involving two students (one with mild developmental delays and one without disabilities), the participants were shown to successfully generalize catheterization skills and self-catheterize after receiving simulation training with dolls (Neef, Parrish, Hannigan, & Iwata, 1989). These skills were grouped into four components:

1. Preparation
2. Mirror use
3. Catheter insertion and removal
4. Clean-up

Detailed task analyses of these components were delineated, and prior to the first training session, the instructor described and demonstrated the procedures. The student was then asked to perform the procedures. If an error was observed, the instructor used a cue hierarchy for correction. Data indicated that both students successfully learned to self-catheterize.

The decision to teach self-administration of procedures is one that should be made by the student's IEP team, including the child's physician. In some cases, close medical supervision is necessary, which would require observation by a trained adult (Altshuler, Meyer, & Butz, 1977). Objectives must be individualized, based on the health and the physical and communicative skill abilities of each individual child. Objectives selected should be based on careful discussion among team members.

Normalizing Education

Students with special health care needs are first of all children (Lehr, 1990a). Programs providing services to children with special health care needs must develop procedures that permit development or maintenance of this perspective. Key to this success are the skills and the quality of the educational services these children receive. Consequently, concentrated efforts must be made to maximize the full inclusion of these children into all educational activities. Students dependent on technology have often been met by less than receptive school officials. When these students have enrolled in schools, accompanying concerns for the students' health care needs have been translated into treating students as patients rather than students or, more importantly, as children (Lehr, 1990a).

To assist children with special health care needs to feel more comfortable with other students, health care services should be delivered in a manner that minimizes the disruption of the student's involvement in the class. Consider the following case example:

> Tasha, a first grader at Sudbrook Elementary School, is fingerpainting with the rest of her class. She indicates to the regular classroom teacher that she needs to be suctioned. The teacher signals to her well-trained teacher's assistant who calmly removes Tasha from the group, assists her in turning on the suction machine, inserts the suctioning tube, observes Tasha for a signal that she is ready for the suctioning to stop, and then returns Tasha to her fingerpainting.

What does this case example convey? Tasha is learning to manage her own care. She is not sick, but needs to be suctioned to remain healthy. Also, Tasha is learning to perform the suctioning by herself so that she can be entirely responsible for her own care, in all, a very positive situation for all concerned.

CONCLUSIONS

The need to provide education to students with special health care needs is increasing. More students with ongoing needs for assistive medical technology are surviving the neonatal period. Additionally, more children are being born with HIV. The implications are obvious. Comprehensive policies that guide the development of practice resulting in safe, healthy environments in which students can receive educational programs that are free of discrimination and respectful of each child's needs as an individual must be formulated. These policies must include an emphasis on increasing students' involvement in their own care. Training and future research on strategies for achieving this end hold the answers to the many unresolved issues regarding how this can be accomplished.

REFERENCES

Altshuler, A., Meyer, J., & Butz, M.K.J. (1977). Even children can learn to do clean self-catheterization. *American Journal of Nursing, 77,* 97–101.

Anderson, R.D., Bale, J.F., Blackman, J.A., & Murph, J.R. (1986). *Infections in children.* Rockville, MD: Aspen.

Council for Exceptional Children. (1988). *Report of the Council for Exceptional Children's ad hoc committee on medically fragile students.* Reston, VA: Author.

Department of Education, State of Hawaii v. Dorr, 727 F. 2d 809 (D.H. Cir. 1983).

Detsel v. Board of Education of the Auburn Enlarged City School District, 820 F. 2d. 587 (2d Cir. 1987).

Detsel v. Sullivan, 895 F. 2d 58 (2d Cir. 1990).

Education for All Handicapped Children Act of 1975, PL 94-142. (August 23, 1977). Title 20, U.S.C. 1401 et seq: *U.S. Statutes at Large, 89,* 773-796.

Golinker, L. (1991, August). *Memorandum re. final settlement agreement in Pullen v. Cuomo.* Washington, DC: United Cerebral Palsy Association.

Graff, J.C., Ault, M., Guess, D., Taylor, M., & Thompson, B. (1990). *Health care for students with disabilities: An illustrated medical guide for the classroom.* Baltimore: Paul H. Brookes Publishing Co.

Hadler, S.C., & McFarland, L. (1986). Hepatitis in day care centers: Epidemiology and prevention. *Reviews of Infectious Diseases, 4,* 548–556.

Hannigan, K.F. (1979). Teaching intermittent self-catheterization to young children with myelodysplasia. *Developmental Medicine and Child Neurology, 21,* 365–368.

Haynie, M., Porter, S., & Palfrey, J. (1989). *Children assisted by medical technology in educational settings: Guidelines for care.* Boston: Children's Hospital.

Hester, H.K., Goodwin, L.D., & Igoe, J.B. (1980). *The SNAP school nurse survey: Summary of procedures and results. Project #1846002587A1.* Washington, DC: U.S. Department of Maternal and Child Health.

Jacobs, R., Samowitz, P., Levy, P., Levy, J., & Cabrera, G.A. (1992). Young Institute's comprehensive AIDS staff training program. In A.C. Crocker, H.J. Cohen, & T.A. Kastner (Eds.), *HIV infection and developmental disabilities: A resource for service providers* (pp. 153–161). Baltimore: Paul H. Brookes Publishing Co.

Joint Task Force for the Management of Children with Special Health Care Needs. (1990). *Guidelines for the delineation of roles and responsibilities for the safe delivery of specialized health care in the educational setting.* Reston, VA: Council for Exceptional Children.

Larson, G. (1988). *Managing the school age child with a chronic health condition.* Wayzata, MN: DCI.

Lehr, D. (1990a). Educating students with special health care needs. In E.L. Meyen (Ed.), *Exceptional children in today's schools.* Denver: Love.

Lehr, D. (1990b). Personnel preparation to serve children with special health care needs. In A. Kaiser & C. McWhorter (Eds.), *Preparing personnel to work with persons with severe disabilities* (pp. 135–151). Baltimore: Paul H. Brookes Publishing Co.

Lehr, D.H., & Haubrich, P. (1986). Legal precedents for students with severe handicaps. *Exceptional Children, 52*(4), 358–364.

Lehr, D., & Noonan, M.J. (1989). Issues in the education of students with complex health care needs. In F. Brown

& D.H. Lehr (Eds.), *Persons with profound disabilities: Issues and practices* (pp. 139–158). Baltimore: Paul H. Brookes Publishing Co.

Martin, R. (1991). *Medically fragile/technology dependent students: Drawing the line between education and medicine*. Unpublished manuscript, Carle Center for Health, Law and Ethics, Urbana, IL.

Martinez v. School Board of Hillsborough County, 692 F. Supp. 1293 (MD FL 1988).

Massachusetts Office for Children. (1990). *Day care regulations* (103 CMR 7.07 [16] [a–k]). Commonwealth of Massachusetts: Author.

Neef, N.A., Parrish, J.M., Hannigan, K.F., & Iwata, B.A. (1989). Teaching self-catheterization skills to children with neurogenic bladder complication. *Journal of Applied Behavior Analysis, 22*, 237–243.

Omnibus Budget Reconciliation Act of 1981, PL 97-35, § 2176.

Orelove, F.P., & Sobsey, D. (1991). Health care problems: Prevention and intervention. In F.P. Orelove & D. Sobsey (Eds.), *Educating children with multiple disabilities: A transdisciplinary approach* (2nd ed.) (pp. 187–231). Baltimore: Paul H. Brookes Publishing Co.

Palfrey, J.S., Haynie, M., Porter, S., Bierle, T., Cooperman, P., & Lowcock, J. (1992). Project School Care: Integrating children assisted by medical technology into educational settings. *Journal of School Health, 62*(2), 50–54.

Pullen v. Cuomo, U.S. District Court for ND of NY, 88-cv-774, August 9, 1991.

Simonds, R.J., & Rogers, F.R. (1992). Epidemiology of HIV infections in children and other populations. In A.C. Crocker, H.J. Cohen, & T.A. Kastner (Eds.), *HIV infection and developmental disabilities: A resource for service providers* (pp. 3–15). Baltimore: Paul H. Brookes Publishing Co.

Sirvis, B. (1988). Students with special health care needs. *Teaching Exceptional Children, 20*(4), 40–44.

Smith, S., & Duell, D. (1989). *Clinical nursing skills*. Englewood Cliffs, NJ: Appleton & Lange.

Snell, M.E. (1993). *Instruction of students with severe disabilities*. Columbus, OH: Charles E. Merrill.

Sobsey, D. (1994). *Violence and abuse in the lives of people with disabilities: The end of silent acceptance?* Baltimore: Paul H. Brookes Publishing Co.

Sobsey, D., & Cox, A.W. (1991). Integrating health care and educational programs. In F.P. Orelove & D. Sobsey (Eds.), *Educating children with multiple disabilities: A transdisciplinary approach* (2nd ed.) (pp. 155–186). Baltimore: Paul H. Brookes Publishing Co.

Sobsey, D., & Varnhagen, C. (1989). Sexual abuse of people with disabilities. In M. Casapo & L. Gougen (Eds.), *Special education across Canada: Challenges for the 90's* (pp. 199–218). Vancouver, Canada: Centre for Human Development and Research.

Tarnowski, K.J., & Drabman, R.S. (1987). Teaching intermittent self-catheterization skills to mentally retarded children. *Research in Developmental Disabilities, 8*, 521–529.

TASH Critical Issue Committee on Individuals with Special Health Care Needs. (1990, December). *Proceedings of Committee on Special Health Care Needs*. Washington, DC: Author.

Tatro v. Irving Independent School District, 468 U.S. 883 (1984).

Taylor, J.M., & Taylor, W.S. (1989). *Communicable disease and young children in group settings*. Boston: Little Brown.

Chapter Six

First-Aid Skills

Nancy E. Marchand-Martella

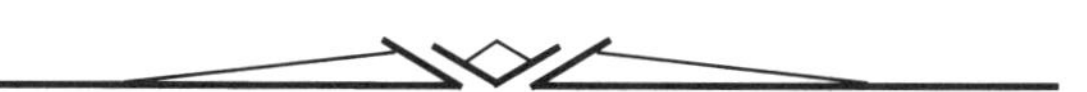

With increased efforts to promote full inclusion for people with disabilities across school, community, and work environments, there will be an increased risk for injuries. Therefore, these individuals should be prepared to respond appropriately to potential problems across a variety of settings. The purpose of this chapter is to assist individuals interested in implementing a first-aid training program for people with developmental disabilities. Preliminary steps that must be carried out prior to beginning a first-aid program are discussed, effective training programs are presented, specific training strategies are offered, and ways to promote generalization of first-aid skills to novel situations and suggestions for encouraging maintenance of skills over time are also addressed. Finally, future research directions in this curricular area are examined. All student age groups (from preschool to young adult) as well as older adults are represented; abilities vary. This chapter expands on the first-aid skills targeted in published research; it does not cover all injury and illness areas in which first-aid training would be needed. However, successful training programs are highlighted to assist readers in planning for more comprehensive skills assessment and training.

FIRST-AID TRAINING FOR PEOPLE WITH DEVELOPMENTAL DISABILITIES

Injury rate data for people with developmental disabilities are not available, but it is reasonable to assume that these rates are probably as high as those for persons without disabilities (Matson, 1980). People with developmental disabilities are at risk for accidents and emergency situations due to such potential characteristics as "poor judgment; lack of awareness of danger; impulsiveness and restlessness; inability or difficulties in communicating; low pain threshold; abnormal muscle functioning causing difficulties in chewing, swallowing, standing, or walking, and impaired vision and/or hearing" (Bryan, Warden, Berg, & Hauck, 1978, p. 88). Also, such health problems as seizures, vulnerability to infection (Blackman, 1984), and other chronic health-related conditions (Lorr & Rotatori, 1985) may increase their risk for emergencies and accidents. The following sections address how to teach needed first-aid skills to people with developmental disabilities.

Preliminary Steps

Identifying Needed Skills Two surveys were conducted by Collins, Wolery, and Gast

(1991, 1992) (see also chap. 2, Table 1, this volume), in which respondents (including parents and/or educators) were asked to indicate the safety skills they considered important for individuals with disabilities to acquire. Respondents indicated that preschoolers and elementary-age children should learn to get help from an adult when injured, and adolescents should learn signs of illness and infection, treatment of burns, knowledge of first-aid materials, how to clean and cover scrapes, and how to get help from an adult. Over 50% of the respondents in each of the two surveys cited first-aid as a necessary skill across age groups.

Stem and Test (1989) reported that those wishing to implement first-aid training should consult the American National Red Cross manual, *Standard First Aid and Personal Safety* (1988). This manual provides operational definitions and step-by-step instructions for treating a variety of injuries, recognizing health-related problems, and providing lifesaving assistance when needed. In addition, a nurse or doctor should be consulted whenever possible to provide assistance in targeting needed skills and modifying existing treatment procedures, if warranted. Finally, educators and careproviders should analyze the environment to identify necessary first-aid skills. For example, if an individual works in a kitchen, he or she may frequently encounter cuts and burns.

Developing Task Analyses Once skills have been identified and defined, task analyses should be developed. Stem and Test (1989) recommend that a representative from the American National Red Cross, a nurse, or a doctor should be consulted to ensure that the task analyses are accurate. Definitions of injuries and other health-related problems, along with the task analyses necessary for treating such problems, are presented in Table 1.

Organizing First-Aid Training Materials After task analyses have been developed, first-aid materials should be assembled. It is recommended that participants be supplied with a first-aid kit identical to the one used in training to keep in their homes. This kit should include the following:

- Soap
- Paper tape
- 5.08 centimeter square sterile pads
- Rolled cling gauze
- Clean cloth or paper towels
- Child-safe scissors
- 5.08 centimeter by 11.43 centimeter adhesive bandage strips

First-aid materials should be contained in a plastic box with a handle and the words, "first aid," and a red cross symbol should appear on the lid. These materials are appropriate for treating abrasions, burns, and cuts. Additionally, Gast, Winterling, Wolery, and Farmer (1992) recommend the inclusion of antiseptic (liquid and cream), calamine lotion, cotton swabs, disposable cleaning towels, tissues, and a plastic bag for treating cuts and burns as well as insect bites. Finally, such first-aid materials as various brands of over-the-counter cough medicine, aspirin, hydrogen peroxide, rubbing alcohol, and a thermometer may also be included (O'Reilly & Cuvo, 1989).

Reviewing Successful Training Programs

Table 2 summarizes some of the studies that have been done on first-aid training programs for children and adults with developmental disabilities and mental retardation. From reviewing the literature, it appears that a combination of instructor modeling, followed by participant practice with feedback appears to be the most effective method for teaching people with developmental disabilities to perform first-aid skills. Additionally, the inclusion of puppets for younger children during the participant practice phase of training is also quite effective.

For participants requiring additional assistance, teachers may combine verbal instructions with modeling (e.g., "You need to wash the wound under cool running water with soap like this."). Participant practice with both positive and constructive feedback is critical. After an error occurs, teachers could use verbal instructions alone or use a combination of modeling and specific instructions. In either case,

Table 1. Injuries and other health-related problems with associated task analyses for carrying out first aid

Abrasions: Scraping of cell tissue from the outer layers of the body that produces limited bleeding (American National Red Cross, 1988)
1. Wash wound under cool running water with soap.
2. Blot dry with sterile gauze or clean, dry cloth.
3. Take out bandage, and peel off adhesive plastic protectors without touching sterile pad.
4. Place bandage pad over wound so that it covers the wound completely.
5. Press adhesive strips so that they adhere to undamaged skin.
6. Show or tell an adult.

Second Degree Burns: Redness of the skin, blisters with swelling, and a wet appearance as a result of the skin touching something hot (American National Red Cross, 1988)
1. Immerse in cold water.
2. Blot dry with sterile gauze or clean, dry cloth.
3. Place sterile nonstick pad onto burned area.
4. Wrap with gauze to secure pad.
5. Tape gauze to secure pad.
6. Show or tell an adult.

Severe Cuts: Incised wounds that occur when body tissue is cut by knives, rough edges, broken glass, or other sharp objects, sometimes causing rapid and heavy bleeding (American National Red Cross, 1988)
1. Cover wound with cloth or sterile gauze pad.
2. Apply pressure to wound.
3. Continue applying pressure and elevate injury above the heart.
4. Continue with steps 1–3 and show or tell an adult.

Insect Bites: Irritations of the skin caused by a variety of insect bites (e.g., flies, mosquitoes, chiggers, spiders) (Green, 1977)
1. Wash and dry hands.
2. Open first-aid kit and remove plastic bag, Q-tips, calamine lotion, and timer.
3. Get two ice cubes from freezer and place in plastic bag.
4. Seal and/or fold plastic bag.
5. Set timer for 1 minute.
6. Place ice bag on bite.
7. Remove ice bag and place on table.
8. Shake calamine lotion, then remove top and place a small amount of calamine lotion on Q-tip and dab on bite.
9. Put top on calamine lotion bottle, empty ice bag, and throw Q-tip and bag in trash.
10. Put materials in first-aid kit and put first-aid kit away.

Choking: An object blocks a person's airway causing an inability to cough, speak, or breathe (American National Red Cross, 1988)
1. Let victim cough to try to get object out of his or her throat.
2. Do not touch victim while he or she is coughing.
3. When victim stops coughing, stand behind him or her.
4. Wrap your arms around victim.
5. Make a fist with one hand, placing the thumb side of the clenched fist against the victim's abdomen slightly above the navel and below the rib cage.
6. Press fist into abdomen with a quick, upward thrust.
7. Repeat steps 5 and 6 as needed.

Seizures: Convulsions that result in a loss of psychomotor control (e.g., kicking, jerking) (Matson, 1980)
1. Catch the person if possible to keep him or her from falling.
2. Slowly lower the person to the ground by holding him or her under the arms (if possible).
3. Turn the person's head to the side and hold it loosely.
4. Do not put objects in the person's mouth.

Colds: One or more of the following: runny nose, unproductive cough, congestion, sore throat, or productive cough (O'Reilly & Cuvo, 1989)
1. Take temperature:
   a. Take thermometer out of medicine box.
   b. Place under tongue until beeping sound is heard.
   c. Read thermometer.
   d. Rinse thermometer.
   e. Return thermometer.

(continued)

Table 1. (*continued*)

2. Perform necessary medical procedures:
   a. Treat worst symptom medically.
   b. Choose correct medicine to treat symptom.
   c. Take correct medicine from medicine box.
   d. Read aloud the right dosage from instructions on medication.
   e. Read aloud at what time intervals to take the medication.
3. Perform necessary nonmedical procedures:
   a. Get extra rest.
   b. Drink plenty of fluids.
   c. If throat is sore, gargle with salt water.

Communicating an Emergency:

1. Locate phone.
2. Pick up receiver.
3. Dial 911.
4. Hold receiver to ear.
5. Listen for operator.
6. Give full name.
7. Give full address.
8. Give phone number.
9. Explain emergency.
10. Hang up after operator has acknowledged your call.

participants should be encouraged to demonstrate their skill independent of instructor prompting. Thus, a retest, in which the participants' skill in using the first-aid procedure without instructor feedback or modeling is examined, is another important component to include in training.

Marchand-Martella and Martella (1990) conducted a training program that was successfully implemented in two studies involving young children with disabilities. This program involved the use of a storytelling manual, puppets, and participant practice. The case example below illustrates how this training program might be conducted. Modifications could be made to the methods described. For instance, each child could practice injury treatment on his or her own puppet, or two children could share a puppet and work together.

Using puppets who are characters in an instructional story provides an interesting alternative to learning a skill through teacher mod-

Bob Johnson, a group home therapist, targeted first-aid instruction as a needed curricular area for three boys (ages 6 and 7) with behavior disorders. These boys lived in the group home during the week and went home on weekends. They were constantly rabble-rousing on the playground at school and at the group home and needed to learn first-aid treatment for potential injuries. Bob selected the safety skills manual, *Mouse Calls* (Marchand-Martella, Martella, & Marchand, 1988), to use in his program. First, Bob had the three boys sit at a table across from him. He read from the storytelling manual, which includes task-analyzed steps and illustrations of two "mouse doctors" who took care of the injuries of their friends. The boys were instructed to listen to the story and to look at the illustrations as they were pointed out by Bob. As the boys listened to the story, Bob asked them to respond in unison to questions he asked to ensure on-task behavior (e.g., "You need to blot the wound dry with a clean cloth. What do you need to do?"). Each boy took turns treating an "injured" puppet who was a character in the story. These puppets had simulated injuries sewn to their arms. During this hands-on demonstration, Bob praised the boys when they performed a step correctly (e.g., "Good job covering the wound with the adhesive bandage.") and provided instructions when the step was incorrect or missing (e.g., "Good try, but you need to blot it dry like this. Show me again."). While one boy practiced injury treatment, the other boys looked at books or worked puzzles. At the end of each session, all the boys earned stickers for their participation.

Table 2. First-aid training programs for people with disabilities

Reference	Participants	Skill(s) taught	Training methods	Generalization	Maintenance monitoring
Christensen, Marchand-Martella, Martella, Fiechtl, and Christensen (1993)	4 children (ages 3–4) with delays in speech and language	Obtain adult help when cut	Instructor modeling, participant practice with feedback, and retest without feedback	Novel settings, removal of first-aid supplies	4 weeks
Gast, Winterling, Wolery, and Farmer (1992)	4 young adults (ages 17–21) with moderate mental retardation	Treatment of cuts, burns, and insect bites	Brief orientation lecture, 5-second time delay with backward chaining, feedback	Peers	Up to 18 weeks
Hauser, Cockson, Redican, and Olsen (1979)	16 adults (ages 23–36) with mild to moderate mental retardation	Basic first-aid course (e.g., care of colds)	Workshop format (i.e., series of films, participant practice and review, completion of workbook)	None	3 weeks
Marchand-Martella and Martella (1990)	4 children (ages 7–11) with mild to severe disabilities	Treatment of minor wounds with continued bleeding and burns	Storytelling manual, puppets, and participant practice with feedback	Novel injury, settings, self/others	Up to 66 weeks
Marchand-Martella, Martella, Agran, Salzberg, Young, and Morgan (1992)	4 children (ages 7–11) with moderate mental retardation	Treatment of abrasions, burns, and cuts	Peer modeling, participant practice with feedback, and retest without feedback	Novel settings, injury locations, novel cues, self/others	Up to 12 weeks
Marchand-Martella, Martella, Christensen, Agran, and Young (1992a)	9 children (ages 7–10) with mild disabilities	Treatment of abrasions, burns, and cuts	Storytelling manual, puppets, and participant practice with feedback	Novel settings, injury locations, self/others	Up to 12 weeks

(continued)

Table 2. *(continued)*

Reference	Participants	Skill(s) taught	Training methods	Generalization	Maintenance monitoring
Marchand-Martella, Martella, Christensen, Agran, and Young (1992b)	4 children (ages 6–12) with mild to moderate disabilities	Treatment of abrasions	Training Program 1: Instructor modeling, participant practice with feedback, and retest without feedback (treatment of puppets) Training Program 2: Same as Training Program 1 (treatment of people)	Injury locations, self/others	None
Matson (1980)	5 adults (ages 25–37) with moderate mental retardation	Treatment of seizures and cuts	Instructor discussion and participant practice with feedback and modeling	None	4 weeks
O'Reilly and Cuvo (1989)	44-year-old adult with anoxic brain injury	Treatment of four classes of cold symptoms	Task analyses (generic, specific, individualized), participant practice with feedback	None	1 week 4 weeks
Spooner, Stem, and Test (1989)	3 adolescents (ages 16–17) with moderate mental retardation	Dial 911, treatment of minor wounds, applying a plastic bandage, and treatment of choking	Group discussion, instructor modeling, participant practice with feedback, and retest without feedback	Novel mock situations	6–12 weeks

eling or discussion. When puppets are paired with colorful illustrations and storytelling, children have a variety of stimuli (visual, auditory, and tactile) to attend to; thus, various learning styles are emphasized. Puppets are aesthetically pleasing, manipulative, easy to clean, and provide a permanent product for educators to judge completion of a first-aid procedure.

Table 3 summarizes studies done on first-aid training programs for children without disabilities. These studies are included in this discussion because some of the methods may be modified for individuals with disabilities. For example, the *Safe-at-Home* manual (Peterson, 1984a) could be used in training, along with instructor modeling of first-aid techniques, participant practice with instructor feedback, and a retest (performed immediately after participant practice or at a later time). Role plays involving the instructor and participant may be used in which both parties take turns treating injuries. The discrimination component of this training (reacting differently to examples and nonexamples) could also be modeled by the instructor with participant imitation immediately following.

Specific Training Strategies

Simulation Because in vivo instruction is usually not possible (i.e., waiting until a child is injured before initiating training), simulated instruction is advocated to approximate the natural environmental context in which the behavior is to be performed (Cuvo & Davis, 1983; Nietupski, Hamre-Nietupski, Clancy, & Veerhusen, 1986). First-aid training programs for children with disabilities have included the following simulations:

- Various cold symptoms simulated in photographs (O'Reilly & Cuvo, 1989)
- Simulated accidents (e.g., cutting vegetables with a knife and pretending to cut finger, applying a red mark for burns and ketchup for abrasions and cuts) (Marchand-Martella & Martella, 1990)
- Costume makeup for cuts, burns, and insect bites and simulated blood (Gast et al., 1992)
- Simulated injuries manufactured by Simulaids™, a company that makes simulated injuries and other first-aid supplies for use in first-aid training programs for healthcare professionals. (Simulated injuries can be purchased from Simulaids™ by writing to the company at P.O. Box 807, Dixon Avenue, Woodstock, New York 12498.)

In addition to the simulations suggested above, Marchand-Martella, Martella, Agran, and Young (1992) used two-way stick tape to adhere the "injuries" to the skin. Simulated blood was used to approximate severe cuts, dirt was applied as abrasions, and embalmer's wax was applied to "burns" to simulate blisters. Educators need to determine their budgetary restrictions when first-aid simulations are considered. If teachers have limited funds, injuries can be simulated using a red mark, dirt, or betadine solution. Red food coloring can be added to corn syrup to produce simulated blood, or vampire blood can be purchased around the Halloween season at relatively low costs.

Measuring Duration of Response The time a person takes to respond to injuries is a critical component of first-aid training programs because most injuries require an immediate response (American National Red Cross, 1979). If a person takes too long to respond to an injury or to care for it, further complications may result. This section presents ways in which first-aid instructors might evaluate the amount of time a participant takes to respond to an injury.

Gast et al. (1992) conducted a training program that included a time element in one task analysis for treating insect bites. Participants were required to set a timer for 1 minute when an ice bag was placed on the injured area and to remove the ice bag after the timer sounded. This time requirement is important for appropriate treatment to occur. Additionally, Gast et al. allowed 60 seconds to complete each step in task analyses for treating cuts, burns, and insect bites; duration errors were recorded for future practice.

Table 4 presents means and ranges of first-aid response duration measures from first-aid

Table 3. First-aid training programs for children without disabilities

Reference	Participants	Skill(s) taught	Training methods	Generalization	Maintenance monitoring
Marchand-Martella, Martella, Agran, and Young (1992)	6 children (ages 6–8)	Treatment of abrasions, cuts, and burns	Storytelling manual, puppets, and participant practice with feedback	Novel injuries, self/others	None
Mori and Peterson (1986)	30 children (ages 3–5)	Treatment of cuts	*Safe-at-Home* manual and participant practice with feedback	None	None
Peterson (1984a)	8 children (ages 8–9)	Treatment of cuts	*Safe-at-Home* manual and participant practice with feedback	Novel setting	52 weeks
Peterson (1984b)	6 children (ages 7–10)	Treatment of cuts	Training Program 1: "Prepared for Today" manual and participant practice with feedback Training Program 2: "Safe-at-Home" manual and participant practice with feedback	Burns	20 weeks
Peterson, Farmer, and Selby (1988)	2 children (ages 6 and 8)	Treatment of cuts	Participant practice with feedback, prompting, shaping through verbal reinforcement, modeling, and praise by parent	Burns self/brother	30 weeks

Peterson and Mori (1985)	8 children (ages 7–9)	Treatment of cuts	Training Program 1: *Safe-at-Home* manual, modeling, praise for correct responses, and extinction for incorrect responses Training Program 2: same as Training Program 1 with Kendall's (1981) problem-solving approach	Burns	20 weeks
Peterson, Mori, Selby, and Rosen (1988)					
Experiment 1	5 children (ages 8–10)	Treatment of cuts	*Safe-at-Home* manual and role plays	Burns	30 weeks
Experiment 2	9 children (ages 7–11)	Treatment of cuts	*Safe-at-Home* manual and role plays	Burns	30 weeks
Experiment 3	24 children (ages 5–11)	Treatment of cuts, burns, and bloody noses	Safety presentations, questions and answers for parents, role play and discussion of safety facts for children	Novel setting	10 days
Peterson and Thiele (1988)	7 children (ages 6–8)	Treatment of cuts and burns	*Safe-at-Home* manual, group discussion, modeling, praise, and group rehearsal	None	None

Table 4. Means and ranges of first-aid response duration measures for students with and without disabilities

Treatment need	Students with disabilities[a]		Students without disabilities[b]	
	Mean	Range	Mean	Range
Abrasions on self	116″	63″–170″	141″	83″–261″
Abrasions on another	117″	70″–205″	101″	49″–168″
Burns on self	137″	63″–182″	112″	60″–163″
Burns on another	111″	54″–274″	88″	72″–105″
Cuts on self	20″	4″–59″	27″	20″–31″
Cuts on another	18″	5″–76″	20″	11″–43″

[a]Adapted from Marchand-Martella, Martella, Christensen, Agran, and Young (1992a).
[b]Adapted from Marchand-Martella, Martella, Agran, and Young (1992).

training programs for students with and without disabilities. Overall, results from the students with disabilities indicated that they could treat most injuries within the established duration ranges obtained by their peers without disabilities. Teachers can use the established duration ranges reported in Table 4 for students without disabilities as a means of comparison when their own students perform first-aid; teachers can also gather duration timings from students in the program or others who are already proficient at completing a first-aid procedure and use these for comparisons.

A standard stopwatch or kitchen timer is useful for collecting duration measures. Response duration should be measured from the time the instructional cue is provided (e.g., "You cut yourself. Show me how to take care of it."). If a student waits to respond until prompted by the instructor to do so, latency measures may be warranted. That is, the instructor would measure the time between the initial instructional cue and the first response emitted by the student. If participants are slow when completing a first-aid procedure, the teacher may need to include fluency training. Such training is critical because dire consequences may result if an individual does not administer the treatment immediately and effectively.

Fluency Training and Modification of Training Materials If participants cannot treat injuries within the established time ranges, fluency training may be warranted to improve their performance. For example, if an individual takes too much time to wash or bandage an injury, additional practice may be needed. Individuals should practice these responses until fluency is achieved (i.e., individuals can perform injury treatment as quickly as proficient peers).

If fluency training does not prove beneficial because of physical or intellectual impairments exhibited by a student, an instructor may need to consider altering the required behaviors or modifying the necessary materials. For example, Marchand-Martella, Martella, Christensen, and Young (1992a) noted that one participant had great difficulty opening bandages due to his lack of fine motor skills. Although fluency training involved additional practice on opening bandages, he still exhibited difficulties. The authors concluded that this difficulty was the main reason for the long durations in his overall treatment of abrasions. Therefore, the bandages were removed from their packages and the first-aid kit was stocked with these unpackaged bandages. This adjustment shortened the participant's response duration.

Another participant had difficulty performing the steps in the appropriate sequence and, consequently, spent a majority of his time attempting to "figure out" what steps to perform and when to perform them. Therefore, the participant was provided a visual cue (cue card) that listed the appropriate steps and sequence for each first-aid skill. This adjustment allowed for a smoother, faster response.

Problem Solving Individuals need to be prepared to respond to actual injuries outside the training situation. The problem-solving strategies illustrated in the following case example are recommended.

Mrs. Myers, a resource room teacher, decided to teach a variety of safety skills, including first aid, to her students. She developed a number of problem scenarios to use with the students of situations they would most likely encounter. When presented with a problem situation, such as "What do you do when you have a badly cut hand?", Mrs. Myers taught the students six problem-solving steps to follow. First, the students had to *stop and think* (e.g., "I've got a bad cut on my hand. What should I do now?"). Second, the students had to *identify the problem and select the goal* (e.g., "I've got to stop the bleeding right away because it is a bad cut. Then I must go and get some help"). Third, the students had to *consider all options* (e.g., "I could wash the cut, shake my hand, run to the neighbors."). Fourth, the students had to *make a plan using the six best things to do* (e.g., "Wrap a clean cloth around the cut, press firmly to stop bleeding, call Mom, put ice on cut, lie down, and elevate hand."). Fifth, the students had to *rehearse the plan* (e.g., practice treating cut, dialing phone to speak with Mom, putting ice on cut, lying down with hand elevated) and demonstrate correct performance three consecutive times. Finally, the students had to *self-reinforce* (e.g., "Good job. I learned to take care of my own cut."). Mrs. Myers praised correct responding and corrected errors when they occurred.

This type of problem-solving training format could easily be used with individuals of all ages and abilities. A group instructional format of four or more students or cooperative learning groups of three or fewer students may be incorporated. Additionally, modifications to these procedures could be made for individuals who need greater assistance. For example, a permanent prompt, such as a poster or cue card, that includes the necessary problem-solving components could be devised to assist learners in remembering all of the requisite steps in solving a problem.

Using Peer Tutors Teaching first-aid skills to students can involve considerable instructional time. However, finding the necessary time is often a problem for teachers. One successful approach to providing students with increased individualized instruction utilizes peer tutoring (Howell & Kaplan, 1978). Marchand-Martella, Martella, Agran, Salzberg, et al. (1992) used peer tutors to assist students with disabilities to learn first aid. These peers were taught to model first-aid techniques, correct errors, praise correct responses, and collect data. Results indicated that the peer tutors successfully learned the instructional techniques and were quite effective in their delivery; they also collected performance data reliably. One positive side effect of the program was that the first-aid skills of the two peer tutors maintained at higher mean levels for up to 12 weeks after their original training as compared to other program participants with similar disabilities (i.e., 86% versus 70% for abrasions, 88% versus 76% for burns, and 93% versus 52% for cuts).

Peer tutors should first be taught to perform the skills accurately and smoothly. Second, they will need to be instructed on how to teach the first-aid skill to the participant, provide positive or corrective feedback to the participant while he or she is practicing injury treatment, and collect performance data on the learner. Educators should periodically observe instructional sessions to ensure that the peer tutor continues to perform the tutoring behaviors and collects performance data reliably. Further information on how to train peers to become first-aid tutors can be found in Marchand-Martella and Martella (1993).

Training Parents The majority of studies have been conducted with children who were still living at home with their parents; therefore, it is crucial that parents be involved in any training program. Parents should be given an orientation on the first-aid skills program before their children receive training, and they should be encouraged to allow their children to treat minor injuries on their own so that independence is promoted. Additionally, parents should receive first-aid training themselves, so that they can effectively remediate any errors that their children demonstrate at home when treating their own injuries. Parents should learn that it is important to provide frequent opportunities for their children to practice first aid. Data sheets that include task-analyzed steps should be left in the parents' home so that parents can refer to the procedures if needed. They should also be provided with a stocked first-aid kit that includes a checklist of supplies so that additional materials can be purchased when depleted, or they should at least be given a checklist of materials so that they can assemble their own kits. Educators should periodically check with parents to determine how well skills are maintaining at home and to provide additional assistance if warranted.

Generalized Responding to Injuries

It is critical that program participants exhibit their acquired first-aid skills in situations other than those used in training, as well as maintain these skills over time. First-aid skills training is useless if participants cannot treat real injuries on themselves or seek adult assistance for injuries, if necessary, once a training program is over. The following sections address ways to promote the transfer of first-aid skills for use in novel situations.

Discrimination Training Discrimination training involves teaching individuals to respond to more than one injury at a time and assessing whether individuals can perform the correct treatment for each type of injury. For example, if an individual is shown a burn and a cut, does he or she provide the correct treatment for each injury or treat *all* injuries using the same first-aid procedure? Marchand-Martella, Martella, Agran, Salzberg, et al. (1992) taught individuals with disabilities to treat three different injuries within the same instructional session. The study included a withdrawal of training components to determine if the participant could care for an injury based on its physical characteristics (e.g., redness of skin, blisters with swelling, a wet appearance for burns) rather than on specific verbal instructions (e.g., modeling and feedback) provided by the teacher. To be sure that characteristics typical to the injury rather than specific verbal cues (e.g., "You cut yourself." or "You burned yourself.") were controlling responding, novel cues (e.g., "You were slicing vegetables and look what happened." or "You touched a hot pan and look what happened.") were used during the 3-month generalization assessment. Results indicated that the participants learned to discriminate among injuries based on their appearance, not on the instructional cues used in training.

The ability to discriminate different types of injuries is critical because individuals will not always have an adult present to specify to the individual whether he or she has been cut, burned, or scraped. In particular, participants should be taught to discriminate those injuries requiring immediate outside help and those they could treat themselves. Such discrimination training includes teaching individuals to discriminate depending on the type, severity, and location of the injury.

Learning to discriminate an injury's physical characteristics may involve training using photographs of examples of the injury (e.g., different sizes/appearances of abrasions), as well as nonexamples (e.g., insect bites, burns). When an individual is proficient at labeling these photographs correctly, first-aid training may proceed so that the individual learns to provide the appropriate treatments in the presence of the appropriate corresponding injuries. The instructor should use the cue, "What kind of injury is this?", and watch to see if the correct treatment is performed.

General Case Programming General case programming promotes generalized responding by focusing on teaching representative examples so that any task in the instructional class can be performed correctly (Pancsofar, Schafer, Blackwell, & Gavron, 1984). Horner, Sprague, and Wilcox (1982) recommend the following steps in implementing general case programming (as cited in Steere, Pancsofar, Powell, & Butterworth, 1989):

1. The instructional universe (the range of situations to which the learner's response must generalize) must be defined. For example, the individual needs to treat abrasions of various sizes on different areas of the body.

2. The relevant stimulus and response variations in the instructional universe should be analyzed. Thus, for instance, the instructor would need to determine the proper procedures for treating abrasions based on their location, size, and stimulus conditions for treatment (e.g., using different faucets, soap dispensers, paper towels, adhesive bandages).
3. Examples for teaching and probe sessions should be selected. For instance, the instructor might select six injuries to use in direct instruction and six untrained injuries to test for generalized responding.
4. The teaching examples must be sequenced. That is, the instructor must juxtapose the six treatment examples so that important differences and similarities become more salient to the learner.
5. The teaching examples need to be taught using behavioral-instructional techniques.
6. Generalization using the examples selected for probes should be tested. For example, the instructor should test to see if the participant can treat the six novel injuries after training has been conducted.

Schafer (1983) validated a general case strategy for the instruction of persons with severe disabilities in applying adhesive bandages. Participants learned to apply a number of different adhesive bandages in this training program. The general case approach seems especially suited to first-aid training because of the multitude of possible injuries of differing sizes, severity levels, and locations on the body that require a variety of treatment methods. Additionally, nonexamples should be included in a training program to determine if a participant incorrectly treats all types of injuries using the same treatment procedure.

Functionally Equivalent Procedures Functionally equivalent procedures are indications of response generalization; that is, participants are taught a traditional method of treating an injury, but utilize another procedure (one that is potentially easier for the participant to perform) that serves the same purpose of protecting the injury from infection or otherwise promoting well-being. For example, putting an adhesive bandage on a burn is functionally the same as putting on a sterile pad, gauze, or tape, which is typically how burns are treated. Conversely, putting a sterile pad, gauze, or tape on an abrasion is functionally equivalent to putting an adhesive bandage on it (again, a more traditional approach to treatment).

The use of functionally equivalent procedures has an important implication for training; namely, as long as the procedure meets the same first-aid goal (e.g., preventing infection) as more traditional techniques, but is easier for program participants to perform, using the procedure will enhance participant success. Another advantage is that functionally equivalent procedures sometimes cost less than traditional techniques. For example, adhesive bandages typically cost much less than sterile pads, gauze, tape, and child-safe scissors. In addition, educators need to consider the response time of various procedures when planning instructional programs. Putting on a sterile pad, wrapping it with gauze, and taping the gauze to the skin takes more time to perform than simply putting an adhesive bandage on an injury.

Educators may need to teach functionally equivalent procedures for use during community activities when individuals will typically not have immediate access to traditional first-aid supplies. For example, because children will not have paper towels or clean cloths on the playground when they are injured, they will need to learn to cover the injury as quickly as possible with their hand and get assistance from an adult (Christensen, Marchand-Martella, Martella, Fiechtl, & Christensen, 1993). That is, covering the injury with a hand and applying pressure is functionally equivalent to covering an injury with a clean cloth and applying pressure. The goal is to stop/slow the blood flow while help is bcing sought.

Treatment of Others Not only is it important for learners to be able to perform first aid on themselves, but they should also be able to treat the injuries of others (Kittleson, 1983). That is, a person who is properly trained is prepared to assist others who are stricken or to give them instructions on how to handle situations involving first aid (American National Red Cross, 1979). Given the results of several studies (Gast et al., 1992; Marchand-Martella, Martella, Agran, Salzberg, et al., 1992; Marchand-Martella, Martella, Christensen, Agran, & Young, 1992a, 1992b; Marchand-Martella & Martella, 1990), it is clear that students can be taught to treat simulated injuries on themselves as well as their peers. This training approach has the added benefit of promoting social skills because it requires that students interact with their peers to find out what type of injury they have, to assist peers in treating the injury, and to help them seek the guidance of the teacher or instructional aide if needed. Students should also learn how to look out for one another and provide assistance when someone is in need of help.

Treatment of Novel Injuries When first-aid skills are being taught, treatment is typically restricted to the hand. Therefore, it is important to assess whether participants exhibit generalized performance when they are injured on differing body locations, receive an injury different than those simulated in training, or experience injuries that are larger or smaller than those taken care of in training.

Two studies incorporated assessments of novel injury treatment. Marchand-Martella and Martella (1990) taught participants to treat injuries on puppets, then simulated injuries during generalization assessments on the hands and fingers of the participants and supervising adults. Injury sizes were larger than those used on puppets, and participants were successful.

Marchand-Martella, Martella, Agran, Salzberg, et al. (1992) taught participants to treat injuries on their hands. During generalization assessments, injury sizes and locations were placed on various body locations (e.g., elbows, knees, fingers, hands, arms). Overall, participants exhibited generalized performance; however, retraining was needed on several injuries across participants.

Generalization to real injuries following first-aid training was noted in several studies. Marchand-Martella and Martella (1990) reported that the parents of three participants indicated that their children had taken care of injuries on their siblings and taught the skill to others. Marchand-Martella, Martella, Agran, Salzberg, et al. (1992) reported that one parent collected data on her son when he treated his knee following a fall off his bicycle. He completed all first-aid steps correctly and independently. Gast et al. (1992) reported that one first-aid training participant fell and cut her hand at Special Olympics. Although she did not have a cloth to cover it, she immediately located her teacher to inform her of the injury.

Spooner, Stem, and Test (1989) reported the successful generalization of one student's response. The student's bedridden mother had scalded herself with hot soup, and the individual appropriately treated the wound, applied a bandage, and dialed 911. Another student in the Spooner study was accidentally left at home alone when his school bus failed to stop to pick him up; he responded by dialing 911, and the police took him to school. Spooner et al. pointed out that although it could be argued that the latter situation was not a real emergency, this was the only option available to the student, and he did demonstrate generalized responding across settings as well as maintenance of learned skills.

When students are injured on the playground or in gym, educators should let them treat their own injuries whenever possible, supervising injury treatment and providing feedback as needed. Parents should also promote independence by letting their children treat injuries on their own. Any time a child independently treats an injury he or she should be immediately reinforced.

Treatment in Novel Settings Educators should assess whether the training program enables participants' newly acquired skills to transfer to nontrained contexts (Kameenui & Simmons, 1990) such as environments different from those used in training (Christensen et al., 1993). For example, if training occurs in the classroom, educators should assess whether children can treat injuries they receive outside, in the gym, in the lunchroom, or at home. Likewise, parents should assess their child's knowledge of injury treatment in a neighbor's house, outside, or in the community.

ASSESSMENTS AND EVALUATIONS

Error Analyses

In order to determine specific patterns of errors in generalized responding, participants' responses should be analyzed so that programs can be refined to eliminate potential problems or to focus on problem-specific training for individuals experiencing difficulties. For example, if a student always completes the first step in a given sequence incorrectly, a teacher should ask himself or herself, "What is the student doing wrong?" or, "What is the student failing to do?" followed by "What can I do to remediate this deficit?". Informal observations can prove beneficial in answering these questions.

Gast et al. (1992) recorded the following as potential areas of error in performing first aid:

- Topography (response does not conform to definition)
- Sequence (step is performed out of order)
- Duration (response not completed within specified time limit)
- No response (failure to initiate response within specified time limit)

Marchand-Martella, Martella, Agran, Salzberg, et al. (1992) reported extensive error analyses during generalization assessments that yielded some interesting findings. For example, participants had difficulty washing abrasions on their knees with soap and water. This difficulty may have been due to the fact that they were trained to wash injuries under running water in the sink. However, after training, the participants often had to improvise (e.g., wash knee in the bathtub; use a wet paper towel with soap on it to wash knee). Participants also had difficulty putting the bandage on their own knees and found it easier to place an adhesive bandage on someone else's knee. It is typically comfortable to stand or sit upright when treating someone else's knee where the injury is in full view. In contrast, treating one's own knee requires some physically awkward positioning.

After performing such an error analysis, educators may decide to prepare students to deal with different kinds of faucets, paper towel dispensers, soap dispensers, and sinks by practicing injury treatment in a variety of bathrooms or kitchens. Training might include how to wash a knee or other types of injuries on parts of the body that cannot be easily inserted into a sink by using a bathtub or a wet cloth with soap, followed by washing the soap off the wound.

Social Validation

Educators should include measures of social validation when first-aid programs are being conducted. Social validation refers to judgments made by professionals, parents, or program participants that provide additional measures of program success beyond those observed during training. In order to determine if a program is socially valid, educators should ask themselves the following questions *before* training begins:

1. Did I consult a professional in the area of first aid about the appropriateness of the treatment procedure?
2. Did I review the American National Red Cross manual (1988) to see if treatment procedures are following the Red Cross guidelines?

Additionally, educators should ask themselves the following questions *after* training is conducted:

1. Did I ask the individual's family and any significant others in the life of the person how well he or she is performing the skill(s) at home? In the community? What changes would they recommend?
2. Did I ask the participant if he or she was satisfied with the first-aid program? Would the participant recommend this program to others? What changes would he or she recommend?

3. Did I ask a professional in the area of first aid to judge how well the individual is performing the first-aid skill once he or she has acquired it?

Maintenance Assessments

Skills that are not practiced on a regular basis tend to atrophy over time; therefore, regular assessments of maintenance of performance are critical (Horner, Williams, & Knobbe, 1985). During training, participants usually practice first-aid treatments daily. During maintenance, however, when participants practice treatment of injuries less often, performance may deteriorate (Marchand-Martella, Martella, Christensen, et al., 1992a; Peterson & Thiele, 1988). Therefore, frequent opportunities to practice first-aid skills with feedback from trainers or others are essential. These opportunities can be scheduled one to two times per month, with more intensive retraining provided if skill level declines.

CONCLUSIONS

Previous first-aid skill training programs have demonstrated success in improving participants' abilities to treat a variety of injuries and to respond to a variety of emergency situations. Despite these demonstrated benefits, further research is needed in a number of areas. First, strategies that promote generalized responding are needed; acquired responses should *not* occur in inappropriate, nontrained stimulus conditions (Horner, Albin, & Ralph, 1986). For example, individuals are typically not taught to respond to and discriminate between examples and nonexamples of various first-aid procedures.

Second, further descriptive research is needed in the area of injury prevention, specifically in determining the antecedents to injuries. For example, if individuals frequently cut themselves when using a knife, they should learn how to prevent this injury by using a knife correctly, as well as how to treat a cut if it occurs. Individuals should be taught that certain behaviors (e.g., picking up a piece of broken glass) increase the chances of injury. Furthermore, individuals should be taught to wear protective gear for certain activities (e.g., knee pads when roller blading, helmets when riding bicycles) that can prevent injuries from happening.

Finally, given the results of the survey conducted by Collins et al. (1992), in which it was determined that only 3% of the respondents taught first-aid skills in their classrooms, educators need to be taught to incorporate first-aid programs into their curricula. Activities that present any possibility of injury (e.g., food preparation, leisure/recreation, cooking) should include a training component in which students are taught the types of injuries that may occur and how to treat them. Providing persons with disabilities the skills to treat their own and others' injuries represents a set of skills that will promote both their well-being and their independence.

REFERENCES

American National Red Cross. (1979). *Standard first aid and personal safety* (2nd ed.). Washington, DC: Author.

American National Red Cross. (1988). *Standard first aid and personal safety* (3rd ed.). Washington, DC: Author.

Blackman, J. (1984). *Medical aspects of developmental disabilities in children: Birth to three.* Rockville, MD: Aspen.

Boy Scouts of America. (1982). *Prepared for today.* Dallas, TX: Author.

Bryan, E., Warden, M.G., Berg, B., & Hauck, G.R. (1978). Medical considerations for multiple handicapped children in the public schools. *Journal of School Health, 48,* 84–89.

Christensen, A.M., Marchand-Martella, N.E., Martella, R.C., Fiechtl, B.J., & Christensen, B.R. (1993). Teaching preschoolers with disabilities to seek adult assistance for simulated injuries. *Journal of Behavioral Education, 3,* 109–123.

Collins, B.C., Wolery, M., & Gast, D.L. (1991). A survey of safety concerns for students with special needs. *Education and Training in Mental Retardation, 26,* 305–318.

Collins, B.C., Wolery, M., & Gast, D.L. (1992). A national survey of safety concerns for students with special needs. *Journal of Developmental and Physical Disabilities, 4,* 263–276.

Cuvo, A.J., & Davis, P.K. (1983). Behavior therapy and community living skills. In M. Hersen, R. Eisler, & P. Miller (Eds.), *Progress in behavior modification* (pp. 125–172). New York: Academic Press.

Gast, D.L., Winterling, V., Wolery, M., & Farmer, J.A. (1992). Teaching first-aid skills to students with moderate handicaps in small group instruction. *Education and Treatment of Children, 15,* 101–124.

Green, M.I. (1977). *A sigh of relief: The first-aid handbook for childhood emergencies.* West Stockbridge, MA: Bantam.

Hauser, C., Cockson, A., Redican, K.J., & Olsen, L.K. (1979). First aid and the mentally retarded. *Health Education, 10,* 3–4.

Horner, R.H., Albin, R.W., & Ralph, G. (1986). Generalization with precision: The role of negative teaching examples in the instruction of generalized grocery item selection. *Journal of The Association for Persons with Severe Handicaps, 10,* 172–175.

Horner, R.H., Williams, J.A., & Knobbe, C.A. (1985). The effect of "opportunity to perform" on the maintenance of skills learned by high school students with severe handicaps. *Journal of The Association for Persons with Severe Handicaps, 10,* 172–175.

Howell, K.W., & Kaplan, J.S. (1978). Monitoring peer tutor behavior. *Exceptional Children, 45,* 135–137.

Kameenui, E.J., & Simmons, D.C. (1990). *Designing instructional strategies: The prevention of academic learning problems.* Columbus, OH: Merrill.

Kendall, P.C. (1981). Cognitive-behavioral interventions with children. In B.B. Lahey & A.E. Kazdin (Eds.), *Advances in clinical child psychology* (pp. 53–90). New York: Plenum Press.

Kittleson, M.J. (1983). Teaching the four C's of first aid. *Health Education, 14,* 44–45.

Lorr, C., & Rotatori, A.F. (1985). Who are the severely and profoundly handicapped? In A.F. Rotatori, J.O. Schween, & R.A. Fox (Eds.), *Assessing severely and profoundly handicapped individuals* (pp. 38–48). Springfield, IL: Charles C Thomas.

Marchand-Martella, N.E., & Martella, R.C. (1990). The acquisition, maintenance, and generalization of first-aid skills by youths with handicaps. *Behavioral Residential Treatment, 5,* 221–237.

Marchand-Martella, N.E., & Martella, R.C. (1993). Evaluating the instructional behaviors of peers with mild disabilities who served as first-aid instructors for students with moderate disabilities. *Child and Family Behavior Therapy, 15*(4), 1–17.

Marchand-Martella, N.E., Martella, R.C., Agran, M., Salzberg, C.L., Young, K.R., & Morgan, D. (1992). Generalized effects of a peer-delivered first-aid program for students with moderate intellectual disabilities. *Journal of Applied Behavior Analysis, 25,* 841–851.

Marchand-Martella, N.E., Martella, R.C., Agran, M., & Young, K.R. (1992). Assessing the acquisition of first-aid treatments by elementary-aged children. *Child & Family Behavior Therapy, 13*(4), 29–43.

Marchand-Martella, N.E., Martella, R.C., Christensen, A.M., Agran, M., & Young, K.R. (1992a). Assessing the duration of first-aid treatments by elementary-aged students with disabilities. *Child & Family Behavior Therapy, 14*(3), 33–52.

Marchand-Martella, N.E., Martella, R.C., Christensen, A.M., Agran, M., & Young, K.R. (1992b). Teaching a first-aid skill to students with disabilities using two training programs. *Education and Treatment of Children, 15,* 15–31.

Marchand-Martella, N.E., Martella, R.C., & Marchand, A.G. (1989). *"Mouse calls": A storytelling approach to teaching first-aid skills to children with handicaps.* Logan: Utah State University, Outreach, Development, and Dissemination Division, Center for Persons with Disabilities.

Matson, J.L. (1980). Preventing home accidents: A training program for the retarded. *Behavior Modification, 4,* 397–410.

Mori, L., & Peterson, L. (1986). Training preschoolers in home safety skills to prevent inadvertent injury. *Journal of Clinical Child Psychology, 15,* 106–114.

Nietupski, J., Hamre-Nietupski, S., Clancy, P., & Veerhusen, K. (1986). Guidelines for making simulation an effective adjunct to in vivo community instruction. *Journal of The Association for Persons with Severe Handicaps, 11,* 12–18.

O'Reilly, M.F., & Cuvo, A.J. (1989). Teaching self-treatment of cold symptoms to an anoxic brain injured adult. *Behavioral Residential Treatment, 4,* 359–375.

Pancsofar, E.L., Schafer, S., Blackwell, R., & Gavron, S. (1984). Utilization of general case programming for teaching health education behaviors to students with severe handicaps. *Journal of School Health, 54,* 435–436.

Peterson, L. (1984a). The "safe at home" game: Training comprehensive prevention skills in latchkey children. *Behavior Modification, 8,* 474–494.

Peterson, L. (1984b). Teaching home safety and survival skills to latchkey children: A comparison of two manuals and methods. *Journal of Applied Behavior Analysis, 17,* 279–293.

Peterson, L., Farmer, J.G., & Selby, V. (1988). Unprompted between subject generalization of home safety skills. *Child & Family Behavior Therapy, 10,* 107–119.

Peterson, L., & Mori, L. (1985). Prevention of child injury: An overview of targets, methods, and tactics for psychologists. *Journal of Consulting and Clinical Psychology, 53,* 586–595.

Peterson, L., Mori, L., Selby, V., & Rosen, B.N. (1988). Community interventions in children's injury prevention: Differing costs and differing benefits. *Journal of Community Psychology, 16,* 188–204.

Peterson, L., & Thiele, C. (1988). Home safety at school. *Child & Family Behavior Therapy, 10,* 1–8.

Schafer, S.M. (1983). *The validation of a general case strategy for the instruction of a safety behavior with the severely handicapped.* Unpublished master's thesis, Bowling Green State University, Ohio.

Spooner, F., Stem, B., & Test, D.W. (1989). Teaching first-aid skills to adolescents who are moderately mentally handicapped. *Education and Training in Mental Retardation, 24,* 341–351.

Steere, D.E., Pancsofar, E.L., Powell, T.H., & Butterworth, J. (1989). Enhancing instruction through general case programming. *Teaching Exceptional Children, 22,* 22–24.

Stem, B., & Test, D.W. (1989). Teaching first-aid skills in the classroom. *Teaching Exceptional Children, 22*(1), 10–12.

Stokes, T.F., & Osnes, P.G. (1988). The developing applied technology of generalization and maintenance. In R.H. Horner, G. Dunlap, & R.L. Koegel (Eds.), *Generalization and maintenance: Life-style changes in applied settings* (pp. 5–19). Baltimore: Paul H. Brookes Publishing Co.

Chapter Seven

Fire Safety Skills

Diane Bannerman Juracek

Residential fires result in thousands of deaths each year and present an especially serious problem for people with developmental disabilities who do not know how to respond safely during fire emergencies (Levin & Nelson, 1981). To address this problem, living environments must be fire safe and people with disabilities must learn to respond effectively in such fire emergencies as nighttime house fires, stove-top fires, and fires in the workplace or at school. Historically, the number of fire fatalities among people with developmental disabilities has been limited due to residential living in highly supervised, large institutional facilities equipped with such fire safety features as sprinkler systems, fire alarms, round-the-clock supervision, and, sometimes, on-campus fire departments. During the last decade, a national commitment to community inclusion has led most states to encourage the development of small homes and supervised apartments that house four or fewer individuals within a family or with a roommate without disabilities. These small community residential settings are a favorable alternative to larger institutions because they facilitate community inclusion and are typically less expensive.

Smaller residences, however, may pose a critical fire safety risk for residents who do not know how to evacuate safely and promptly during a fire emergency. This is because residences that can be classified as "single-family dwellings" do not require more protective fire safety features, such as fire alarms, sprinkler systems, and self-closing doors (National Fire Protection Association, 1991). Fewer fire safety requirements decrease the cost of housing, thereby increasing the attractiveness of these residential alternatives.

The National Fire Protection Association (NFPA) (1991) statistics indicate that the greatest fire loss and the most fatalities have been within single-family dwellings. This statistic is surprising to many. Much more media attention has been given to the few disastrous multiple-death fires that have occurred in high-rise buildings, dormitories, and nursing homes. For example, an early morning kitchen fire that killed 10 people with developmental disabilities in a three-story Detroit boarding house made headline news in 1992 ("Ten Killed," 1992). This multiple death fire was catastrophic, but not typical. Single-family home fires occur daily, causing tremendous financial loss, injury, and death. The NFPA (1991) reports that 5,000 Americans die every year in home fires. Because more people with disabilities are moving to single-family homes, fire safety in these homes is a critical concern.

The NFPA does not specifically track the number of people with disabilities who have died or been injured in fires. Data do show, however, that many of the multiple-death fires have occurred in community residences (including group and foster homes) that house people who require care and supervision (Jones, 1980; NFPA, 1991) and that fatalities in residential fires are typically a result of people not knowing how to evacuate (Skurat, 1985). Teaching fire emergency skills is a critical step in addressing this dilemma.

Learning what to do during a fire emergency is not a simple task. One must learn to assess the conditions of the fire and make decisions based on that assessment. For example, one of the most common fire emergencies is a nighttime fire that occurs while people are sleeping (Yuill, 1983). If a smoke or fire alarm should alert an individual during this type of emergency, the recommended response is to check the bedroom door for temperature. If the door is cold, the person should attempt to exit. If, however, the door is warm and/or warm air is felt underneath the door, then the individual should go to the window and yell for help.

Case studies of various fire emergencies have shown that people without disabilities have difficulty avoiding panic, assessing the conditions, and making sound decisions. People with developmental disabilities often have even greater difficulty with these skills. Additionally, people with physical disabilities are often limited in their physical capacity to engage in the recommended responses.

Teaching how to respond safely during a fire is especially difficult because fires occur infrequently. Fire emergency skills are almost never practiced during the actual conditions of surprise, smoke, fire, and panic. Rather, simulations of fire emergencies are used in training. This training is helpful; however, because the conditions that exist during a real fire cannot be realistically and safely replicated, generalization of the skills to real situations is never assured (Bertsch, Fox, & Kwiecinski, 1984).

This chapter discusses the challenges of deciding what fire emergency skills to teach and how to teach them. The first section helps the reader to make informed decisions as to what specific fire emergency skills to teach. The second section presents a brief review of the literature on teaching fire emergency skills and draws several conclusions about the most effective teaching procedures. The third section provides curricula for teaching three fire safety response skills. The final sections describe critical issues with regard to teaching and future directions and research.

The recommendations made in this chapter are based on the body of research literature examining the acquisition and use of fire safety skills by people with developmental disabilities of all age ranges, including those with sensory impairments and physical disabilities. Individualized teaching strategies and adaptations are recommended for people with severe disabilities (e.g., those with no receptive or expressive language skills and substantial physical challenges) as well as for those with less severe disabilities. Individuals with learning disabilities may also benefit from the strategies suggested. Adaptive equipment is described to assist people with physical disabilities to evacuate safely.

WHAT FIRE EMERGENCY SKILLS SHOULD BE TAUGHT

The answer to the question of "what to teach" is not an easy one. Unfortunately, no national fire safety education programs have been developed for people with developmental disabilities. There are several widely used public fire safety education programs disseminated by NFPA for use with school-age children. Preschoolers and kindergartners are taught to "stay low and go, go, go," and then are taught simple discriminations for choosing the safest exit. Higher grade–level children learn a "stop-drop-and-roll" curriculum that teaches several conditional responses.

There are also fire education programs for people with physical disabilities and their families. These programs teach how to prepare for fire emergencies, such as how to install adequate fire safety features and how to practice an escape plan. Although all of these programs contain useful fire safety information, none address the special learning difficulties and/or physical challenges that people with developmental disabilities may have.

One important factor in deciding what to teach is to look at which fire emergencies are most common. The NFPA statistics show that fires occur most often in homes, that injuries and fatalities typically take place at night when people are sleeping, and that a large percentage of home fires begin in the kitchen. An additional common cause of fires is the misuse of matches, lighters, and smoking materials (Lavoie, 1988; Yuill, 1983). Based on these statistics, professional fire safety experts agree that a critical teaching priority should be to teach people who live in single-family dwellings to respond safely to nighttime fire emergencies, cooking fires, and other daytime fire emergencies and to learn how to use smoking materials appropriately.

After finding out which fire emergencies are most likely to occur, the next step is deciding what the responses to those emergencies should be. Unfortunately, there is much debate among experts concerning this matter. To illustrate, the research literature shows that a variety of different responses to home fires have been validated by experts. For example, Jones, Kazdin, and Haney (1981a) obtained consensus from 14 firefighters as to the nighttime fire responses that should be taught to 6- and 7-year-old children without disabilities who lived with their families in community homes. The responses entailed a series of fairly complex decisions based on the conditions of the fire emergency. For example, steps to follow during one type of nighttime fire emergency included:

1. Slide to the edge of the bed;
2. roll out of bed;
3. crawl to door;
4. if door is cool, proceed to exit unless blocked by fire or smoke;
5. if door is hot, push the rug in the crack;
6. crawl to the window;
7. open the window; and
8. yell and signal for help. (Jones, Kazdin, & Haney, 1981b, p. 254)

In another study, Bannerman, Sheldon, and Sherman (1991) indicated that the fire safety responses recommended by firefighters were very different from those suggested by Jones et al. (1981a). In this study, the participants had mental retardation and required high levels of assistance. They lived in a group home equipped with advanced fire safety features, including a fire alarm that sounded at the fire department and a sprinkler system. Under these conditions, fire experts agreed that it was best that the participants simply be taught to promptly evacuate from the nearest exit during day or nighttime fires.

It is reasonable to conclude that there is no set answer to the question of what to teach. Rather, the decision must be based upon analysis of four critical variables:

1. The fire safety features of the residence
2. Capabilities of the individuals involved
3. Availability of trained staff or roomates
4. Predicted conditions of the most likely fire emergencies

These four variables may be assessed as follows. First, analysis must be made of the structure, layout, and fire safety features of the facility or home in which the individual resides; the fewer the fire safety features, the fewer the available response options and the less time available to deal with the situation and/or escape. Recommended fire safety features include the following:

- Sprinkler systems
- Fire and smoke alarms (some of which can automatically notify the fire department)
- Self-closing, solid-core doors
- Easily accessible emergency exits
- Firesafe construction
- Round-the-clock awake staffing

Second, abilities of the individual(s) to be taught must be considered. People with no physical disabilities, but with developmental disabilities requiring low levels of assistance, may be able to learn more complex response discriminations, whereas people with severe physical and developmental disabilities may require adaptive equipment and special teaching procedures to learn a single emergency response, such as exiting through a targeted door.

Third, the availability of staff, roommates, or other supervision must be assessed. Fewer fire safety skills will be needed by an individual living in a home in which at least one trained staff person or roommate is available to assist in responding safely to an emergency. In a home without nighttime supervision, additional training and fire safety equipment may be required.

Finally, the conditions of the most probable fire emergency situations for the particular dwelling must be considered. For instance, what type of fire is most likely to occur, and how much smoke and fire could accumulate before detection? NFPA statistics may be used to delineate the most likely types of fires. The probable conditions may be ascertained by analyzing the most typical activities, the structure, and the fire safety features of a particular residence. For example, one could predict the conditions of a fire started by a hot cooking oil spill on the stove burner in a kitchen equipped with a smoke alarm.

After analyzing these variables, decisions can be made about what to teach, and social validation of these decisions can be solicited from the local fire marshall or other fire safety experts. To aid one in making decisions about what to teach, the research literature was reviewed to determine what safety responses have been most consistently taught based on the four critical variables and on social validation. These conclusions are in the paragraphs to follow. Instructors should analyze the fire safety needs of learners on an individual basis and validate their decisions with fire safety experts, rather than solely relying on the information provided here.

Safe Responses to Nighttime and Daytime Fires

Individuals housed in highly fire-safe residences, including the recommended fire safety features previously mentioned, are likely to be safe if taught to exit the building at the sound of the alarm. If possible, individuals should be taught to crawl while exiting to avoid smoke inhalation and to gather at a preset meeting place once outside. If learners have not been successful in learning to exit at the sound of the alarm, they should be taught to stay in their room, remain calm, and wait for help.

If neither staff nor well-trained roommates are available to help and supervise at night, but the residence is equipped with all other fire safety features (i.e., a sprinkler system, self-closing, solid-core doors, fire-safe construction, and an alarm system that sounds at the fire station), teaching individuals to stay in their rooms and calmly wait for help may be the safest behavior to teach. Because most home fires originate in common living areas (e.g., kitchens, living rooms) and not in bedrooms, it may be safer for an individual with disabilities to remain in his or her bedroom with a closed, solid-core door until help arrives, rather than attempt to exit and make decisions about the safest routes out of the building.

Typical homes and apartments equipped with smoke alarms, but with few other safety features, require that residents are trained in more sophisticated fire safety responses or that adequate staff/roommate supervision is available at all times. People with disabilities who live in residences such as these should be taught the safety responses described in the research of Jones et al. (1981a). That is, individuals should be taught to crawl to the bedroom door at the sound of the smoke alarm, check the door for temperature, and then either exit or signal for help at the bedroom window, depending on whether the door was cool or hot. The individual should also be taught to use an alternate exit if the first exit attempted is blocked by fire or heavy smoke. Again, if a resident is unable to learn these fire safety responses, he or she might be taught to wait at the window for the help of a trained staff member or roommate.

Responding to daytime fires requires much of the same instruction as previously mentioned. In all types of residences and public school or work settings, individuals should be taught to leave the building from the nearest safe exit at the sound of the alarm. They should also be taught to gather at a preset meeting place after exiting. Individuals who cannot learn this skill require trained staff, teachers, roommates, or employees to aid them should a fire emergency arise.

Safe Responses to Contained Fires

Individuals with developmental disabilities may also be taught how to extinguish contained fires (e.g., fires in a pan on the stove, fires in a wastebasket). They will need to learn to quickly obtain and operate the materials needed to extinguish the fire and to do so from a safe distance, with their back to a viable exit (in case of failure to put out the fire). Such materials should be easily accessible.

If an individual cannot be taught to extinguish a contained fire, and staff or trained roommates are always available in the residence, it is best to teach them to immediately get staff or roommates to help. If staff/roommates are not always available, then it may be best to teach that individual to exit the residence and call for help, or simply exit if the individual cannot call for help.

Preventive Fire Safety Skills

A critical step in avoiding injuries and deaths due to fire emergencies is teaching skills to prevent such emergencies from occurring. Because fires caused by cooking and smoking materials are common, preventive skills in these areas, should definitely be taught. Individuals should be taught general cooking skills, as well as how to prepare particular foods in a safe manner. Among the skills to teach are the following: proper use of stove, oven, and microwave; use of potholders; keeping flammable objects away from stove; remaining in the kitchen while the stove or microwave is in use; using a timer when the stove, oven, or microwave is in use; and wearing close-fitting clothing while cooking on the stove, so that shirtsleeves do not catch fire. (See chap. 3, this volume, for more on teaching cooking skills.)

The Ventura County Association for the Retarded (1990) suggests some possible topic areas for teaching individuals how to prevent fires caused by tobacco smoking:

- Safe lighting of cigarettes and pipes
- Where to dispose of ashes
- Making sure ashes are out prior to disposal and that cigarettes or pipes are properly extinguished after smoking
- Refraining from smoking when tired or in bed
- Refraining from throwing away cigarettes while riding in a car

Individuals who have not learned preventive skills should engage in smoking or cooking only when closely supervised. Residences providing services for individuals who have not learned safe smoking skills should consider prohibiting smoking within the residence.

EFFECTIVE TRAINING PROGRAMS

Table 1 summarizes a review of the research literature on fire safety skills training programs for individuals with developmental disabilities and mental retardation. Out of this review, several conclusions can be drawn. It appears that a teaching package including modeling, assistance, correction, practice, reinforcement, and sometimes verbal rehearsal and props to simulate fire emergencies has been used successfully to teach fire safety responses to children and young adults with developmental disabilities requiring lower levels of assistance. These fire safety responses include exiting safely during a fire emergency by making conditional responses based on the presence of heat, flames, and smoke (e.g., see Jones et al., 1981b); calling 911; and extinguishing flames on oneself.

Less success has been shown in teaching conditional fire safety responses to people with more severe disabilities (Haney & Jones, 1982; Rae & Roll, 1985). In three studies, however (Bannerman et al., 1991; Cohen, 1984; Holburn & Dougher, 1985), people with severe or profound mental retardation were taught to exit at the sound of an alarm using a shaping procedure where participants learned to stand up at the sound of thc alarm and walk increasingly longer distances until each was walking from different locations to and through the exit door. The problem with teaching the exiting response is that it does not include conditional responding based on the presence of heat and flames

Table 1. A review of fire safety training programs for people with developmental disabilities

Reference	Participants	Skill(s) taught	Teaching methods	Results	Generalization	Maintenance monitoring
Bannerman, Sheldon, and Sherman (1991)	Three adults with severe to profound mental retardation	Walk out exit door to meeting place when fire alarm sounds	Prompts, modeling, practice, and reinforcement used to shape increasingly longer distances to the exit door; training schedules, exit doors, and trainers varied to promote generalization	All three learned to exit independently in unannounced fire drills.	Exited from five areas of the house from which training was not done; little generalization to nighttime drills	Up to 16 months after teaching
Cohen (1984)	One adult with profound mental retardation and blindness	Walk out the exit door at the sound of the fire alarm	Brief instructional prompts, practice, and rewards used to shape increasingly longer distances to the exit door	Participant learned to exit at the sound of the alarm in unannounced fire drills.	None	For 12 months after teaching
Haney and Jones (1982)	One child with moderate mental retardation and three with severe mental retardation	Multi-step safe responses to four types of fire emergencies, including how to check door for heat and go to window if door is hot or if hot air rushed through when opened, how to crawl out after opening a cool door and seeing smoke, and what to do if fire is blocking path	Modeling, correction, assistance, practice, rewards, and props used to simulate fire emergencies; praise and rewards faded, three participants taught to self-reinforce, and two participants taught from two different rooms	In unannounced fire drills, one child learned all steps to all four fire emergencies; one child learned all steps to three fire emergencies, and two children learned 83% of steps to two types of fire emergencies.	Two children who were taught in two rooms generalized skills to their own bedrooms. Other two showed some generalization.	For 6 months after teaching, two children maintained at post-teaching levels, and two children maintained 57%–83% of the steps learned.

Jones and Thorton (1987)	Four adults with mild mental retardation	Responses (steps) to four types of fire emergencies listed in Haney and Jones (1982) and safe response to nighttime emergencies; props used for simulation	Skills taught in community apartments using instructions, modeling, behavioral rehearsal, feedback, and reinforcement; after acquisition, a 30-day period occurred where situations were randomly presented and participants were asked to respond and self-evaluate; nighttime responses taught at night	All participants performed the four responses at close to 100% criterion after teaching and during the 30-day period. Nighttime tests showed inconsistent demonstration of skills.	None	5–8 months later, participants averaged 85.6% correct steps on the four emergencies. 2–5 months later, nighttime performance remained inconsistent.
Holburn and Dougher (1985)	One adult with severe mental retardation	Walk out the exit door when the fire alarm sounds	Prompts, practice, and reward used to shape increasingly longer distances to the exit door; training schedules, exit doors, and trainers varied	Participant exited in one minute or less during 9 of 10 unannounced fire drills.	Participant exited from different locations, at different times, and with different individuals initiating the drills.	For 18 months after teaching
Jones, Kazdin, and Haney (1981a)	Four third-graders with mild mental retardation	Responses (steps) to descriptions of nine types of fire emergencies (e.g., "what would you do if you were awakened by smoke?")	Skills taught in a simulated bedroom in a school gym using modeling, correction, assistance, practice, and rewards	All children displayed all steps in simulated bedroom after teaching.	None	5 months later, performance dropped to a mean of 46% correct steps

(continued)

Table 1. *(continued)*

Reference	Participants	Skill(s) taught	Teaching methods	Results	Generalization	Maintenance monitoring
Jones, Kazdin, and Haney (1981b)	Same participants as in Jones, Kazdin, and Haney (1981a)	Retrained steps to nine types of fire emergencies from Jones, Kazdin, and Haney (1981a)	Same as in Jones, Kazdin, and Haney (1981a), with the addition of extra review sessions	All children displayed all steps in simulated bedroom after teaching.	None	4 months later, performance dropped to a mean of 53% correct steps
Jones, Sisson, and Van Hasselt (1984)	Eight adolescents with blindness and mild mental retardation, three of whom were successfully taught four safe responses in Jones, Van Hasselt, and Sisson (1984)	Three adolescents from Jones, Van Hasselt, and Sisson (1984) were retaught to exit at the sound of the alarm and then taught to cue their five roommates to evacuate	Same as in Jones, Van Hasselt, and Sisson (1984)	Three adolescents displayed the exiting skill at the sound of the tape-recorded fire alarm and cued the other five to exit in roleplays after teaching.	Seven of eight adolescents exited correctly during one nighttime fire drill.	None
Jones, Van Hasselt, and Sisson (1984)	Four adolescents with blindness and mild mental retardation	Responses (steps) to four types of fire emergencies, listed in Haney and Jones (1982), simulated with props	Skills taught in dormitory using modeling, correction, assistance, practice, and rewards; to promote generalization, self-evaluation, fading of rewards, mastery of combined emergency situations, and extra practice	Three of four adolescents performed all steps correctly at the sound of the tape-recorded alarm during roleplays in dormitory.	No generalization to nighttime fire drills	4 months later, the three adolescents who had learned the skills maintained at between 82% and 100% mastery.

Katz and Singh (1986)	Nine adults with mild mental retardation	Steps to safe exiting, reporting a fire, and extinguishing flames on themselves when props were used to simulate	Skills taught in individuals' group home using modeling, assistance, correction, practice, and reward	All participants learned all steps to all three skills after teaching.	None	6–18 weeks later, all individuals displayed almost all steps in three to five tests.
Matson (1980)	Five adults with moderate mental retardation	Taught to describe how to exit safely during a fire	Practice, using a cardboard home model and figures depicting the participants, verbal rehearsal, and reward	After teaching, all five learned to describe exiting procedures.	None	7 months later, participants could still describe exiting procedures.
Rae and Roll (1985)	Ten adults with profound mental retardation	Exit apartment at the sound of the verbal cue "fire drill"	Prompting and praise used during daily fire drills at varied times	After 48 weeks of daily practice, none learned to exit independently. Fewer physical prompts were required and more verbal prompts were used; time taken to exit decreased.	None	After 8 weeks of weekly fire drills, lower levels of assistance were maintained.
Risley and Cuvo (1980)	Three adults with mild mental retardation	Steps to calling and reporting an emergency to the fire station, police station or doctor, depending on the nature of a verbally presented situation	Modeling, prompts, feedback, practice, and reinforcement	After teaching, all three correctly completed all steps to making all three types of emergency calls.	After training on one emergency call, skills generalized to the other two types of emergency calls.	None

and, therefore, may not always be safe. The only safe use of this skill for individuals with severe disabilities would be in a facility with adequate staff supervision and protective fire safety features to ensure immediate detection and extinguishment of a fire.

Generalization of Skills

Generalization of fire safety skills outside the instructional format is critical because fire emergencies occur infrequently, without warning, and vary as to how, when, and where they occur. Because of this, it is essential that fire safety skills be used accurately at a moment's notice, at any time and place, and long after instruction is completed. A number of procedures used successfully in the research literature are recommended.

First, fire safety response training should be conducted within the setting conditions in which the learner is most likely to be faced with such an emergency. For example, training should be conducted in a variety of rooms, with different people present, during the day and night, and at different times of the year. The variance of setting conditions will increase the likelihood that individuals will be able to respond safely across a wide range of situations.

Second, stimuli common to emergencies, such as the sound of the fire alarm and the element of surprise in a fire emergency, should be replicated in training and testing (Bertsch et al., 1984). If used consistently, these common stimuli are likely to cue individuals to engage in the correct response. Third, probes (testing without reinforcement) may be interspersed among reinforced teaching trials to create an intermittent reinforcement schedule (as opposed to continuous). This schedule will set the occasion for better responding in future nonreinforced opportunities (Bertsch et al., 1984; Jones & Haney, 1984; Jones et al., 1981b, Katz & Singh, 1986).

Finally, systematic fading of reinforcers during training may increase the likelihood of skill performance in the absence of reward (Jones & Haney, 1984; Jones, Van Hasselt, & Sisson, 1984). If, after programming for generalization, the skill does not generalize to a particular target situation, then further training within the context of that situation is necessary. Such is the case with exiting in nighttime fire emergencies. The research indicates that this critical skill may have to be trained at night, from bed, with the elements of a fire emergency closely simulated.

Maintenance of Skills

Occasional testing and review of skills appears to be the best means of encouraging fire safety skill maintenance (Bannerman et al., 1991; Cohen, 1984; Jones & Thornton, 1987; Katz & Singh, 1986; Matson, 1980). A combination of overlearning and self-evaluation may also facilitate maintenance. However, the self-evaluation technique can only be used with individuals who have adequate receptive and expressive language skills.

RECOMMENDED TEACHING STRATEGIES

Conclusions based on the research literature indicate that people with disabilities requiring low levels of assistance can learn many critical fire safety skills, including conditional exiting responses based on the presence of fire, smoke, and heat. Additionally, although people with more severe disabilities (including those with poor receptive and expressive language skills) may have a difficult time learning conditional fire safety responses, they can learn to exit at the sound of a fire alarm. Generalization and maintenance of fire safety skills remains a significant challenge due to the infrequency and variety of fire emergencies.

In considering the above factors, three curricula are suggested. The first involves safely exiting a typical home during a nighttime fire emergency. The second involves extinguishing contained fires. The third includes evacuation procedures for those residing in highly protective settings (including sprinkler systems, fire alarms, automatically closing, solid-core doors, and fire-safe construction).

Teaching strategies include direct instructions, rationales, modeling, practice, feedback, reinforcement, and self-evaluation (consisting of a "yes" or "no" learner response to questions as to whether or not each step of the skill was completed). Teaching should be conducted without the presence of real fire until a stringent criterion of correct responding is met, then with the controlled use of fire or smoke until a second stringent criterion is met. Because of the potential for injury and emotional response when real fire is used to teach, appropriate precautions should be taken to ensure safety, and informed consent should be obtained from the individual and his or her parent(s) or guardian.

During the teaching sessions, the instructor should begin by reviewing each step in the task analysis and explaining why it is important. Next, the steps should be modeled by the teacher and practiced by the learner. The real conditions of fire emergencies should be simulated as closely as possible without risk of endangerment. Simulation could include controlled smoke, hot air from a blow dryer, and burning timbers in a bucket. Learners should practice the skill several times during a session and the instructor should provide positive and corrective feedback throughout.

After the learner meets a stringent criterion of independent performance, surprise fire drills, with feedback and prompting (if necessary), should be conducted. Initially, the learner should be forewarned of the impending surprise drill. After several drills with warnings, no forewarning should occur so that a more realistic fire emergency situation is replicated. Surprise drills with prompting and feedback should be conducted until a stringent criterion is met.

To enhance generalization and maintenance, occasional testing (at least once a month) and review of fire safety responses should be conducted with the elements of a real fire emergency closely simulated. Participants should not be forewarned of the tests. During testing and review, correct performance should be reinforced and retraining should be implemented if errors are made. The following sections present task analyses of three different fire safety skills, along with illustrative case examples.

Exiting Safely During a Nighttime Fire Emergency

Because Jones and colleagues have conducted the majority of research in this particular area, the following fire safety responses and teaching procedures are heavily based on their findings. Teaching should occur during the day until a stringent criterion is met, then teaching at night should occur. The following is a task analysis of critical nighttime exiting skills:

1. If while in bed you hear a smoke alarm or smell smoke, roll out of bed to the floor.
2. If your eyes are burning and you are coughing, go to the window and either wave for help or climb out.
3. If your eyes are not burning and you are not coughing, crawl to the door and feel it for warmth.
4. If the door is hot, go to the window to exit or wave for help.
5. If the door is cool, open it slightly.
6. If hot air is rushing through, close the door and go to the window.
7. If hot air is not rushing through, open the door wider.
8. If, by this time, you are coughing and your eyes are burning, crawl out of the house and go to the designated meeting place.
9. If your eyes are not burning, walk out of the house and go to the meeting place.
10. If upon walking or crawling out of the house you encounter fire, leave the house via an alternate route.

The case example on page 114 illustrates how to teach nighttime fire safety response skills.

Extinguishing Contained Fires

The following task analysis may be used for extinguishing a contained fire:

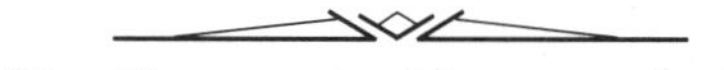

1. Identify a contained fire as one that has begun in a container, such as a wastebasket

Miguel recently moved from home to a brand new group living situation with five other friends. He appeared to enjoy his new home, communicating with his friends via his picture board and helping with all home maintenance tasks. Miguel was learning to bathe himself, put on his own clothes, brush his teeth, and communicate effectively with others using his communication board. He was progressing well in the home, but had difficulty with one required safety skill: exiting at the sound of the fire alarm.

The home was required to have an alarm that alerted the fire department when activated, and the individuals in the home were required to practice exiting at the sound of the alarm at varied times during the day and night. Miguel's particular problem with the alarm was at night. When the alarm sounded, he would jump out of bed screaming, run everywhere, and scratch everyone and everything in sight. Though he was also frightened by the alarm during daytime fire drills, nighttime drills were by far the worse. Miguel upset others with his reaction as well, hindering their practice of good fire safety skills.

To address Miguel's fear, the home began a desensitization program. They made a tape recording of the fire alarm and at first turned the volume way down. Miguel began daily practice of exiting at the barely audible sound of the tape-recorded alarm. Before each practice, he would go through the steps without the alarm and choose a special reward that he would earn when he completed the exiting with the tape-recorded alarm. At first, prompts and modeling were used to help him learn to exit. His teachers were able to fade the prompts as Miguel became more and more tolerant of the alarm. When he mastered exiting at the sound of a barely audible fire alarm, the sound was turned up slightly and he was again prompted and reinforced for exhibiting the exiting behavior. As Miguel learned to exit and became tolerant of the sound of the alarm, the volume was turned higher and higher, until it was almost as loud as the real alarm that was slowly faded in. Going from the tape-recorded alarm to the house alarm in unannounced fire drills was the hardest step for Miguel, but with a little help, he was able to master the exiting.

Miguel is still uncomfortable with fire drills, especially at night. However, he can now exit safely and quietly. Monthly drills are used to maintain his skills.

or a pan, and has not caught anything else in the vicinity on fire.

2. Quickly obtain the materials recommended to extinguish the particular fire:
   a. Extinguish a grease fire on the stove with baking soda.
   b. Extinguish a grease fire in a pan or an oven fire by turning off the source of heat and carefully securing the lid to the pan or closing the oven door.
   c. Extinguish a paper fire in a wastebasket with water.
   d. Extinguish an electrical fire in a kitchen appliance by unplugging the appliance and using a fire extinguisher.
3. Extinguish fire from a safe distance, with one's back to a viable exit (in case of failure to extinguish the fire).
4. If the fire spreads to other items outside of the container (e.g., a towel, wallpaper, wall decoration), leave the house and call for help.

The case example on page 115 presents a sample contained fire safety response curriculum.

Fire Emergency Evacuation Procedures in Highly Protective Settings

As discussed previously, individuals who have difficulty learning the complex conditional responses required to evacuate safely during a fire will need more protective safety features and the assistance of staff, teachers, or roommates. Individuals who live, work, or go to school in highly protective settings (where fire detection, containment, and extinguishment are quick) may be taught to exit the facility upon hearing the fire alarm. Similarly, the safest response to a nighttime fire in a highly protected home with self-closing, solid-core doors

Four weeks ago, Donna had the opportunity to move out of a group home into a nice townhome with three roommates, one who was her friend and teacher. It was fun, and Donna was learning a lot. Cooking, however, was not her strong point. One day, in attempting to make popcorn on the stove, she left the oil heating in a pan for too long and it burst into flames, catching a nearby dishcloth on fire. Donna jumped backwards and screamed as the fire began to blacken the adjacent wall and consume the dishcloth inch-by-inch. Fortunately, Donna's teacher was in the next room and ran in at the sound of her screams. She quickly reached for baking soda in the refrigerator and doused the fire, extinguishing it. Donna was upset for the rest of the day.

Although Donna was practicing every day on learning to cook, clean, shop, and work her new job at the grocery store, she and her teacher had not thought about learning fire safety skills. Donna and her teacher started the day after the accident on practicing how to extinguish a small grease fire. First, Donna's teacher described the steps to putting out a grease fire and they discussed rationales as to why each step was important. Donna learned that if a pan has a lid on it and a fire is suspected, she should leave the lid on and turn off the heat source. She also learned to use baking soda to extinguish a fire in an open pan. After Donna displayed these skills perfectly during role play, a candle or small burning piece of paper was used to help Donna practice in more realistic situations. When Donna mastered extinguishing small fires during teaching sessions, her teacher began using the element of surprise to test Donna's skills at extinguishing fires that occurred without warning. The first few surprise fires were scary and difficult for Donna, but she quickly learned to handle the challenge.

After mastering the skill of extinguishing small grease fires, Donna and her teacher worked on practicing responses to other types of fire emergencies. Because Donna occasionally practices these other skills in realistic conditions, she is probably more equipped to handle a fire emergency than most people. Donna is also learning to prevent fires from occurring by being a careful cook.

may be to remain in the bedroom on the floor and wait for help. It is critical to gain the opinion of fire safety professionals as to the safest fire emergency responses to teach different individuals in particular settings.

The following task analysis is appropriate for a trainee who must learn to exit at the sound of the fire alarm, but has trouble learning this skill with the use of a typical teaching package. It is recommended that the individual learn to crawl out of the house during a fire emergency to avoid smoke inhalation. However, if the individual cannot crawl or is prohibitively slow, then walking may be substituted.

1. Upon hearing the fire alarm, crawl or walk to the nearest exit door and walk outside.
2. Go to the preset outside meeting place.

The following paragraphs describe a shaping procedure where a learner is taught to stand at the sound of the fire alarm and walk increasingly longer distances each day until he or she can walk from any room to and through the exit door and stop at a designated outside meeting place. In preparation for instruction, approximately five teaching locations, each increasingly further from an exit door, should be designated. The first should be approximately 6 feet from and in view of the exit door. The final location should vary each trial to include wherever the learner is seated or standing at the beginning of the teaching session and two other locations frequented by the learner (e.g., a favorite chair). A high-quality audiotape of the building's fire alarm (with a 10-second lead) and a variety of preferred rewards for the purpose of reinforcement should be obtained.

Teaching sessions should be held at different times of the day and evening, in varied weather conditions, and in the presence of varying combinations of people. Learners should be taught in two phases from each teaching location. Phase I entails teaching with a model, and Phase II entails teaching without a model. After criterion is met for both teaching phases at a teaching location, the learner may be taught from the next location in the sequence.

Phase I of Instruction In Phase I, learners are taught to go to the door and then to a designated meeting place at the sound of the recorded alarm after the teacher models the behavior. The teacher begins each trial by bringing the learner to the teaching location, turning on the hidden tape recorder, and returning to the learner. When the alarm sounds, the teacher jogs to the exit door. If the participant walks to the door, the teacher praises. If the learner does not start walking, the teacher prompts using the least intrusive prompt. Prompts are used in the following sequence:

1. Verbal ("[name of learner], fire, go out.")
2. Gestural (point to the door)
3. Light physical contact (one brief touch or gentle push toward the door)
4. More involved physical prompting (the least amount of physical assistance required to get the learner out; e.g., gently escort the person to the door)

Regardless of the level of prompting necessary, the learner should be praised as he or she exits the building. With the alarm continuing to sound, the same modeling and prompting procedure should be used to get the individual from the exit door to the meeting place. Decreases in the level of required prompting should be rewarded with preferred items or edibles. When the learner walks from the teaching location out the door and to the meeting place without prompts (but with a model) in a prescribed "safe" amount of time on three consecutive trials, the teacher can proceed to Phase II teaching from that location.

Phase II of Instruction In Phase II teaching, learners are taught to exit without a model. The teacher begins each trial by bringing the learner to the location, leaving the room, and turning on the tape recorder. The tape-recorded alarm should not sound until the teacher is out of sight. If, after the alarm sounds, the teacher sees that the learner is walking toward the door, the teacher proceeds to the meeting place. If about 10 seconds pass (this depends on the time it takes for the learner to stand up from a chair, his or her walking speed, and the distance from the particular teaching location to the door), and the learner is not proceeding toward the door, the teacher should come into the room and prompt using the same prompting sequence as used in Phase I. Again, praise should be given when the learner reaches the door, regardless of the level of prompt required.

With the alarm continuing to sound, the same procedures are used to help the learner get to the meeting place. A previously chosen reward should be given if no prompts are required to get the learner from the teaching location to the meeting place. When the learner walks from a teaching location out the door to the meeting place with no model, no prompts, and in the prescribed amount of time in three consecutive trials over three consecutive teaching sessions, instruction should continue from the next teaching location in the sequence until teaching is completed at all five locations.

Generalization and Maintenance Occasional testing and review (at least monthly) should be conducted. Tests should be unannounced, and correct performance should be reinforced. Retraining, using Phase II teaching, should be implemented if errors are made. If generalization to nighttime fire emergency tests is not shown, then nighttime instruction using Phase I and Phase II procedures should be implemented. If an individual is unsuccessful in learning to exit at the sound of the alarm, it may be advisable to teach the person to remain in his or her location (especially at night) and wait for help from a trained teacher, staff, or roommate.

CRITICAL ISSUES

Assistive Devices

As more individuals with disabilities move into the community to live and work, continued effort should be focused on keeping people safe

In September of 1985, Community Living Opportunities (CLO), Inc., an agency providing community-based home living and habilitation to individuals with severe disabilities, received a letter from the Kansas Department of Health and Environment stating that eight of the individuals living at Marty and Lane Houses would have to move out because they could not exit at the sound of the house fire alarm. The homes were equipped with many fire safety features, such as a fire and smoke alarm system that alerted the fire department, fire-safe construction, and self-closing, solid-core doors. Unfortunately, the hall widths were several inches too narrow to meet the Life Safety Code regulations (National Fire Protection Association, 1991) for housing individuals who could not evacuate.

Parents and staff were extremely upset over the situation, as they had advocated for many years to be able to provide community residential services to individuals with severe disabilities. Danny's mother was especially exasperated. She had cared for Danny for 22 years prior to his moving into Lane House. He was happy, well cared for, and was learning new skills at Lane. The threat of having him leave was incomprehensible. At that time, Danny was about 23 years old. He was small in stature, with a winning smile and bright eyes. He loved to interact with people using vocalizations and hugs. He did not have expressive language, except for use of adapted signs for "food" and "drink." Dan could follow some simple requests, but needed almost total assistance with all of his self-care needs. He had difficulty walking and did so with poor balance and a labored gait. Danny also had great difficulty standing when seated on the floor or in a chair.

CLO responded to the threat of expulsion of Danny and his housemates in two ways. First, they initiated negotiations with the Department of Health and Environment and with the state fire marshall. Second, CLO did what they do best—teach. An intervention team, including two professors from the University of Kansas, came up with a teaching strategy. It was a shaping procedure, where individuals would learn to exit the house at the sound of the fire alarm from locations that were increasingly further from the exit doors. For example, Dan began practicing at a location 6 feet away from the exit door. After being seated at the location, a tape recording of the house alarm was sounded. After a few seconds, if Dan did not start to walk toward the door, the teacher modeled the exiting behavior and, if necessary, used a sequence of prompts to help Dan walk to the door and to the outside meeting place. Dan was praised upon reaching the door and was given a candy that he had previously chosen as a reward when he reached the meeting place. When Dan mastered exiting from the 6 feet location without modeling or prompts, the distance from the door was increased. As Dan continued to learn, he mastered exiting from numerous locations in different rooms, through a variety of exit doors, at different times of day, and with varying members of staff. Danny's training took many months. Other individuals were trained in shorter periods of time (e.g., a few weeks or a couple of months), depending on their abilities and motivation.

Happily, long before the training was completed, negotiations with Health and Environment resulted in a waiver, enabling Danny and his friends to remain at Marty and Lane.

from harm. Teaching fire safety skills and increasing the quality of fire safety features built into residences are not the only solutions to this problem. Innovative, assistive devices can make the difference between whether an individual can or cannot live safely and independently in the community. Some assistive devices that enhance fire safety are described in Table 2.

Peer Assistance

Assistance during a fire emergency can also come from peers or neighbors. Jones, Sisson, and Van Hasselt (1984) showed that trained roommates can cue untrained individuals to evacuate safely during a fire. Neighbors can also be helpful in securing fire safety. For example, the fire alarm of a person with disabilities could also be wired to sound at a neighbor's house. The trained and willing neighbor can often respond much faster in a fire emergency than can the fire department. The neighbor could be compensated in some way for his or her services. The neighborly support system would certainly be a positive way to aid an individual to live independently in the community.

Table 2. Assistive fire safety devices

1. A timer on a stove or rangetop with an "automatic off"; if the stove or range is left on after the time has elapsed, the heat source is disengaged
2. Appliances, such as irons, space heaters, or curling irons, with an "automatic off" that disengages them after elapse of a specified time period or if they are knocked off balance
3. A sensitive smoke alarm next to the bed of an individual who is apt to smoke in bed
4. Stickers on bedroom windows of individuals who cannot evacuate independently, so that neighbors and firefighters will be able to easily discover who needs help
5. Mechanical "lifts" to aid individuals in independently transferring from bed to wheelchair in the event that they might have to escape from their bedrooms without assistance
6. Auditory monitoring devices to be used to call for help
7. Flashlights placed in strategic locations to use as a beacon or a source of light during a fire emergency
8. Kitchen towels, curtains, and bedclothes treated with a fire retardant
9. Fire alarms for persons with auditory impairments that vibrate the bed during a nighttime fire emergency or engage strobe lights during a daytime emergency
10. Escape windows to increase safety during nighttime fire emergencies

Self-Monitoring

People with or without disabilities who have successfully mastered fire safety responses and who have effective fire safety features and assistive devices installed in their homes still may not be safe. The research literature indicates that individuals must practice their skills in order to maintain them. Fire safety equipment must be checked and maintained in order to function properly when needed. Self-monitoring may help to address this issue. Pictured or written checklists may be used to help individuals to review fire safety responses and see that equipment is checked once per month.

CONCLUSIONS

With the benefits of including individuals with disabilities in community living also come the risks. Fire safety risks are increased because typical community residences do not require the protective fire safety features, like sprinkler systems and fire alarms, that have traditionally protected people who cannot respond safely in a fire emergency. The solution to this problem is to increase safety by: 1) ensuring needed fire safety features and roommate/staff assistance in residences housing people with disabilities, 2) being aware and prepared for the most likely fire emergencies, and, most importantly, 3) teaching people with developmental disabilities the fire safety responses that they need to live safely in the community using the recommendations provided in this chapter.

Future research is needed in at least two areas with regard to the fire safety of individuals with disabilities. First, further research is needed regarding the teaching and maintenance of nighttime fire safety skills. Research continues to show that fire safety responses are not consistently demonstrated during nighttime fire drills. Frequent testing and review of skills may be the solution to this problem.

Investigation is also needed to discover what combinations of fire safety features, assistive devices, staff or roommate assistance, and fire safety response skills are most effective. The National Fire Protection Association could spearhead this research by formatting their national database with a means for tracking information about fire emergencies that involve people with disabilities. Presently, there are no data on fire incidence among this population. With this information, people with disabilities will be better protected and their independence in the community will increase.

REFERENCES

Bannerman, D.J., Sheldon, J.B., & Sherman, J.A. (1991). Teaching adults with severe and profound retardation to exit their homes upon hearing the fire alarm. *Journal of Applied Behavior Analysis, 24,* 571–578.

Bertsch, B., Fox, C.J., & Kwiecinski, J. (1984). Teaching developmentally disabled persons how to react to fires. *Applied Research in Mental Retardation, 5,* 483–497.

Cohen, I.L. (1984). Establishment of independent responding to a fire alarm in a blind, profoundly retarded adult. *Journal of Behavior Therapy and Experimental Psychiatry, 15,* 365–367.

Haney, J.I., & Jones, R.T. (1982). Programming maintenance as a major component of a community centered preventative effort: Escape from fire. *Behavior Therapy, 13,* 47–62.

Holburn, C.S., & Dougher, M.J. (1985). The fire-alarm game: Exit training using negative and positive reinforcement under varied stimulus conditions. *Journal of Visual Impairment & Blindness, 79,* 401–403.

Jones, J.C. (1980). 1979 Multiple-death fires in the United States. *Fire Journal, 74*(4), 58–69.

Jones, R.T., & Haney, J.I. (1984). A primary preventative approach to the acquisition and maintenance of fire emergency responding: A comparison of external and self-instruction strategies. *Journal of Community Psychology, 12,* 180–190.

Jones, R.T., Kazdin, A.E., & Haney, J.I. (1981a). A follow-up to training emergency skills. *Behavior Therapy, 12,* 716–722.

Jones, R.T., Kazdin, A.E., & Haney, J.I. (1981b). Social validation and training of emergency fire safety skills for potential injury prevention and life saving. *Journal of Applied Behavior Analysis, 14,* 249–260.

Jones, R.T., Sisson, L.A., & Van Hasselt, V.B. (1984). Emergency fire-safety skills for blind children and adolescents: Group training and generalization. *Behavior Modification, 8,* 267–286.

Jones, R.T., & Thornton, J.L. (1987). The acquisition and maintenance of emergency evacuation skills with mildly and moderately retarded adults in a community living arrangement. *Journal of Community Psychology, 15,* 205–215.

Jones, R.T., Van Hasselt, V.B., & Sisson, L.A. (1984). Emergency fire-safety skills: A study with blind adolescents. *Behavior Modification, 8,* 59–78.

Katz, R.C., & Singh, N.N. (1986). Comprehensive fire-safety training for adult mentally retarded persons. *Journal of Mental Deficiency Research, 30,* 59–69.

Lavoie, K.R. (1988). Overview of the fire protection system. In R.J. Coleman & J.A. Granito (Eds.), *Managing fire services* (2nd ed.) (pp. 30–48). Washington, DC: International City Management Association.

Levin, B.M., & Nelson, H.E. (1981). Fire safety and disabled persons. *Fire Journal, 75,* 35–40.

Matson, J.L. (1980). Preventing home accidents: A training program for the retarded. *Behavior Modification, 4,* 397–410.

National Fire Protection Association. (1991). *Life safety code.* Quincy, MA: Author.

Rae, R., & Roll, D. (1985). Fire safety training with adults who are profoundly mentally retarded. *Mental Retardation, 23,* 26–30.

Risley, R., & Cuvo, A.J. (1980). Training mentally retarded adults to make emergency telephone calls. *Behavior Modification, 4*(4), 513–525.

Skurat, D.J. (1985). Are we gambling with our retarded citizens' lives? *Fire Journal, 79*(3), 47–49.

Ten killed in Detroit fire. (1992, June 1). *Journal World,* p. 2.

Ventura County Association for the Retarded, Inc. (1990). *Training for independent living* (4th ed.). Camarillo, CA: Author.

Yuill, C.H. (1983). Fire losses: A needless waste. In C. Rapkin (Ed.), *The social and economic consequences of residential fires* (pp. 27–42). Lexington, MA: D.C. Heath.

Chapter Eight

Safety Skills on the Job

Ronald C. Martella and Martin Agran

The increased involvement of persons with disabilities in competitive and supported employment represents one of the most significant changes in service delivery in the last decade. One result of this movement, however, is that persons with disabilities are less closely protected from the hazards of working. Thus, individuals must learn to identify work risks and avoid potential injuries on the job.

Work safety must be an important concern of both the special educator and the employment specialist (Lazar, 1980). Mueller, Wilgosh, and Dennis (1989) reported the results of a province-wide survey concerning work safety conducted in Alberta, Canada. The researchers found that employers in competitive industries rated safe work behavior and safety awareness as most important for the job survival of all employees. Heath (1983) pointed out that "not only are workers entering the work force with a minimum of job safety and health knowledge and skills, many of them receive little or no instruction on job risks upon entering the workforce" (p. 22).

McLoughlin, Garner, and Callahan (1987) noted that virtually every work environment is potentially dangerous. To minimize the possibility of injury, employment specialists may seek to place individuals with disabilities in jobs where the risk of injury is relatively low. Such placements would, of course, restrict the types and availability of work opportunities for people with disabilities, as well as prevent them from engaging in work they otherwise would be able to perform. Furthermore, denying persons with disabilities the opportunity to respond to potentially risky situations endangers their dignity and prevents them from experiencing the risk taking of ordinary life (Wolfensberger, 1972). To prepare persons with disabilities for normative functioning at work, they must not be shielded from the risks of their jobs, but taught to handle such risks adaptively.

The purpose of this chapter is to review recommended practices for teaching work safety skills to people with disabilities. Specifically, this chapter focuses on teaching safety skills in the workplace to individuals with developmental disabilities from secondary to postsecondary age. The chapter does not address safety skills for individuals under employment age.

Other disabilities not covered in this chapter may be addressed by modifying the training procedures. For example, for individuals with visual impairments, the written cues used during training can be printed in large type and/or presented verbally to each participant. Investigations with individuals with head injuries, chronic mental illness, or emotional problems have shown that the training procedures described in this book (see chap. 1, this volume) are effective in teaching a variety of community living skills (Foxx & Bittle, 1989). Thus, the recommendations made in this chapter are generalizable to individuals with other disabilities and require minor, if any, adaptations.

JOB-RELATED INJURIES

Accidents are defined as unanticipated, chance occurrences in a progression of events that come about through a combination of causes. They produce unintended harm (i.e., injury, disease, death) to an individual, damage to property, or any combination of these effects (Stern & Gathercoal, 1987). An injury may be defined as a harmful condition endured by the body as a result of an accident and "can take the form of an abrasion, a bruise, a laceration, a fracture, a foreign object in the body, a puncture wound, a burn, or an electric shock" (Anton, 1979, p. 2). For purposes of this chapter, the accidents and injuries discussed are restricted to work environments.

Causes of Job-Related Injuries

There are two categories of work injuries: those produced by an individual (behavioral) and those produced by the environment (environmental). Behavioral causes relate to the inappropriate actions of an individual or the lack of an appropriate response to an injury-causing situation; in either case, they are preventable. Such behaviors as throwing things, not wearing protective equipment, or fighting with others may cause injuries to the individual and/or his or her co-workers. Environmental hazards are situations in the workplace that can cause an injury (e.g., items laying in an aisle, exposed electrical wiring, dangerously hot materials).

Because many injuries are behaviorally produced, specific behaviors that will prevent injuries need to be identified and taught. According to Anton (1979), safety behavior is not a state of the mind, but a cluster of behaviors that differ across a variety of settings. Thus, safety skills training programs need to focus on actual, measurable change in a targeted behavior, rather than just on a change in attitude.

Martella, Marchand-Martella, and Agran (1992) surveyed a sample of employers from various industries. Respondents were given a list of potential environmental and behavioral causes of work-related accidents and asked to rate both their seriousness (i.e., their believed potential for causing an accident) and the actual frequency or number of accidents produced by each situation on the list. Tables 1 and 2 indicate the survey findings.

All causes were rated on a scale of 1 to 5, with 3 corresponding to "somewhat serious" and 2 corresponding to "a serious cause." For frequency, all causes were rated as "sometimes" to "rarely occurred" on a scale of 1 to 5. Interestingly, employers' ratings of seriousness and frequency did not correlate significantly. Thus, causes that are present more frequently were not necessarily rated as having a greater potential for injury than those causes that occur less frequently. It is clear that because of the seriousness of their injury-causing potential, both low and high frequency causes represent important training targets. In all, the investigation validated the evidence that accidents result from both environmental and behavioral causes and suggests a potentially useful repertoire of work safety skills for employees with disabilities. A well-trained worker should know how to behave safely and be able to identify potentially risky workplace conditions (Martella, Marchand-Martella, & Agran, 1992).

Incidence of Job-Related Injuries

Although a large percentage of injuries involve automobiles or are related to home environments, many injuries also occur in the workplace (Heath, 1983; Stern & Gathercoal, 1987). The price to society for these injuries is apparent given the following statistics. According to the United States Department of Commerce (1990), 10,600 workers were killed and 1,800,000 disabled due to work-related injuries in 1988. Additionally, the National Safety Council (1991) reported that in 1990, 60,000 workers received permanent impairments and approximately 1,700,000 received temporary disabilities on the job as a result of an injury sustained while at work.

Table 1. Mean ratings of seriousness for all survey items presented by business type and behavioral category[a]

Accident causes	Mean seriousness ratings by industry type				
	Service	Manufacturing	Wholesale/ retail	Food	All industries combined
Environmental causes					
Slippery floor	2.28	2.64	2.71	2.06	2.34
Flammables	2.67	1.19	2.29	2.76	2.34
Exposed wires	2.50	2.45	3.14	2.71	2.64
Poisonous substances	2.67	2.82	3.29	2.47	2.72
Hot materials	2.89	3.00	3.00	2.65	2.85
Objects on floor	2.78	3.18	3.00	2.76	2.89
$\bar{X}$	2.63	2.55	2.91	2.56	2.63
Behavioral causes					
Inappropriate use of machines or appliances	2.39	2.64	2.86	2.82	2.64
Fighting	2.72	2.18	3.29	2.65	2.66
Not wearing protective equipment	2.50	2.72	2.71	2.85	2.69
Lifting heavy objects	2.56	2.82	2.14	3.00	2.70
Lack of knowledge of tool use	2.84	2.82	2.71	3.06	2.89
Wearing loose or inappropriate clothing around power tools	2.95	2.64	3.00	3.00	2.91
Fatigue	3.11	2.73	3.29	2.65	2.91
Tool misuse	3.11	2.73	3.00	2.94	2.96
Throwing objects	3.11	2.91	3.14	3.06	3.06
Play behavior	3.17	2.82	3.14	3.06	3.06
Lack of attention span	3.22	2.82	3.29	3.24	3.15
$\bar{X}$	2.88	2.71	2.97	2.94	2.87

[a]These numbers are weighted averages based on the total number of respondents from each industry type. The following ratings were used for seriousness: 1 = a very serious cause (an accident definitely would occur); 2 = a serious cause (a high likelihood that an accident would occur); 3 = a somewhat serious cause (a moderate likelihood that an accident would occur); 4 = not a serious cause (a small likelihood that an accident would occur); and 5 = not a cause (unlikely that an accident would occur).

Work-related accidents are classified as follows:

- Near-injury accidents in which an injury does not occur but may occur in the future, given the same conditions
- Minor-injury accidents that require first aid or doctor's care
- Disabling-injury accidents, including fatality, permanent total disability, permanent partial disability, or temporary total disability
- Material damage, including the damage of products or equipment (DeReamer, 1961)

Near misses, minor, or slight injuries are rarely reported (Duenk & Burke, 1991). Although the obvious priorities would be to reduce or eliminate fatalities or permanently disabling injuries, the need to reduce or eliminate accidents in each of these categories is warranted. In particular, near-injury accidents or minor-injury accidents warrant attention, as individuals experiencing these types of accidents could have far more serious injuries in the future if not provided appropriate instruction.

Prevalence of Injuries Among Workers with Disabilities

Data on work injuries are based on accident figures for persons without disabilities. At present, there is no available data base on the number or types of injuries sustained by people with disabilities involved in supported employment. While such data are not available, injury rates may be as high for persons with disabilities as rates for persons without disabilities be-

Table 2. Mean ratings of frequency for all survey items presented by business type and behavioral category[a]

Accident causes	Mean seriousness ratings by industry type				
	Service	Manufacturing	Wholesale/ retail	Food	All industries combined
Environmental causes					
Slippery floor	3.06	3.82	4.00	2.47	3.15
Objects on floor	3.28	3.36	3.43	2.88	3.19
Hot materials	3.22	3.64	3.00	3.18	3.27
Poisonous substances	3.89	4.09	4.29	4.00	4.02
Flammables	4.17	4.09	4.57	3.88	4.11
Exposed wires	4.05	4.27	4.86	4.24	4.26
$\bar{X}$	3.61	3.88	4.03	3.44	3.67
Behavioral causes					
Lifting heavy objects	2.94	3.64	2.86	3.00	3.10
Not wearing protective equipment	3.39	3.55	3.43	3.88	3.57
Tool misuse	3.83	3.73	3.86	3.59	3.67
Lack of attention span	3.61	3.45	4.14	3.47	3.69
Fatigue	3.72	3.36	4.00	3.12	3.71
Lack of knowledge of tool use	3.89	3.82	4.29	3.76	3.88
Play behavior	3.78	4.00	4.71	3.88	3.98
Inappropriate use of machines or appliances	3.83	3.82	3.86	4.06	4.08
Fighting	4.28	4.18	5.00	4.41	4.11
Throwing objects	4.05	4.09	4.57	4.24	4.18
Wearing loose or inappropriate clothing around power tools	4.11	4.09	4.14	4.24	4.20
$\bar{X}$	3.77	3.80	4.08	3.79	3.82

[a]These numbers are weighted averages based on the total number of respondents from each industry type. The following ratings were used for frequency of occurrence: 1 = always (at least one a day); 2 = often (two to four times a week); 3 = sometimes (once a week); 4 = rarely (less than three times a month); and 5 = never.

cause of a number of physical and adaptive difficulties (Matson, 1980). Such characteristics may put them at greater risk for emergencies and accidents. With the increased efforts to provide supported employment services, more injuries may occur.

In such work placement options as an industrial enclave or a mobile work crew, the prevalence of work injuries may be understandably low because of the intensive involvement of the employment specialist; however, this remains an empirical question. In individual placements where the employment specialist ultimately withdraws from the site, it is uncertain as to how many consumers may sustain injuries (mild or serious). Heinrich (1959) suggested that of 350 work accidents, 29 will be minor on the average and one will be serious. It is uncertain if this formula would apply equally to individuals with disabilities. In any case, it is reasonable to assume that as more employees with disabilities are prepared for employment in less restrictive work environments, their chances for work-related injuries are higher.

SAFETY ON THE JOB

Safety may be defined as the mitigation of personal injury or property damage through the prevention of accidents (Bever, 1984). Lazar (1980) noted the following in regard to safety skills training:

> There is a vital need for research and curriculum development by special educators and others in this new emerging area as it relates to career education and vocational education. The time for ca-

reer safety awareness as part of career education has come. (p. 3)

The purpose of safety skills training is to teach workers how to discriminate when safety hazards exist "during the working day, as well as how to perform their jobs without endangering themselves or their fellow employees" (Re Velle, 1980, p. 22). Safety skills training, then, involves instructing the individual on how to minimize injury and loss from such nondeliberate acts as accidents.

Assessing Individual Training Needs

Based on the aforementioned findings, there are several needs that must be addressed in order to ensure a successful training program. First, employees need to be taught both generic and job-specific safety skills (Martella, Marchand-Martella, & Agran, 1992). For example, the most serious environmental cause of accidents in the service and food industries is a slippery floor, while flammables are the most serious cause in manufacturing. What this suggests is that, in addition to the generic safety skills that all employees must acquire (e.g., how to lift heavy boxes, paying attention to what you are doing, not running in the work area), skill development must be directed to the risk situations that are specific to the particular workplace setting.

Social validation methodology can be helpful in this respect (Agran, Martin, & Mithaug, 1987). Job trainers should make every effort to ask employers, supervisors, and co-workers what are the types and causes of work injuries at their particular jobs. Instruction should then be provided in identifying these situations, as well as responding appropriately to them.

Second, to ensure the successful work placement of a person with disabilities, a job analysis needs to be conducted (Rusch & Mithaug, 1980). Such an analysis will identify the demands of a job and reveal stimuli in the work setting that may hinder or facilitate work performance (e.g., "rush" times, co-worker support). Although most job analyses include information about the physical conditions of the work environment, few job analyses include detailed information about work risks. Therefore, a job safety analysis, such as the one presented in Table 3, is recommended.

Typically, a job analysis includes the desired task responses and the environmental cues that control the responses. Employment specialists may also want to include potential safety hazards for each job step. Work supervisors and co-workers may be helpful in providing this information. Such hazards may involve environmental stimuli (e.g., excessive levels of noise, dust, or fumes) or behavioral events (e.g., misusing tools, not wearing safety glasses). Thus, for each step in a task, trainers may wish to identify hazards that may be present. Additionally, the appropriate and safe response to execute to prevent an injury should be included.

With this information, employees can be alerted to the problems that may exist in a given task. For instructional purposes, trainers may include these hazardous stimuli in the work setting when teaching the task so the employee learns how best to respond to them. Such an analysis should be standard practice in employment preparation or safety programs (Re Velle, 1980).

Third, attention must be directed to the individual needs and requirements of workers. For

Table 3. Sample job safety analysis

Task steps	Environmental cue	Potential safety hazard	Safe procedure
Cut wood to a specified length. 1. Take out wood. 2. Put on goggles. 3. Measure and mark wood to be cut. 4. Turn on power saw. 5. Move the wood across the blade. 6. Turn off machine.	Power tools running	Behavioral: Wearing loose clothing while using power tools	Wear tight fitting clothes or tie down loose clothing.

example, if a worker has poor motor behavior skills, an intervention may target injury prevention skills that are directly related to problems posed by these deficits. Suppose a worker has difficulty grasping a particular tool, such difficulty helps prevent the individual from meeting the production quota and also causes undue muscle strain and frustration. In such a case, a prosthetic grip on the tool may be appropriate. If a worker has poor mobilization or sensory impairments, training may focus on safe maneuverability within the confines of the workplace. The individual could be shown the most efficient way to move through the work setting while being exposed to any of a number of hazardous stimuli (e.g., large box or loose tools on the floor, spilled liquids, trash). Such instruction may be as vital to an employee's well-being as his or her job performance.

Fourth, the assessment of an individual's work safety skills should be a standard component in any work performance evaluation. Several vocational assessments include working safely as a criterion item (e.g., see Rusch, Schutz, & Agran, 1982), but fail to specify the specific responses desired. Also, behaviors related to work safety may be included, but not operationally defined (e.g., a vague statement such as, "employee knows how to work safely"). The assessment of work safety skills should not be thought of as an attitudinal or global construct, but rather, as a set of specific and observable work skills.

Finally, work safety competence is measured paradoxically by what the participant both does and does not do. For example, such motor skills as handling tools appropriately or dressing oneself can be measured by the frequency of occurrence of these responses. However, other responses such as not fighting or not engaging in play behavior (e.g., horseplay) may be equally as important in terms of preventing accidents. Regarding the latter, *nonoccurrence* represents the important measure. The nonoccurrence of an undesirable behavior does not by itself suggest that the behavior is not part of the worker's repertoire. Instead, it may just mean that the undesirable behavior was not sufficiently cued. If it were cued—say, two co-workers are clowning around—the participant may join them by exhibiting the same behavior.

In this respect, trainers are encouraged to provide feedback to trainees for engaging in desirable behaviors, especially those behaviors that are incompatible with undesirable behaviors. Ideally, this should be done in the natural work setting. If this is not possible, both examples and nonexamples should be presented in role plays.

Existing Training Practices

There are two types of injury prevention training approaches: nonsystematic and systematic. Nonsystematic training involves attempting to reduce the incidence of work injuries by consequating safe work behaviors; however, the behaviors to be learned and/or reduced in order to prevent injuries are not specifically defined and targeted. Additionally, the schedule of rewarding individuals for safe work behaviors (e.g., every month) and the form of this reward (e.g., money or prizes for low injury rates) are not always specified. Finally, a nonsytematic program may not be structured to track improved behaviors in order for an assessment of the program effects to be measured. For these reasons, nonsystematic training represents an inadequate approach to the teaching of work safety skills.

A behavior analytic approach, in which the work behaviors of employees are systematically modified so that they are less likely to sustain an injury, has been found to be successful in reducing work-related accidents (Denton, 1982; Hendrick, 1990; Komaki, Barwick, & Scott, 1978). This approach not only seeks to target certain behaviors for change, but also to provide a means for motivating employees to perform their jobs in a safe manner by rewarding safety-related behaviors (Hendrick, 1990; Komaki et al., 1978). For example, rewarding employees through public acknowledgment and feedback has been found to be an effective and acceptable procedure to use for both employees and employers (Hendrick, 1990; Komaki, Heinzmann, & Lawson, 1980). Systematic training programs specify the behavior to be targeted and the reward system, then implement a system for tracking employee behavior. Finally, and possibly most important, a systematic training program is consistent in the implementation of the program's critical variables (e.g., target behavior definition, rewarding target behavior).

Although behavior analytic safety skills programs have been found to be effective in reducing the occurrence of injuries for persons without disabilities, few systematic safety skills programs for persons with disabilities have been published. Many employers may assume that an employee already knows safe work behavior and, thus, do not think that safety skills training is necessary. The situation for persons with disabilities is even that much more critical. Therefore, safety skills training is critically needed for these individuals in the work environment.

Instruction in work safety needs to focus on preparing workers to discriminate the nature and magnitude of work-related hazards in their work environment (Bever, 1984) and to identify these safety hazards and determine how to avoid, eliminate, or reduce them (Finn, 1979; Ridley, 1986). In addition, Pryor (1983) indicated that individuals should be assessed on their knowledge of safety, be encouraged to report unsafe conditions, and understand the importance of working safely for their own interests and for those of the people around them.

Problem-Solving Skills Several studies support the assumption that the ability to recognize and resolve commonly occurring problem situations has a positive impact on successful work and community placement (e.g., Alper, 1985; D'Zurilla & Goldfried, 1971; Foxx, Martella, & Marchand-Martella, 1989; Froland, Brodsky, Olson, & Stewart, 1979; Platt & Spivack, 1972a, 1972b, 1974). One method of problem solving that has been demonstrated to be effective is the modified generation of alternatives approach (Foxx & Faw, 1990; Foxx et al., 1989). In this approach, participants are taught to provide solutions to problem situations using predetermined criteria. For instance, in the Foxx et al. (1989) study, participants with closed head injuries were taught to respond to problem situations using the following four criteria:

1. When will the problem be solved?
2. Where would you look for help?
3. Who would you talk to?
4. What would you say?

Participants were given a problem situation, and then asked to respond by first following the criteria as they were presented to them on a cue card and then by responding from memory. During training, each participant was required to provide either an initial solution or an alternative one to each problem situation. For example, a problem situation at a restaurant could be presented to the trainee such as: "A co-worker tells you that toast is stuck in the toaster. She says that she will take it out with a knife, even though the toaster is still plugged in. What should you do?" The participants' responses to the four criteria presented above might be as follows: 1) when will the problem be solved? (e.g., "when the toaster is unplugged before the toast is removed"); 2) where would you look for help? (e.g., "a co-worker or supervisor"); 3) who would you talk to? (e.g., "the woman who is pulling out the toast"); and 4) what would you say? (e.g., "unplug the toaster before you take out the toast").

The results of the Foxx et al. (1989) study indicated that the experimental group's mean increased from pre- to posttest assessments, and the participants' responses generalized to actual community setting situations for both similar and dissimilar situations as compared to those presented in class. Foxx and colleagues also employed a memory strategy that featured vocal rehearsal to both facilitate the retention of new material and to determine if the participants had actually learned the problem-solving strategy. In other words, what was taught was not *what* to think, but *how* to think (Meichenbaum & Asarnow, 1979).

The value of teaching problem-solving skills to supported employees is clearly apparent. In most work environments, any of a number of work hazards may exist. Teaching appropriate responses to all of these stimuli may be too costly and difficult to accomplish. Thus, providing employees with skills for responding to hazards in both trained and untrained environments represents a potentially more useful approach.

Training Involving Persons with Disabilities To date, there are two published studies on training injury prevention behaviors to individuals with disabilities while on the job. Martella, Agran, and Marchand-Martella (1992a) used a modified generalization of alternative problem-solving strategies to teach individuals in supported employment how to prevent work-related injuries. The percentage of criterion components present in a problem situation was measured. Criterion components were specific responses required for each solution. The four components were as follows:

1. How would an accident happen?
2. When would an accident be prevented?
3. Who would you talk to?
4. What would you do or say?

During training sessions, the trainer recorded whether or not all of the component responses were present and appropriate in each solution. Results indicated that the participants' newly acquired problem-solving skills generalized to situations similar and dissimilar to those presented in training.

Martella, Marchand-Martella, Agran, and Allen (in press) taught a modified generalization of alternative problem-solving strategies to nine sheltered workshop employees to prevent work-related injuries. The percentage of criterion components present in a problem situation was measured. The criterion components were the same as those used by Martella et al. (1992a).

Training was conducted across three groups of three participants. Results indicated that all participants used the targeted problem-solving strategy to respond to situations that could cause injuries. In addition, the generalization results indicated that the participants' newly acquired problem-solving skills generalized to situations similar and dissimilar to those used in training. In addition to the assessments listed, participants were also assessed on their ability to discriminate between safe and unsafe work behaviors. The results (see Table 4) indicated that the participants learned to discriminate between situations that could cause injuries during the assessments. Although the number of investigations of the effects of training programs to teach work safety skills to persons with disabilities remain limited, the findings reported suggest that persons with disabilities can successfully achieve a repertoire of work safety skills.

TEACHING WORK SAFETY SKILLS

The following is a description of a work safety program developed by Martella, Agran, and Marchand-Martella (1992b) based on the problem-solving approach proposed by Foxx and associates (see previous section, "Existing Training Practices"). This problem-solving ap-

Table 4. Percentage of correct discriminations for nonexamples during simulated generalization probe assessments

	Group 1	Group 2	Group 3	Total
Baseline (P-1)[a]	71%	50%	58%	59%
Training:				
with cue (P-2)[b]	75%	58%	88%	74%
without cue (P-3)[c]	75%	54%	81%	68%
Maintenance:				
2-week	69%	59%	79%	69%
8-week	100%	92%	88%	93%

[a]P-1 indicates generalization assessments after baseline condition.
[b]P-2 indicates generalization assessments after training with cue cards.
[c]P-3 indicates generalization assessments after training without cue cards.

proach provides a means for individuals to generate solutions across a variety of problem situations. It is designed to be implemented in either a group or one-on-one format, wherein each participant takes turns providing an initial solution to a problem that relates to a potential injury-causing situation. After a solution is provided, participants are given feedback by their trainers. The trainer determines, on an individual basis, a certain number of correct solutions that are needed to earn a reward. Participants remain in training until they have mastered the problem-solving strategy.

Training Responses to Problem Situations

In training the ability to problem solve, simulated injury-causing situations must be developed that involve either injuries caused by environmental hazards or injuries resulting from inappropriate worker behavior. Table 5 lists the problem situations identified in the survey conducted by Martella, Marchand-Martella, & Agran (1992). These situations are grouped as either environmental hazards or behavioral causes. For each of these potential causes, one training and two probe situations were generated. For example, when teaching a learner how to respond appropriately when a pool of water is on the work floor, the individual will also be asked how to respond appropriately when there is grease on the work floor; or, the learner might be asked how to respond appropriately to a patch of slippery ice on the sidewalk if working outdoors in the winter. These probe situations are designed to promote generalization.

The participant who is taught how to generate alternative responses (problem solve) is more likely to respond effectively to novel situations in various settings. If a participant is not taught problem-solving skills, but is instead taught specific responses to specific situations in the same settings, he or she will be restricted in their ability to respond to nontrained situations and settings.

Two primary methods are used to evaluate responding. First, participants are asked to respond verbally to hypothetical situations during an interview generalization assessment. This evaluation provides a measure of the participant's skill competency before he or she is exposed to actual situations in the work environment. During the interview assessment, the participant is asked to generate a solution to situations that are either similar or dissimilar to those used in training. Similar situations require the same response as a parallel training situation. For example, in training, a learner might be given the following problem: "You are working and notice a box lying in the middle of the aisle. What should you do or say?". In the interview, a similar problem might be posed to the learner, such as, "You are walking to your work station and see a piece of metal lying on the floor in the aisle. What should you do or say?". Dissimilar situations require a different response than the one in the training situation (e.g., training: "You are working and notice a box laying in the middle of the aisle. What should you do or say?"; dissimilar: "You are working in the kitchen and need to take a hot pan from the oven. What should you do or say?").

Table 5. Problem situation list

Environmental hazards	Behavioral causes
Obstacle in passageway	Lifting heavy box
Slippery floor	Fighting
Flammables near heat source	Horseplay
Exposed electrical wires	Running in work area
Broken glass	Inappropriate tool use
Sharp objects	Inappropriate work clothing
Spilled gasoline and/or leakage	Not attending to work task
Protruding objects	Throwing objects
Unlabeled fluids	Not wearing goggles
Frayed cord of appliance or power tool	

The second measure for evaluating responding involves a staged assessment. During a staged assessment, the participant is exposed to problem situations in his or her natural work environment. These situations are set up by the trainer in a manner in which the participant is unaware of what is taking place. For example, the trainer may leave broken glass in the middle of the aisle and observe how the participant reacts. This assessment measures how well the participant responds to an actual work situation. Therefore, if training has the desired effect, the participant will respond to the situation in an appropriate manner. Again, these situations are either similar or dissimilar to those used in training.

Scoring and Recording Response Data

Data should be collected on the participant's solutions to problem situations. These solutions are then compared to the ones provided by employers and job coaches. For scoring purposes, the percentage of problem-solving criterion components present in a learner's response is calculated. Problem-solving criterion components are specific response elements required in each solution. For example, a participant might be asked to respond to the following: "You are at work and notice another employee wearing loose clothing while working with a power tool. What would you do or say?" If the participant states the clothing could get caught in the power tool and the person could get hurt (*how*), that tighter clothing should be worn (*when*), and that the participant would tell the supervisor (*who*) that the other employee was wearing loose clothing (*what*), all components would be scored as correct.

The percentages of criterion components completed correctly for training and probe sessions are obtained by dividing the number of correct criterion components by the total num-

Carl is a 35-year-old employee with mental retardation who works at a local department store as a custodian. His primary job responsibilities include cleaning the bathrooms, sweeping floors, and taking out trash. He was involved in a number of accidents when he first started the job, and his supervisors were concerned that he may become seriously injured if he did not receive accident prevention training. Carl had completed training on how to avoid injuries while at work; however, his training had only involved providing verbal responses to problem situations. The investigators were not only interested in Carl's verbal responses to situations during training; they were also interested in whether his ability to respond to training situations generalized to his actual work environment.

Generalization assessments were conducted in two primary ways. First, an individual who had not interacted with Carl previously met with him and read situations to him that could cause an injury. The interviewer then requested Carl to tell her how he would prevent an accident. The situations read to Carl were similar to those used during training by the trainer (i.e., required the same or similar motor response) and dissimilar to the situations used in training (i.e., required a different motor response). The interviewer found that Carl could indicate appropriately what he would do when faced with situations similar and dissimilar to those used in training.

A second type of generalization assessment was also used. Teaching Carl what to say when faced with a situation was one thing, but making sure that he actually prevented injuries was another. A job coach who regularly worked with Carl set up situations that could potentially cause an injury while Carl was at work. For example, the job coach placed broken glass in the middle of an aisle where someone could step on it and cut themselves. (The job coach stayed near the glass and prevented someone from actually stepping on it.)

These staged situations were approved by a university human rights committee and by Carl's employer. After the situations were set up without Carl's knowledge, the job coach observed how Carl actually responded when confronted with a potentially injury-causing situation. As in the interview assessment, these real situations were either similar or dissimilar to the hypothetical situations presented in training. The job coach indicated that Carl was able to prevent injuries much better after training in the actual context of his workplace.

ber of criterion components possible and multiplying by 100. For example, suppose a participant responded to the box lying in the middle of the floor by stating that someone could trip over the box (*how*), the box should be moved (*when*), and he or she would talk to the supervisor (*who*). In this response, the *what* component was not present. Therefore, the participant's level of performance would be 75% (3 correct criterion components divided by four possible components).

Training with Cue Cards

Training can involve either environmental hazards or worker behaviors that may cause an accident in the work place. First, the trainer explains the purpose of the program, then gives each participant a cue card that lists the criterion components:

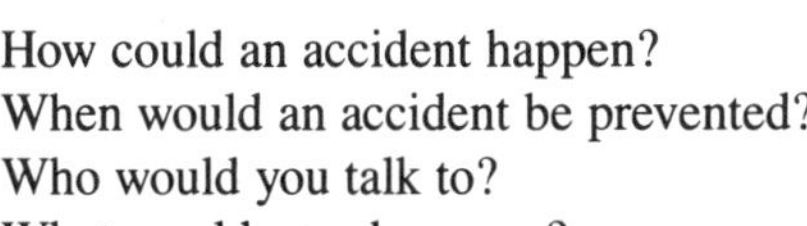

How could an accident happen?
When would an accident be prevented?
Who would you talk to?
What would you do or say?

The cue card prompts a participant to remember the criterion components. The participants are instructed to refer to the cue card when formulating a response to a problem situation.

In addition to the cue card, the trainer gives each participant a scorecard (see Figure 1). The scorecard allows the learner to follow his or her progress by marking off the number of times he or she responded correctly to all four criteria. The trainer circles the number of correct solutions needed for each participant to respond appropriately. The scorecard not only shows how many correct solutions are needed to earn a reward (in this case, nine) but also allows the participant to track his or her performance throughout the training sessions. The following case example illustrates how these cards may be utilized in training.

Setting Individualized Criteria

Individualized criteria are established based on a predetermined number of solutions to problem situations in order to earn a reward. At the beginning of each session, the trainer informs each participant how many correct solutions are required in order for him or her to earn a reward. Initially, the criterion can be set at one correct solution. After a participant reaches or surpasses this initial criterion, there are any number of methods to set the next session's criterion. For example, the criterion can be increased by 33% after it is met by the participant. (Thus, if a participant correctly responded to six situations, the criterion can be set at eight in the next session.) Another method of determining the individualized criterion is to simply increase each session's criterion by a predetermined number (e.g., two solutions) each time the last criterion is successfully met.

Training without Cue Cards

When training without cue cards, all training conditions remain the same except that the cue cards are removed. The trainer instructs the participants to remember the components when they are generating a solution. The withdrawal of cue cards can usually occur with most participants at some point in the training. However, if a participant (or participants) is lagging behind others in the group, the participant(s) who is behind can retain his or her cue card. The cue card training ceases when all

Place a mark (/) through each box when you state all four components in a solution.
Participant ________________
Session ________________ w/cue w/out cue

1	2	3	4	5	6	7	8	9

Figure 1. Scorecard for safety skills training.

Joan is a 22-year-old employee of the city parks service. Her job duties include cleaning the bathrooms and the area around the bathroom sites at a number of local parks. Joan was considered to be prone to accidents and had suffered a number of cuts and scrapes while on the job. She was referred to accident prevention training by her job coach. Joan had mental retardation and required high levels of assistance. She began training with two other participants, Ben and Maria. Ben and Maria both worked at a university cafeteria cleaning dishes and tables. They were referred to the training by their supervisors. Ben, age 60, and Maria, age 19, also had mental retardation, but required lower levels of assistance.

During training, Joan, Ben, and Maria sat at a table with the trainer. They were each given cue and scoring cards. On the cue cards, components to be taught were listed; the scoring cards contained nine numbered boxes. The participants were told to listen to each problem situation when read aloud by the trainer and were instructed to think of possible solutions. Each participant took turns providing an initial response to the situation. For example, during the first training session, Maria provided the first solution. After Maria's solution, Ben was asked to provide an alternative solution, followed by Joan. The alternative solutions had to include different responses to the *who* and *what* components. Thus, Joan, Ben, and Maria each provided three initial solutions and six alternatives to problem situations.

After each participant provided a solution, the trainer determined if the solution was correct. This determination was aided by a scoring matrix (see Table 6). A correct solution was considered to be one that included all of the problem-solving components indicated for that particular situation. For example, when Maria was provided with the problem of an exposed electrical wire, she answered that someone could get shocked, that the wiring needed to be covered up, and that she would talk to her supervisor. However, Maria could not think of what to say to her supervisor. Therefore, the trainer told Maria that she made a good effort and answered the first three components correctly, but that the last component was not present in her response. Maria was then asked to tell everyone what she could say to her supervisor. Maria still could not think of what to say, so the trainer told her she could say, "There is an exposed electrical wire. Let me show you where it is." Maria was then asked to repeat what the trainer had said. After this, Ben was requested to provide an alternative. He was given feedback in the same manner as Maria. Finally, Joan was asked to provide another solution and was also given feedback.

After all participants provided a solution, the next situation was read. When all problem situations were addressed, the trainer checked each participant's scorecard to determine if he or she had met the individualized criterion. If the participant had met the criterion, he or she received a reward. If he or she failed to meet the criterion, the trainer explained to the participant that he or she did a good job and with continued effort could receive a reward the next time if the criterion was met.

participants have reached a preestablished criterion. For example, one criterion might be taking away the cue cards when all participants have responded correctly at greater than 80% for three consecutive sessions.

For participants who are unable to read, the trainer should prompt (e.g., "What is the first, second, third, and fourth component?"). If the participant(s) is unable to state each component, the trainer should read each criterion component aloud and ask the participant(s) to repeat what he or she has said. The trainer should discontinue reading each component to the participant(s) after he or she can verbalize each component after the initial prompt to do so. It is important to have the participant(s) restate each component after the trainer in order to help him or her remember them once the cue card is withdrawn. It is also important to make sure the participant(s) can state each component without prompts so that he or she is not taught to rely on the trainer for assistance while formulating a solution.

This program represents a promising means of teaching individuals with disabilities to prevent work-related accidents. We believe that the use of this program will be beneficial for those individuals who are being prepared for supported or competitive employment. The program is also helpful for those individuals

Table 6. Scoring matrix for safety skills training

Problem situation	How could accident happen?	When would accident be prevented?	Who would you talk to?	What would you do/say?
You are working and notice a box lying in the middle of the aisle. What should you do or say?	People could trip over it and hurt themselves.	When the box is moved and out of the way	Supervisor Other workers	Can I move the box out of the way? Are you using the box? Move the box from the aisle.

presently in supported or competitive employment, but who lack the requisite skills to prevent accidents on the job.

CONCLUSIONS

Although work safety in supported employment is an issue that is beginning to receive more attention, it is clear that additional research is needed. Because work environments may have potential risks and employment specialists may not be present to correct risky situations, employees with developmental disabilities need to be taught strategies to respond appropriately. Failure to provide them with such skills not only limits their employability, but it may also put them in a potentially dangerous situation.

Knowledge about the types of safety skills training programs provided to supported employees remains limited. Specifically, what is the content of such training? How is mastery assessed? Are individuals being taught a generalizable repertoire of safety skills for a variety of work conditions, or is their training limited to learning to respond only to the most obvious risk conditions in their current work environments? Are they being taught to provide feedback to co-workers after observing a potentially dangerous action? Are they being taught to correct or modify potentially risky situations, or are they instructed instead just to tell a supervisor, co-worker, or employment specialist that a risk situation is present? Last, is ensuring safety considered to be the responsibility of the trainer, not the trainee?

The accident causes identified in the Martella, Marchand-Martella, and Agran (1992) investigation represent potentially useful information for employment preparation programs. However, the generalizability of the study's findings are restricted to the causes listed and the employers sampled. Additional study is needed on other potential accident causes across a greater diversity of occupations. Last, and perhaps most importantly, although a list of potential causes of accidents was revealed in this investigation, no data were obtained on the number of accidents that occurred or the types of injuries sustained by workers in competitive or supported employment. Consequently, it is unknown how many accidents are directly attributable to the causes suggested. Such information is crucial in our efforts to identify potential causes and develop appropriate stategies to teach individuals with disabilities safe work behaviors.

McLoughlin et al. (1987) indicated that employees should not be excluded from jobs that contain risks, but that unsafe working conditions are an absolute "no go" criterion for employment. In many places of employment, trainers can identify potential risks. Do employees receive corrective feedback when they don't wear safety glasses or when they engage in horseplay? Are electrical circuits overloaded? Are there guards for power tools? With this information, trainers can alert employers to potential hazards and have them corrected. However, trainers may not always be available to do this troubleshooting. Thus, employees need to have skills so that they can evaluate both the safety of their work environments and their own behavior. There is general agreement that employees with disabilities must learn a set of vocational survival skills—skills that are essential for their entry into and maintenance of employment. Safety skills represent a set of work survival skills in the truest sense.

REFERENCES

Agran, M., Martin, J.E., & Mithaug, D.E. (1987). Transitional assessment for students with mental retardation. *Diagnostique, 12,* 173–184.

Alper, S. (1985). Comparing employer and teacher identified entry-level job requisites of service occupations. *Education and Training of the Mentally Retarded, 20,* 89–96.

Anton, T.J. (1979). *Occupational safety and health management.* New York: McGraw-Hill.

Bever, D.L. (1984). *Safety: A personal focus.* St. Louis, MO: Times Mirror/Mosby College.

Denton, D.K. (1982). *Safety management: Improving performance.* New York: McGraw-Hill.

DeReamer, R. (1961). *Modern safety practices.* New York: John Wiley & Sons.

Duenk, L.G., & Burke, S.R. (1991). Greater accident awareness can help prevent injuries. *School shop/tech directions, 50,* 13–14.

D'Zurilla, T., & Goldfried, M. (1971). Problem solving and behavior modification. *Journal of Abnormal Psychology, 78,* 107–126.

Finn, P. (1979). Stimulating occupational health and safety concerns. *Health Education, 10,* 8–9.

Foxx, R.M., & Bittle, R.G. (1989). *Thinking it through: Teaching a problem-solving strategy for community living.* Champaign, IL: Research Press.

Foxx, R.M., & Faw, G.D. (1990). Problem-solving skills training for psychiatric inpatients: An analysis of generalization. *Behavioral Residential Treatment, 5,* 159–176.

Foxx, R.M., Martella, R.C., & Marchand-Martella, N.E. (1989). The acquisition, maintenance, and generalization of problem-solving skills by closed head-injured adults. *Behavior Therapy, 20,* 61–76.

Froland, C., Brodsky, G., Olson, M., & Stewart, L. (1979). Social support and social adjustment: Implications for mental health professionals. *Community Mental Health, 15,* 32–93.

Heath, E.D. (1983). Youth and safety for the world of work. *Vocational Education, 58,* 23–24.

Heinrich, H.L. (1959). *Industrial accident prevention.* New York: McGraw Hill.

Hendrick, K. (1990). *Systematic safety training.* New York: Marcel Dekker.

Komaki, J., Barwick, K.D., & Scott, L.R. (1978). A behavioral approach to occupational safety: Pinpointing and reinforcing safe performance in a food manufacturing plant. *Journal of Applied Psychology, 63,* 434–445.

Komaki, J., Heinzmann, A.T., & Lawson, L. (1980). Effects of training and feedback: Component analysis of a behavioral safety program. *Journal of Applied Psychology, 65,* 261-270.

Lazar, A.L. (1980). Exceptional persons, careers and health hazards. *Journal for Special Educators, 17,* 2–3.

Martella, R.C., Agran, M., & Marchand-Martella, N.E. (1992a). Problem solving to prevent accidents in supported employment. *Journal of Applied Behavior Analysis, 25,* 637–645.

Martella, R.C., Agran, M., & Marchand-Martella, N.E. (1992b). *Teaching individuals with disabilities how to prevent accidents in the work place.* Unpublished manuscript, Utah State University, Department of Special Education.

Martella, R.C., Marchand-Martella, N.E., & Agran, M. (1992). Work-related accident causes: A neglected transitional area. *Canadian Journal of Rehabilitation, 6,* 117–122.

Martella, R.C., Marchand-Martella, N.E., Agran, M., & Allen, S. (in press). Using a problem-solving strategy to prevent injuries due to unsafe worker behaviors. *British Columbia Journal of Special Education.*

Matson, J.L. (1980). Preventing home accidents: A training program for the retarded. *Behavior Modification, 4,* 397–410.

McLoughlin, C.S., Garner, J.B., & Callahan, M. (1987). *Getting employed, staying employed: Job development and training for persons with severe handicaps.* Baltimore: Paul H. Brookes Publishing Co.

Meichenbaum, D., & Asarnow, J. (1979). Cognitive-behavioral modification and metacognitive development: Implications for the classroom. In P.C. Kendall & S.D. Hollon (Eds.), *Cognitive-behavioral interventions: Theory, research, and procedures.* New York: Academic Press.

Mueller, H.H., Wilgosh, L., & Dennis, S. (1989). Employment survival skills for entry-level occupations. *Canadian Journal of Rehabilitation, 2,* 203–221.

National Safety Council. (1991). *Accident facts.* Chicago: Author.

Platt, J.J., & Spivack, G. (1972a). Problem-solving thinking of psychiatric patients. *Journal of Consulting and Clinical Psychology, 39,* 148–151.

Platt, J.J., & Spivack, G. (1972b). Social competence and effective problem-solving thinking in psychiatric patients. *Journal of Clinical Psychology, 28,* 3–5.

Platt, J.J., & Spivack, G. (1974). Means of solving real-life problems: Psychiatric patients versus controls and cross cultural comparisons of normal females. *Journal of Community Psychology, 2,* 45–48.

Pryor, R.O. (1983). The importance of safety instruction. *Vocational Education, 58,* 24.

Re Velle, J.B. (1980). *Safety training methods.* New York: John Wiley & Sons.

Ridley, J. (1986). *Safety at work* (2nd ed.). London: Butterworths.

Rusch, F.R., & Mithaug, D.E. (1980). *Vocational training for mentally retarded adults: A behavior analytic approach.* Champaign, IL: Research Press.

Rusch, F.R., Schutz, R.P., & Agran, M. (1982). Identification of job requisite skills to facilitate the entry of the mentally retarded. *Journal of The Association for the Severely Handicapped, 7*(3), 54–59.

Stern, S., & Gathercoal, F. (1987). Our field's most basic basic: Developing safe attitudes. *School Shop, 46,* 22–23.

United States Department of Commerce. (1990). *Statistical abstract of the United States: The national data book* (110th ed.). Washington, DC: Author.

Wolfensberger, W. (1972). *The principle of normalization in human services.* Toronto, Ontario, Canada: National Institute on Mental Retardation.

Chapter Nine

Preventing Substance Use

Daniel Morgan

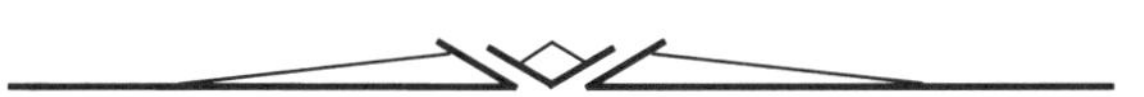

This chapter focuses specifically on preventing the substance use of young students with disabilities. In doing so, several key issues are addressed. First, the extent of the substance use problem among students with disabilities is examined. Second, the reasons why children and young adults use alcohol and illegal substances is explored. Third, the different types of prevention programs and their effectiveness are reviewed and school-based curricula that have potential for students with disabilities are highlighted. Finally, special attention is devoted to addressing the training needs of professionals, involving parents in prevention efforts, and understanding the legal issues associated with substance use among students with disabilities.

The use of illegal drugs is a widespread problem throughout American society. Illegal drug use is defined as follows:

- Use of legally prohibited drugs such as marijuana, cocaine, PCP, and "designer drugs" (e.g., "ecstasy")
- Use of prescription drugs for purposes other than as prescribed
- Use of substances such as glues or aerosols that can be inhaled to produce drug-like effects
- Use of legal drugs including alcohol and tobacco by legally underage persons

The United States has the highest rate of teenage drug use of any industrialized country in the world. One of the more extensive surveys of alcohol and other drug use is the federally funded High School Senior Survey that has been administered since 1974 to approximately 16,000 seniors in over 100 different schools across the United States (Johnston, O'Malley, & Bachman, 1991). Significant findings from this survey and other data are presented in Table 1.

SUBSTANCE USE AND PEOPLE WITH DISABILITIES

Is alcohol, tobacco, and other drug use more or less of a problem for students with disabilities as compared to students without disabilities? It is difficult to answer this question precisely. The High School Senior Survey does not specifically identify students with disabilities as a subgroup in its analyses. Similarly, other large-scale national surveys and/or small-scale regional and local surveys, also do not specifically identify students with disabilities in their results. It is even doubtful whether students

Substance use research discussed in this chapter is oriented around type of disability because that is how research in this area has typically been conducted.

Table 1. Substance use among school-age children and youth in the United States

1. More boys than girls use illegal substances, although the gender gap is closing.
2. Use is higher in larger cities, although suburban and rural use rates are also unacceptably high.
3. Initial use of alcohol and other drugs occurs at an increasingly early age; one in six 13-year-olds have used marijuana and 26% of fourth graders have used alcohol.
4. A third of all high school seniors state that on at least one occasion during the prior 2-week interval they drank heavily (i.e., five or more drinks in a row). Nearly all students have tried alcohol at least once.
5. Cigarettes, the most lethal commercial product sold in the United States and also the most heavily promoted, are smoked by 19% of high school seniors on a daily basis. Almost two-thirds of students have tried cigarettes at least once.
6. Illicit drugs most widely used by teenagers include marijuana, followed by stimulants, inhalants, and cocaine. Crack cocaine has been used at least once by 3%–5% of seniors; hallucinogens have been used by almost 10% of seniors.
7. Half of all traffic fatalities are alcohol-related; two out of five Americans will be involved in an alcohol-related vehicle crash sometime during their lives.
8. 70% of all youths attempting suicide were frequent drug and/or alcohol users.
9. Of youths age 16–19, half were more likely to have sex if they and their partner had been drinking.
10. Many students purchase their drugs (other than alcohol) at school.

Data adapted from Johnston, O'Malley, and Bachman (1991); U.S. Department of Education (1989); Utah State Division of Substance Abuse (1991).

with disabilities are even included in schoolwide surveys of substance use because many of them are frequently served in special education programs that are often excluded as a source of data.

There are several studies published, however, that provide a clearer picture of substance use rates among students with disabilities. The following sections summarize the findings from these surveys.

Students with Learning Disabilities

A major problem in reviewing the substance use prevalence literature for students with learning disabilities is that learning disabilities are often discussed synonymously with attention-deficit/hyperactivity disorders (ADHD). However, many special education professionals disagree as to whether learning disabilities and ADHD are one and the same, a subset of one another, or clearly distinct disabilities. Confounding the issue further is another body of literature that argues that ADHD, with its accompanying impulsiveness, noncompliance, and aggression, may be more closely related to a serious emotional disturbance/behavior disorder.

This debate is so significant that Congress mandated a special 3-year study in 1990 to determine whether ADHD is sufficiently and identifiably distinct from other disabilities as to warrant a separate designation under the Individuals with Disabilities Education Act of 1990 (IDEA) (PL 101-476). This issue is too vast and complex to resolve in this chapter. Consequently, to accomplish the purpose of this section, we will first review the prevalence literature on learning disabilities not directly connected with ADHD and conclude with a review of the prevalence literature specifically addressing substance use rates among students with ADHD.

Only two studies were located that addressed substance use in individuals with learning disabilities. Bruck (1985) conducted a study of young adults diagnosed as having learning disabilities and a comparison group without disabilities. The study examined the academic, occupational, social, and emotional status of the two groups. No differences in alcohol or other drug use were discovered.

Elmquist, Morgan, and Bolds (1992) surveyed substance use among junior and senior high students without disabilities and students with learning disabilities or behavior disorders. The students with learning disabilities reported the lowest use rates of the three groups; the rates were somewhat lower than rates for youth reported in large-scale national surveys of substance use such as the High School Senior Survey referred to earlier. However, when ADHD is considered to be a learning disability, substance use prevalence studies reveal that children and youth diagnosed as ADHD tend to use illegal substances at higher rates than students without disabilities (August, Stewart, & Holmes, 1983; Hartsough & Lambert, 1987). Moreover, longitudinal studies of students with ADHD have also documented the persistence of substance use into young adulthood (e.g., Gittelman, Mannuzza, Shenker, & Bonagura, 1985).

A confound in many of these studies is the lack of a consistent, standard definition of ADHD. Usually, when studies have revealed an association between ADHD and substance use, the subjects' characteristics also invariably include a strong pattern of conduct disorder behaviors including aggression, noncompliance, and other antisocial behaviors (Prendergast, Austin, & deMiranda, 1990). As will be discussed later, conduct disorder is a strong predictor of substance use and is also a primary characteristic of students classified as having a serious emotional disturbance/behavior disorder. Until substance use prevalence studies resolve these definitional issues and other methodological problems, a clear understanding of the extent of the problem of substance use among students with learning disabilities and students diagnosed as having ADHD will be lacking (Moore & Polsgrove, 1991).

Students with Mental Retardation

Few investigations have studied substance use patterns among individuals with mental retardation, and most of the research has involved adults, as opposed to school-age children and youth (Delaney & Poling, 1990). The findings from these studies suggest that children and adults with mental retardation use substances at rates equal to, or slightly less than, people without disabilities (Edgerton, 1986; Halpern, Close, & Nelson, 1986; Huang, 1981; Krishef, 1986). It also appears that the problem of substance use may be more problematic among individuals with mental retardation who require lower levels of assistance (Moore, 1991).

Students with Behavior Disorders

Two studies have specifically examined substance use rates among school-age students with behavior disorders. Leone, Greenberg, Trickett, and Spero (1989) examined drug use by students with mental retardation or learning disabilities receiving special education services in general junior high, middle school, and senior high school settings. Another 55 students with behavior disorders in special school settings for adolescents with severe emotional disturbance/behavior disorders were also included in the sample. The results suggested that the students with behavior disorders in special school settings used substances at much higher rates than the other students in the sample who were placed in special education programs within general school settings.

Substance use among junior and senior high students with either behavior disorders or learning disabilities was assessed by Elmquist et al. (1992). A comparison group of students without disabilities was also included in the study. Students who classified as having behavior disorders and placed in a special school reported 43% more alcohol use and 32% more marijuana use than their peers without disabilities. Other prevalence studies with this population have revealed higher use rates among children and adolescents with psychiatric disorders (Brook, Gordon, Whiteman, & Cohen, 1986; Needle, Su, Doherty, Lavee, & Brown, 1988; Pandina & Schuele, 1983), suicidal behavior (Crumley, 1990; Garfinkel, Froese, & Hood, 1982), and depression (Shedler & Block, 1990).

Students with Sensory Impairments

There has been little published research concerning substance use rates among students with hearing and/or visual impairments. The research reported in this area has included adult subjects, and, for the most part, is woefully out-of-date. What scant literature exists seems to indicate that substance use rates among individuals of all ages with hearing and/or visual impairments are probably at least equal to those without these impairments (Leone, 1991; Prendergast et al., 1990).

Students with Physical Disabilities

There is also little published research that reliably documents the prevalence of substance use among school-age students with physical disabilities. A body of substance use prevalence research is forming, however, that includes college-age students with physical disabilities. The results of these studies suggest that substance use (primarily alcohol) among college-age students with physical disabilities is essentially comparable to use rates among college-age students without physical disabilities (Moore & Siegal, 1989).

Students with Spinal Cord or Traumatic Brain Injuries

There is clear evidence that alcohol and other drug use is implicated in at least half of all cases of spinal cord or traumatic brain injuries (Heinemann, Doll, & Schnoll, 1989; Jones, 1989). That is, the accident or trauma that directly led to the specific injury-caused disability was often precipitated by alcohol or other drug use. For these individuals, it also appears that the use of alcohol and other drugs is not eliminated or decreased as a result of the injury and, in fact, may present significant problems and impediments during rehabilitation (Moore & Siegal, 1989).

Summary of Findings

The following statements can be drawn from the preceding sections:

1. Students with behavior disorders and/or attention-deficit/hyperactivity disorders use substances at higher rates than the general student population.
2. Students with mental retardation use substances at lower rates than the general student population, with the exception, perhaps, of those students requiring lower levels of assistance.
3. Students with sensory impairments use substances at rates comparable to students without such impairments. The same can be said of students with physical disabilities, although it appears as if students who have either a spinal cord or traumatic brain injury may have experienced a significant problem with alcohol or other drugs prior to their disability-causing accident or event.

The overwhelming conclusion from this literature is inescapable; that is, the problem of substance use among students with disabilities has been grossly undocumented and, therefore, largely undetected. To assume, in the absence of data, that there is no problem or that the problem is trivial in contrast to students without disabilities does a serious injustice. Even if the evidence suggests that the use of alcohol, tobacco, and other drugs may be no higher for students with disabilities than for other students, that comparable rate is far too high to be ignored.

RISK FACTORS

Why do children and youth use illegal substances? Attempts to identify the etiology of substance use among children and youth has resulted in a plethora of empirical studies that point to a multitude of factors that increase risk for using alcohol, tobacco, and other drugs. These efforts have led to the identification of certain conditions and characteristics that statistically occur more often in children and youth who use illegal substances than they do in other students.

In an attempt to better understand these risk factors, Johnston and O'Malley (1986) analyzed data collected by the *Monitoring the Future* project, a large scale survey of representative samples of high school seniors. In addition to self-reporting use of various illegal substances, students were also asked to name the most important reasons for why they were taking a certain drug. Reasons for use were found to vary considerably by substance and by degree of involvement with a particular substance (e.g., experimental use, occasional use, heavy use). While social/recreational reasons seemed to predominate, experimentation and relaxation reasons were also commonly mentioned. The rank ordering of the most frequently cited reasons for use of any drug is listed below:

1. To have a good time with my friends
2. To experiment and see what it's like
3. To feel good or get high
4. To relax or relieve tension
5. Because it tastes good
6. Because of boredom, nothing else to do
7. To get away from my problems or troubles

8. Because of anger or frustration
9. To fit in with the group I like

Reviews of research have identified several key risk factors that tend to predict illegal substance use (Austin, 1992; Brook et al., 1986; Hawkins, Lishner, & Catalano, 1985; Hawkins, Lishner, Catalano, & Howard, 1985; Jessor, 1987; Newcomb, Maddahian, & Bentler, 1986; Newcomb, Maddahian, Skager, & Bentler, 1987). These risk factors include:

- Family management problems such as poor communication, vague expectations, inconsistent discipline, lack of monitoring, and excessively harsh discipline
- Failure at school
- Hyperactivity and socially aggressive behavior in early elementary school
- Friends who use illegal substances
- Parent(s) who abuse alcohol or illicit drugs
- Rebellion against and alienation from school, family, and other social institutions
- Emotional distress

Another definition of "high-risk" is presented in Table 2. As can be seen, this definition is consistent with the individual, family, school, and community factors referenced above. It should also be noted that the presence of a single risk factor does not automatically lead to the conclusion that an individual will use illegal substances. However, the more risk factors present, especially the key risk factors noted here, the more likely it will be that the child or youth will use substances.

Table 2. High-risk youth

The Anti-Drug Act of 1988 (PL 100-690) defines high-risk youth as: any individual who has not attained the age of 21 years, who is at high risk of becoming or who has become a drug user or alcohol abuser, and who:

1. is identified as a child of a substance abuser
2. is a victim of physical, sexual, or psychological abuse
3. has dropped out of school
4. has become pregnant
5. is economically disadvantaged
6. has committed a violent or delinquent act
7. has experienced mental health problems
8. has attempted suicide
9. has experienced a long-term physical pain due to injury
10. has experienced chronic failure in school

In the 1980s and 1990s, researchers studying the etiology of substance use have expanded the scope of their efforts from a sole concentration on identifying risk factors that *predict* use, to include a concentration on identifying *protective* factors, or those characteristics and conditions that increase the probability that an individual will *refrain* from substance use (McIntyre, White, & Yoast, 1992). The concept of the "resilient child" who refrains from drug use is often discussed in the alcohol and other drug prevention literature (Benard, 1991). Also known as "invulnerable," "hardy," or "invincible," a resilient child is able to avoid the impact of the negative risk factors that may be present in his or her life and grow and develop in comparatively healthy ways. Table 3 details those factors strongly identified in the literature as protective against alcohol, tobacco, and other drug use (McIntyre et al., 1992). A sense of attachment and commitment to family, school, peers, and community appears to be a significant protective factor (Fetro, 1991).

Are there specific factors that place students with disabilities at greater risk for substance use? Again, information and data are lacking. In a comprehensive review of this area, Prendergast et al. (1990) concluded that, for the most part, people with disabilities are influenced by the same risk factors for substance use as people without disabilities. Among the individuals with disabilities identified by Prendergast et al. as being most at risk are the following:

> 1. Those who become disabled after the onset of adolescence, especially through a traumatic injury;
> 2. Those who have made the least positive adaptation to their disability;
> 3. Those who demonstrate the least self-esteem and most problem behavior;
> 4. Those who have a family history of abuse (parental or sibling); and
> 5. Those who have been exposed to the most risk factors found to influence people in the [general] population, especially exposure to peer influences and ready availability. (p. 17)

Prendergast et al. point out three specific factors that place students with disabilities at higher risk. First, the stressors experienced by some individuals with disabilities may affect

Table 3. Protective factors

Positive self-esteem
Internal locus of control
Personal and social competence
Effective coping skills
Independence and autonomy
Commitment to societal norms about substance use
Positive social bonding to social institutions
Accurate perceptions of peers' use of alcohol and other drugs
Effective family management patterns
Family cohesion and intactness
Emotional support for children
Clear and consistently enforced norms regarding use of alcohol and other drugs

Adapted from McIntyre, White, and Yoast (1992).

substance use. For example, some individuals may have difficulty with relatively simple tasks such as eating, dressing, and communicating. These difficulties may create extra stress, lower self-esteem, and loneliness related to social isolation. If the individual lacks the necessary skills to deal with these feelings, and if there is little support in the community in terms of relieving physical obstacles, the stressors may result in increased use of alcohol and other drugs as a means of coping.

Second, professionals, family members, and other caregivers involved with people with disabilities may actually facilitate the use of illegal substances by engaging in certain *enabling behaviors* and/or by avoiding the problem altogether. A person who enables another makes it easier for the person to use alcohol or other drugs by various means (e.g., providing excuses, condoning use, or actually providing access). The rationale offered for enabling behavior is rather specious (e.g., "She has a right to feel sorry for herself," or "He deserves to have some fun."). Furthermore, there is also evidence to suggest that adult caregivers tend to avoid the entire issue of substance use by simply ignoring it, often until it becomes too late.

The third risk factor that Prendergast et al. focus on is the evidence that suggests a marked absence of prevention programs specifically geared toward students with disabilities. For example, over 200 special education teachers in Utah were asked about the nature of prevention efforts for the students they served in both self-contained classrooms and resource room programs (Morgan, Cancio, & Likins, 1992). While agreeing that prevention programs in the area of substance use were very important, the vast majority of the teachers stated that only a very small percentage of their students received any kind of prevention education. Thus, although research points to a significant risk of substance use among students with disabilities, the risk may be even greater due to their lack of exposure to meaningful prevention education.

SUBSTANCE USE PREVENTION EDUCATION

Just as there are a variety of approaches used to teach students how to read, spell, or behave appropriately in school, so too are there a variety of approaches used in the area of substance use prevention education. The developers or proponents of the various approaches all share a similar overall goal (i.e., preventing the use of illegal substances). However, differing views concerning the etiology of substance use, human development, and other psychological and sociological variables have led proponents to prefer one approach over another.

Jaker (1985) described four basic approaches to substance use prevention education: 1) the information approach, 2) the affective education approach, 3) the social competencies approach, and 4) the alternative approach. In the information approach, the primary goal is to increase an individual's knowledge about the harmful effects of using illegal substances in the hope that unfavorable attitudes will develop, resulting in a reduced probability of substance use. The affective education approach focuses on increasing the individuals' self-esteem and self-awareness as low self-esteem predisposes one to substance use. Increasing social skills is the goal of the social competencies approach whereby enhanced social competence will enable the individual to resist peer pressure to use substances. The alternative model emphasizes the creation of desirable activities or options for individuals as an alternative to using illegal substances.

Hansen (1990) developed a more fine-grained analysis of substance use prevention education programs. Within this conceptual framework, 12 distinct types of prevention education approaches were identified:

1. *Information:* Targets facts about substances, consequences of substance use, and myths associated with substance use
2. *Decision making:* Teaches how to make rational decisions about substance use
3. *Pledge:* Solicits personal commitments not to use substances
4. *Values clarification:* Clarifies personal values and identifies relationship between one's own personal values and the use of illegal substances
5. *Goal setting:* Teaches how to set and achieve positively oriented goals
6. *Stress management:* Teaches how to cope with and manage stress in everyday life, particularly in situations that may involve pressures to use substances
7. *Self-esteem:* Focuses on increasing personal feelings of worth by identifying one's strengths and weaknesses
8. *Resistance skills:* Teaches students how to resist peer pressure
9. *Life skills training:* Teaches students communication skills, interpersonal skills, and conflict resolution skills;
10. *Norm setting:* Establishes conservative opinions about substance use by clarifying the actual prevalence of substance use among one's peer group
11. *Assistance:* Provides peer support to at-risk students through peer counseling and tutoring
12. *Alternatives:* Offers experiences and activities that are incompatible with substance use, thereby decreasing exposure to situations in which substance use has a higher probability of occurring.

Few prevention programs employ only a single approach. In fact, most combine multiple approaches in their programming. The different levels of effectiveness of these approaches is reviewed in the following sections.

Effectiveness of Substance Use Prevention Education

How to determine and assess effectiveness are among the most pressing concerns now facing researchers examining prevention education. For example, does assessing gains in knowledge, attitudes, self-concept, and social skills provide a valid indicator of success? Many of the published reports include one or more of these mediating variables, yet far fewer studies include actual substance use rate data as a primary dependent variable. However, as prevention researchers become more aware of the various methodological shortcomings of prior efforts, more quality evaluations of substance use prevention programs are being published. This section reviews a selected small sample of these studies.

The effectiveness of a 20-session cognitive-behavioral approach to substance use prevention was tested on 1,311 seventh grade students from 10 suburban New York junior high schools (Botvin, Baker, Renick, Filazzola, & Botvin, 1984). The program was a multicomponent package designed to increase basic life skills and personal competence, with special attention devoted to dealing with the pressures and influences of drug use. The intervention package included the following: 1) didactic instruction and information on illegal substances and the consequences of using them, 2) decision-making skills, 3) stress management skills, 4) social and resistance skills training, and 5) self-management training.

An interesting aspect of this study was that it also investigated the relative effectiveness of peer-led versus teacher-led instruction. Results indicated that the peer-led program had a statistically significant positive impact on reducing or preventing cigarette smoking, excessive drinking, and marijuana use. Furthermore, changes were also observed for several other risk factors including attitude, cognitive understanding, and personality. Interestingly, there was almost a complete lack of effectiveness for the teacher-led condition when compared to the control group. The authors attributed this finding to "implementation failure"; that is, the teachers did not implement the program in the manner in which it was intended.

Ellickson and Bell (1990) reported the results of Project ALERT, a well-designed longitudinal experiment to curb drug use among seventh and eighth grade students. Project ALERT's approach involves helping students to develop their own reasons for not using drugs, recognize pressures to use drugs, learn skills to help them resist these and other pressures, and recognize the benefits of non-use. Project ALERT's instructional procedures included discussion, role playing, and skills practice. Eight lessons were taught one week apart for seventh graders, and three boosters were taught to eighth graders.

The program's impact was assessed at 3-, 12-, and 15-month follow-ups. The results indicated that the program was effective in delaying first use or reducing current use of cigarettes and marijuana for both low- and high-risk students. The impact of Project ALERT was more short-lived for use of alcohol, where modest reductions in drinking occurred in seventh grade, but were not maintained during eighth grade. The authors of the study attributed this problem to the fact that the "widespread prevalence of alcohol use, in society at large, as well as in the schools that participated in our experiment, undermined curriculum messages about resisting pressures to drink" (p. 1304).

In another longitudinal study, a comprehensive community-wide approach to substance use prevention was evaluated with high-risk and low-risk adolescents (Johnson et al., 1990). The program components, delivered over a 3-year period, included: 1) a school-based program, 2) a parent involvement and training program, 3) a community-wide drug abuse prevention task force, and 4) involvement of the community's mass media. The school-based program was a 10-session program delivered to sixth and seventh graders that addressed such topics as consequences of substance use, information about the actual prevalence of substance use, identifying and dealing with various pressures to use substances, ways to assertively resist pressures to use, methods of solving difficult problems involving the use of drugs, and making a commitment to avoid illegal substances. The instructional methods involved discussion, role playing, and practice of the skills and concepts taught in the program. Findings demonstrated that a community-wide approach was effective in reducing tobacco and marijuana use for both high- and low-risk adolescents. There were no statistically significant effects, however, for alcohol use.

Finally, Hansen and Graham (1991) investigated the effectiveness of a prevention approach referred to as normative education or establishing conservative norms. This approach was described by the authors as follows:

> The roots of this strategy are derived from the propensity of young people to overestimate actual prevalence of all forms of substance use. This overestimation may lead young people to expect use to be normative when, in fact, it is not. This may create an internally generated expectation that the reference group will find use of substances to be desirable and appropriate. To counter this, programs provide students with feedback about actual rates of use and publicize the conservative attitudes toward substance use that exist in the peer group. (p. 415)

Junior high school students exposed to this approach were pretested prior to program implementation and were post-tested 1 year following program completion. The authors concluded that differences found in the effectiveness of the normative education approach to reducing or preventing alcohol, tobacco, and marijuana use were related to their availability and the expectations or pressures concerning the acceptability of their use:

> Among young adolescents, alcohol, marijuana, and tobacco are consumed primarily in social settings, particularly at parties and informal get togethers. Among groups of students where underlying conservative beliefs have been revealed, the availability of alcohol at social functions will be reduced since hosts will feel providing alcohol will be unacceptable to guests. Offers to use substances in all settings will be reduced due to a perceived intolerance toward such offers. (p. 426)

After reviewing these studies, one might conclude that it is extremely difficult to eliminate altogether the use of alcohol, tobacco, and other drugs by children and young adults. Alcohol, in particular, has been very resistant to prevention efforts. There is a great deal of societal support for alcohol consumption, and this support makes it more difficult to communicate to young people that it is inappropriate for them to consume alcoholic beverages. Most of the studies that have demonstrated a positive impact on substance use have only been able to reduce the expected rate of increase of illegal substance use. While this realization may seem disheartening, it also sheds light on the magnitude and scope of the problem.

General Principles

What we are learning from studies such as those discussed here has contributed to the establishment of a knowledge base that enables prevention educators to design programs that are responsive to the needs of students who are at varying degrees of risk. Unfortunately, no study has yet been reported that specifically addresses the effectiveness of prevention programming for students with disabilities. However, given the findings that have emerged from the empirical literature and the contributions that have resulted from several meta-analyses of the prevention literature (see, e.g., Bangert-Drowns, 1988; Moskowitz, 1989; Rundall & Bruvold, 1988; Schaps, DiBartolo, Moskowitz, Palley, & Churgin, 1981; Tobler, 1986), the following principles for effective prevention programming are generally accepted as sound strategies for both low- and high-risk students, including students with disabilities:

1. Focus should be on teaching behavioral skills that influence the use of alcohol, tobacco, and other drugs. Programs that focus only on information, attitude change, or self-esteem enhancement produce few, if any, meaningful outcomes. The skills that should be the focus of a prevention program extend far beyond learning to "just say no." Effective programs teach such life skills as interpersonal communication, problem solving, self-management, stress management, assertiveness, and how to get along with others.
2. Students should be taught: 1) the short-term consequences of substance use, and, to a lesser extent, the long-term consequences; 2) external and internal pressures to use substances; 3) adaptive ways of responding to those pressures; and 4) accurate information about the actual prevalence of alcohol, tobacco, and other drug use among their peer group.
3. Using peers in prevention programming either as a peer instructor or teaching assistant is a promising approach. It is critical that, regardless of whom the key instructional leader is, the program is implemented in the manner in which the program's designer intended it to be taught.
4. Parents and the community need to be involved. Parents must be encouraged and, in all likelihood, trained to take an active interest in their child's behavior and to provide a good model for their children regarding the use of alcohol, tobacco, and other drugs. Law enforcement, social services agencies, and the business community must work together with the schools and each other to promote and achieve the goals of a comprehensive prevention effort.
5. Prevention programming must be viewed as a long-term effort. One-shot or short-lived efforts will not make an appreciable difference in students' use of alcohol, tobacco, or other drugs. Intensive interventions must be implemented by knowledgeable individuals over an extended period of time if positive outcomes are to be achieved.

A model of a program to prevent substance use is displayed in Figure 1. This model addresses the many risk and protective factors related to the problem of substance use among all students, including those with disabilities. The model acknowledges the need for a compre-

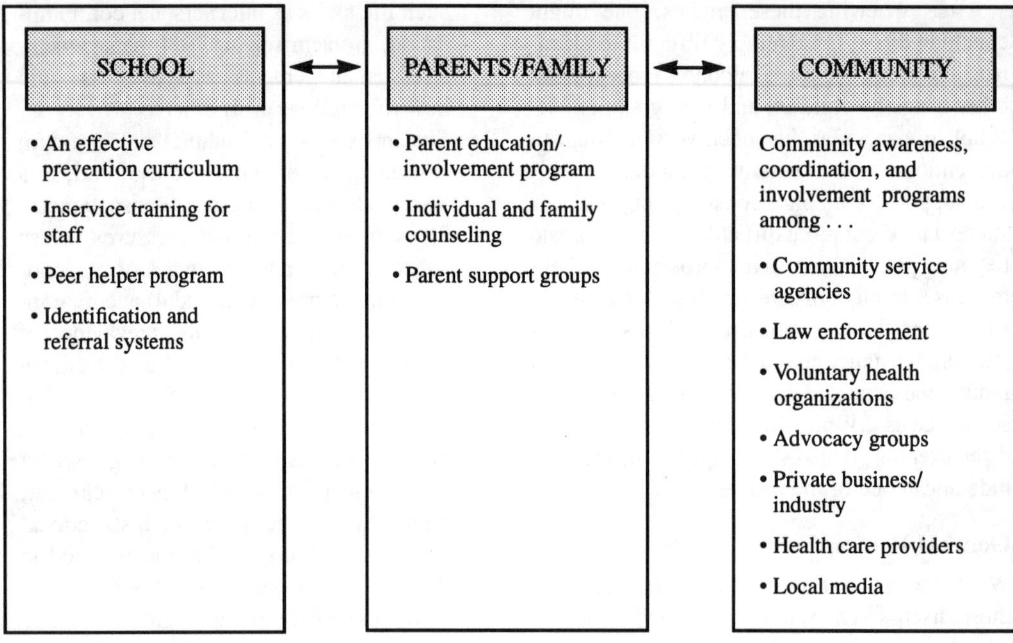

Figure 1. A comprehensive model to prevent substance use among students with disabilities.

hensive approach to the problem by highlighting roles and responsibilities for the school, parents, and communities. Given the seeming intractability of the problem of substance use, it appears as if only a truly integrated and comprehensive approach to the problem will have a meaningful, positive impact on the health of all students.

SUBSTANCE USE PREVENTION EDUCATION CURRICULA

Although it is clear that a comprehensive, multi-faceted approach to substance use prevention is required, schools are frequently the focus of the overall effort. Thus, educators interested in implementing substance use prevention in their schools find themselves searching for appropriate curricular materials to use with their students. Finding curricular programs is not a big problem; however, locating sound programs is somewhat difficult if one is not familiar with substance use prevention education. The purpose of this section is to offer a set of guidelines that educators should employ in selecting curricular programs in the area of substance use prevention. Special emphasis will be placed on reviewing two essential questions: 1) what should be taught?, and 2) how should the content be taught? It is important to note that curricular content and objectives need not differ between programs for students without disabilities and programs designed for students with disabilities. However, several significant modifications or adaptations may be necessary to effectively address concerns unique to these students.

The U.S. Department of Education (1990) has published a set of guidelines for schools selecting from among the available materials. These guidelines are as follows:

1. Prevention curricula should emphasize the fact that most youths do not use drugs.
2. Prevention curricula should clearly and unequivocally communicate the message that illegal drug use is wrong and harmful for everyone.
3. Prevention curricula should be implemented early before pressures to use in-

crease dramatically. The best time is between the fourth and ninth grades.

4. Prevention curricula should not provide information on how to obtain, prepare, or consume illegal substances.
5. Concepts such as social use, responsible use, and controlled use are unacceptable. The only appropriate message to be communicated throughout the program is "no use."

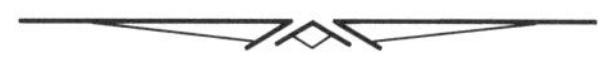

In addition to these guidelines, the Department of Education also attaches a great deal of importance to school policies that discourage substance use. The following is a summary of the basic content of a model school policy:

> School policies should clearly establish that drug use, possession, and sale on the school grounds and at school functions will not be tolerated. These policies should apply both to students and to school personnel, and may include prevention, intervention, treatment, and disciplinary measures.
>
> School policies should have the following characteristics:
>
> 1. Specify what constitutes a drug offense by defining (a) illegal substances and paraphernalia; (b) the area of the school's jurisdiction . . . ; and (c) the types of violations (drug possession, use, and sale).
> 2. State the consequences for violating school policy; punitive action should be linked to referral for treatment and counseling. Measures . . . found effective in dealing with first-time offenders include the following:
>
>   —A required meeting of parents and the student with school officials, concluding with a contract signed by the student and parents in which they both acknowledge a drug problem and the student agrees to stop using and to participate in drug counseling or a rehabilitation program.
>
>   —Suspension, assignment to an alternative school, in-school suspension, after-school or Saturday detention with close supervision, and demanding academic assignments.
>
>   —Referral to a drug treatment expert or counselor.
>
>   —Notification of police. (U.S. Department of Education, 1989, p. 23)

Several aspects of this policy, especially as it relates to disciplinary consequences, have legal implications for students with disabilities; these implications are discussed later in this chapter.

K–12 Prevention Curriculum Guidelines

In addition to school policy recommendations concerning the use of drugs on the school campus, the U.S. Department of Education (1990) also breaks down substance use prevention curriculum into general guidelines for designing a K–12 curriculum. Table 4 presents some of these recommendations. The guidelines are broken down into appropriate information for children and youth in grades K–8.

A somewhat more in-depth set of criteria is offered by the Stanford Center for Research in Disease Prevention in a monograph entitled, *What Works? A Guide to School-Based Alcohol and Drug Abuse Prevention Curricula* (Rogers, Howard-Pitney, & Bruce, 1989). Focusing on the what and how of prevention curricula, Rogers et al. recommend that the skills taught in a K–12 prevention curriculum should include problem solving, decision making, coping with peer pressure, communication, assertiveness, and stress reduction skills. The instructional strategies and practices that should be used to teach these skills include such preferred instructional techniques as role playing and behavioral rehearsal, cooperative learning and peer tutoring, and ample practice opportunities. Among other recommended guidelines are: 1) the information presented must be accurate and up-to-date, 2) the scope and sequence of the content should be appropriate, 3) the program should not require extensive training or specialized instructional skills, and 4) accessible materials and information need to be available to teachers to support their implementation efforts. The following are additional recommendations for substance use prevention curriculum content for students in grades K–12 (U.S. Department of Education, 1990).

Students in grades K–3 should:

- Understand that alcohol, tobacco, marijuana, and other drugs are harmful
- Know that using drugs can lead to dependence and damaged health

Table 4. Substance use prevention curriculum recommendations for grades K–8

K–3	4–6	7–8
Keep information simple and direct Focus on life skills, such as decision making and problem solving. Neither glamorize, nor instill inappropriate fear, about drugs. Emphasize that most people do not use drugs. Encourage the development of self-confidence and responsibility for self and others. Stress information over evaluation and testing.	Focus on the drugs children are apt to use first (i.e., tobacco, alcohol, and marijuana). Encourage open and frank discussions of concerns about drugs and drug use. Focus on life skills, such as problem solving, resisting peer pressure, developing friendships, and coping with stress. Deglamorize drug use by rejecting the drug-using behaviors of some folk heroes (e.g., rock stars, actors, and athletes). Emphasize that most people, including the vast majority of people their own age, do not use drugs. Encourage the development of good self-esteem and personal and civic responsibility. Focus on the development of healthy leisure activities, such as sports, music, art, clubs, and volunteering.	Encourage frank discussions about concerns related to drugs and drug use. Emphasize the establishment of positive life goals, such as continuing education and developing work skills that will permit a legal income source. Emphasize the law and its consequences.

Adapted from United States Department of Education (1990).

- Understand the difference between medicines and illegal drugs
- Be able to determine from whom they may accept medicine

Students in grades 4–6 should:

- Be able to identify alcohol, tobacco, marijuana, cocaine, inhalants, hallucinogens, and stimulants in their various forms
- Understand that use of alcohol, tobacco, and other drugs is illegal at their age
- Realize that laws about drug use and sales are designed to protect people
- Understand what addiction is and how it affects individuals and their families
- Recognize that smokeless tobacco and wine coolers are also drugs that are both harmful and illegal for children
- Understand that the effects of drugs vary from person to person
- Know how drugs affect different parts of the body, and why drugs are dangerous for growing bodies and developing minds
- Understand how drugs interfere with the performance of physical and intellectual tasks
- Realize that social influences, such as media advertising, peer pressure, family influences, and community standards may encourage drug use
- Develop life skills such as problem solving, resisting peer pressure, developing friendships, and coping with stress

Students in grades 7–8 should:

- Recognize that experimenting with drugs is still using drugs and thus carries significant risks
- Understand how drugs are pushed and how society fights the drug supply problem
- Know the extent of the problem locally and the efforts of authorities to control it
- Understand how steroid use can damage the body and brain
- Know how drugs affect the circulatory, respiratory, nervous, and reproductive systems

- Understand how drugs and the AIDS virus are related

Students in grades 9–12 should:

- Know how drug use is related to certain diseases and disabilities, including AIDS; learning disorders; birth defects; and heart, lung, and liver disease
- Understand that taking a combination of drugs, whether illegal or prescription, can be fatal
- Know how alcohol, tobacco, and other drugs affect the developing fetus and the breastfeeding infant
- Know the effects and consequences of operating equipment, driving vehicles, and performing other physical tasks while using drugs
- Know that drug use can affect opportunities for personal growth and professional success
- Be familiar with treatment and intervention resources
- Understand that they are role models for younger youths

Modifying Curricula for Students with Disabilities

Great caution and care needs to be exercised by teachers as they select prevention curricula because no single program has been shown to be effective with all students in all situations. This is even more true of programs for students with disabilities. In general, the guidelines for substance use prevention education described thus far may be followed for those educating students with disabilities. However, several modifications may need to be made. The following is a list of suggested adaptations.

1. For students with cognitive impairments, the prevention program must contain instructional activities that are concrete and structured.
2. The readability level of the material must be targeted to the reading level of the students. Unfortunately, many prevention programs, especially those intended for use in secondary school settings, are written for the typical student in those grades. That is, reading levels of 10th or 11th grade are not uncommon. This may be acceptable for many students, but students who have mental retardation, learning disabilities, or other disabilities that can affect learning may find this level of difficulty too high.
3. Teaching for mastery is a critical need for all students, especially students with disabilities. Prevention programs must provide ample opportunities for repetition, practice, and spaced reviews. Fluency and accuracy are no less important in prevention curricula than in mathematics curricula.

Characteristics that should *not* be present in a prevention program are also important to recognize. For example, the program should not:

1. Focus primarily on knowledge or attitudes. As mentioned throughout this book, changes in actual behavior are most valuable, thus skills and strategies necessary to remain substance-free should be the primary focus of a prevention program.
2. Be designed and structured in such a way that students with disabilities cannot succeed at an acceptable level (e.g., 80% accuracy).
3. Be devoid of applications to real-life situations. The ultimate purpose of a school-based prevention program is to provide skills that students can use outside of the classroom situation.
4. Be taught in isolation. Integration and infusion in a variety of natural situations and settings is important.

CURRENTLY AVAILABLE PREVENTION PROGRAMS

There are many substance use prevention programs available to school personnel and others planning prevention programs. Many have been published and marketed on a commercial basis; others have been prepared by local or regional school districts or other public agencies. Few, however, have been developed specifically for use with students with disabilities. This section reviews a selected group of these programs and comments on their suitability for use with students who have disabilities.

Table 5 presents a sample listing and brief description of two categories of prevention programs. The first category in the table represents generic programs and identifies only a few of the many programs that have been developed for use with both high- and low-risk students without disabilities. The second category in the table represents programs for students with disabilities.

The generic programs listed in the table have been extensively field-tested and reported in professional journals (see, for example, Botvin

Table 5. Selected substance use prevention programs

Program title	Description
I. Generic programs	
Here's Looking At You, 2000 (1986)	A K–12 curriculum that is one of the most widely used prevention programs; goals are to reduce risk factors and increase protective factors by increasing knowledge, social skills, and bonding with school and family; over 150 lessons with extensive support and supplementary materials
Life Skills Training Program (Botvin, 1990)	Targets alcohol, marijuana, and tobacco use among junior high school students; utilizes cognitive-behavioral approach; emphasizes a broad range of life skills and interpersonal competence; three levels to be taught over 3 years
Minnesota Smoking Prevention Program (1989)	Targets students in grades 6–8; sessions focus on understanding the short- and long-term physiological and social consequences of tobacco use and developing resistance skills and awareness of pressures; implemented by peer leaders
Project SMART (Self-Management and Resistance Training) (Hansen, Graham, Johnson, Flay, & Pentz, 1988)	Teaches how to deal with pressures to use substances by becoming aware of pressures and by learning skills to resist; targets grades 6–9; 13 1-hour lessons over 1 school year; implemented by peer leaders; contains booster lessons
II. Programs for students with disabilities	
LifeFacts 3—Substance Abuse (1990)	Nineteen lessons present basic information about drugs and their consequences; impact on family and work is stressed; lessons also deal with addiction and seeking help; worksheets and other support materials provided
Prevention Curriculum Guide for Looking at Alcohol and Other Drugs—Special Education 7–12 (undated)	Contains 51 lessons for students with mental retardation; focuses on issues and problems faced by these students
Prevention Time (1985)	Designed for students with mild retardation and learning disabilities in upper elementary school; focuses on information, understanding and accepting self, understanding self and others, and developing decision-making skills
A Special Message: A Comprehensive Drug Education Curriculum for Learning Disabled and Behavior Disordered Populations Grades 6–12 (1988)	Developed by Project Oz staff; promotes development of coping skills, decision making, self-esteem, assertiveness, and stress management skills; 27 lessons; includes teachers' guides and learning activities, overheads, and parent involvement components

et al., 1984; Hansen, Johnson, Flay, Graham, & Sobel, 1988; Hopkins, Mauss, Kearney, & Wesheit, 1988). In general, the evaluation data reveal positive results, especially as they relate to tobacco use. (Readers may wish to refer to a publication entitled *What Works? A Guide to School-Based Alcohol and Drug Abuse Prevention Curricula* [Rogers et al., 1989] for a more complete listing of prevention programs geared toward students without disabilities.)

Educators interested in using these or similar programs with students with disabilities would first need to make significant modifications and adaptations similar to those recommended in the previous section. For example, the readability level of the content in these programs may be too difficult for many students with mental retardation or learning disabilities. Furthermore, the amount of repetition and practice required to facilitate learning in students with special learning needs is often not present in these programs. Frequently, difficult concepts are explained or demonstrated in a way that even typical students may have difficulty grasping. In short, while the purpose, content, and essential nature of these generic programs are sound, the teacher would need to make changes to make them more appropriate for students with disabilities.

The programs in Table 5 identified as having been developed for students with disabilities address essentially the same content as the generic programs, but present the lessons and activities in a "geared-down" fashion. That is, the pace of instruction is somewhat slower, concepts are simpler and explained more fully, and the difficulty level of the material is more controlled. However, a significant weakness of these programs is the lack of published reports attesting to their effectiveness. Clearly, more attention to this issue needs to be provided by developers of such programs. (A good source of information and descriptions concerning other prevention materials, including video-based programs, is *Substance Use by Youth With Disabilities and Chronic Illnesses* [2nd ed.], available from the National Center for Youth with Disabilities [1990].)

Another program that has been developed for high-risk students with disabilities is the RESIST Program (Resistance Education Strategies and Interventions Systematically Taught) (Morgan, 1992). RESIST's goals are to: 1) decrease the use of alcohol, tobacco, and other drug use among students with disabilities; 2) reduce risk factors associated with the use of illegal substances; and 3) increase protective factors for students and their families. RESIST consists of 12 core lessons and 5 booster lessons that provide information about drugs; teach assertiveness and resistance skills; and promote problem-solving, coping, and decision-making abilities. The lessons include concept teaching, vocabulary lessons, demonstration of skills, behavioral rehearsal, role playing, and homework activities. A workbook correlated with each lesson is also part of the program.

The RESIST program incorporates what is known about effective instructional procedures for students with mental retardation, learning disabilities, and problem behaviors. The basic premise is to maximize student achievement by increasing the time students are productively engaged in instruction. This is accomplished through the following instructional procedures:

1. Active engagement of the students is emphasized over passive seatwork activities. Frequent opportunities are available for student response, either verbally, in writing, or by demonstrating developing skills.
2. Classwide peer tutoring is used to facilitate fluency and accuracy.
3. The difficulty level of the material is carefully calibrated to enhance student success.
4. A brisk instructional pace is encouraged to prevent boredom and to increase the number of student responses.
5. Automatic responses are considered essential learning outcomes to promote initial acquisition and long-term maintenance of skills.
6. A motivation system for reinforcing appropriate behavior is built into the program. Students receive points for acquiring new skills and information, demonstrating a "drug-free attitude," and completing homework assignments.

RESIST is undergoing field-testing in a variety of elementary, junior high, and senior high school special education settings. It has also been used in resource programs and self-contained classrooms within general school settings. The program has been reviewed favorably by students, teachers, and parents. However, its effectiveness in actually decreasing the use of alcohol, tobacco, and other drugs by students with disabilities remains to be demonstrated.

It is important to recognize that no single prevention education curriculum, either generic or specifically designed for students with disabilities, can be regarded unequivocally as the best program. No program has reported findings that state that it consistently prevents, delays, or reduces substance use with all students. It is for this reason that the reader should review available programs carefully to determine their strengths and weaknesses and be prepared to make the necessary adaptations for their own students.

CRITICAL ISSUES IN SUBSTANCE USE PREVENTION

There are several areas of prevention education for students with disabilities that require special attention. These areas include: 1) staff training, 2) parental involvement, and 3) legal issues. These concerns are discussed in the following sections.

Staff Training

The need for knowledgeable and trained school professionals in the area of substance use prevention was recognized by Congress when it appropriated over $20 million per year for use in personnel training activities to be administered by the United States Department of Education under the Drug-Free Schools and Communities Program. This is a significant level of funding that has provided a needed impetus for federal, state, and local prevention initiatives. Well-developed curricula and programs can be rendered ineffective when placed in the hands of teachers and other school personnel who are inadequately prepared. It is imperative that prevention education programs be taught and supported by teachers who are properly trained and committed to the goals of substance use prevention (Allison, Silverman, & Dignam, 1990).

Experts in the area of substance use prevention were surveyed to identify teacher characteristics and competencies that would be beneficial for preventing substance use among students (Jones, Kline, Habkirk, & Sales, 1990). The most important cluster of characteristics that emerged in this survey were those associated with teacher–student relations; these include communication, honesty, trust, and respect. Other important characteristics and competencies included skills in recognition and referral; an understanding of similarities and differences in people; and knowledge of curricula and prevention principles, illegal substances, and the legal issues related to substance use.

Four general content areas can be identified that would serve as the foundation of an inservice, as well as preservice, training program for teachers and other services personnel who will be involved in substance use prevention education for individuals with disabilities:

1. *Information about alcohol and other drugs:* Teachers need to establish credibility as authoritative sources of information about alcohol and other drugs in order to teach their students how to resist offers to use them (Lewis & Doorlag, 1991). This does not simply include information about substances and their effects. It also includes information about why students may use alcohol and other drugs (e.g., the need to belong, rebelliousness, family influences, risk taking, boredom, alienation).

2. *Signs of substance use and appropriate sources of referral and assistance:* Teachers knowledgeable about the signs of alcohol and other drug use serve as excellent backups for parents who may fail to recognize the danger signs. Inservice training should prepare teachers to recognize these signs and to provide specific guidance when a student appears to exhibit them. It is very important for school professionals to understand the referral and intervention process and to be able to refer cases to

trained staff who can evaluate the situation and take the appropriate actions. Table 6 presents a list of signs of alcohol and other drug use.

3. *Validated teaching strategies and interventions:* A common characteristic of many prevention education programs is the use of group discussion and interactive role playing/behavioral rehearsal techniques. It is essential that teachers are competent in the use of these methods. It is also important that teachers be competent with the behavioral-instructional strategies consistently identified in the literature as positively associated with student achievement in other learning domains (see chap. 1, this volume, for more on these procedures). This area also includes strategies and approaches to meaningfully and actively involve parents in the prevention effort.

4. *Staff attitudes and beliefs regarding substance use:* To be effective in prevention education, teachers need to clarify their own feelings about the use of alcohol and other drugs. Teaching students, especially students with severe learning disabilities and/or problem behaviors, about substance use will likely lead to questions and challenges about the instructor's history of alcohol and other drug use, legal issues involved, and so on. Teachers may lose credibility if their responses to these questions and probes reflect an equivocal or, worse, permissive viewpoint concerning the subject.

Table 6. Signs of alcohol and other drug use

Changes in school performance
Distinct drastic drop in grades
Assignments not completed
Constantly late for class
Sits in the back of class
Absenteeism, truancy
Memory loss
Increased discipline referrals, noncompliance
Loss of interest in extracurricular activities
Changes in behavior
Decrease in energy
Hangs out with a new group of peers who are known users
Easily upset, emotional instability, excessively sad or unhappy, mood swings
Extremely negative, unmotivated
Chronic lying, stealing, dishonesty
Secretive
Reacts angrily when confronted with possible alcohol or substance use
Borrows money excessively
Rapid speech
Changes in appearance and environment
Weight loss or gain
Unkempt physical appearance
Smells of alcohol, tobacco, marijuana
Bloodshot eyes
Persistent cough or cold symptoms
Drug-related jewelry or clothing
Alcohol, tobacco, and other drug paraphernalia

Parental Involvement

It has been repeatedly stressed throughout this chapter that a comprehensive approach to prevention education is required. To enhance ultimate effectiveness, prevention programs must meaningfully involve parents in the overall prevention effort. As discussed earlier, there is a strong association between the behavior and attitudes of a youth's parents and whether the student uses illegal substances.

Attempts to involve parents in prevention efforts have taken several forms (Elmquist, 1992a). Parent education and training programs typically focus on developing child behavior management and communication skills. Many school-based programs involve parents by providing them with information about the content of the prevention program that their children are experiencing in school. Other approaches include establishing parent support groups.

Werch et al. (1991) assessed the effectiveness of a "take-home" prevention program on communication and attitudes of parents and their elementary-age children. Four weekly lessons on alcohol, tobacco, and marijuana and the tools to avoid using them contained a brief classroom-based introduction to the topic and five activities to be completed at home by the child and his or her parents. The activities included brief factual quizzes about the topic, listing reasons not to use substances, constructing responses to hypothetical situations involving pressures to use, thinking of ways to avoid or resist the use of substances, and making pledges and signing contracts not to use drugs. The results indicated that the take-home program resulted in better communication between parents and children regarding substances; however, there were no differences in the students' reported intentions to use substances following completion of the program.

Another study of parental involvement specifically targeted parents of students with disabilities (Elmquist, 1992b). The four-session program taught parents: 1) how to listen to their children; 2) how to monitor the whereabouts of their children; 3) how to develop a family policy concerning the use of alcohol, tobacco, and other drugs; and 4) how to teach resistance skills. The results indicated that parents acquired specific information about substance use and, more importantly, learned and used the skills that were the focus of the program.

Parental involvement programs have a great deal of potential and intuitive appeal; however, efforts to keep parents involved have been plagued with lingering problems. One of the primary difficulties is sustaining parents' interest and active participation in training or education. Low participation and high drop-out rates are common (DeMarsh & Kumpher, 1986; Klitzner, 1987). Attrition rates of 45%–50% in parent education and training programs is not unusual (DeMarsh & Kumpher, 1986). Moreover, it seems as if the parents who may be most in need of education and training, that is, parents of high-risk students, are the parents least likely to participate. Conversely, parents who are the most motivated and engaged in the program are the parents of children who are least likely to have problems with substance use (Klitzner, Gruenwald, & Bamberger, 1990).

Another serious problem facing parent education and training programs concerns their effectiveness. Most of the evaluation indices in these types of programs involve consumer satisfaction measures, assessments of knowledge, analogue ratings of skills, and self-reports of behavioral skills. Often, evidence for positive improvements and changes in these areas are reported by investigators (Elmquist, 1992b). However, there is little evidence to suggest that these programs have a positive effect on actual substance use rates (Klitzner et al., 1990).

This fact has not dissuaded program developers from continuing to implement these programs. The potential for increasing protective factors associated with family functioning holds at least the promise of increasing the odds against alcohol and other drug use. To maximize the effectiveness of these efforts, enhancing program content and focusing on recruiting and sustaining parental involvement are recommended.

Program content should include teaching functional and relevant skills that are associated with enhancing family cohesiveness, bonding, structure, and consistency. Table 7 lists skills that should be included as part of parent training. The Office of Substance Use Prevention (1988) has published a brief guide for parents that can serve as the rudiments of a training program. The guide, entitled *10 Steps to Help Your Child Say 'No,'* includes the following suggestions:

1. Talk with your child about alcohol and other drugs.
2. Learn to really listen to your child.
3. Encourage your child to feel good about himself or herself.
4. Help your child develop strong values.
5. Be a good role model or example.
6. Help your child with peer pressure.
7. Create and enforce family rules about alcohol and drug use.
8. Encourage healthy, creative activities.
9. Team up with other parents to form support groups.
10. Know what to do if you suspect a problem.

In addition to enhancing program content, steps need to be taken to recruit and sustain participation in prevention efforts by the parents most in need of education and training. Target specific groups of parents with specific needs and interests (e.g., parents of students with disabilities). If possible, offer incentives for parents to attend, such as small stipends, good refreshments, local merchandisers' discount coupons). Make personal contacts and offer personal invitations, provide free child care, and schedule group meetings at times

Table 7. Recommended content areas for parent education and training programs

Communication and interaction
Listening ability
Nurturing skills
Behavior management
Structure
Consistency
Positive ways of consequating behavior
Enhancing compliance
Monitoring behavior
Substance use information and related skills
Recognizing signs of use
Responding to use
Creating and enforcing family policies concerning use
Teaching resistance skills
Modeling

convenient for parents. See Table 8 for further recommendations.

Few parent programs have been developed specifically for use with parents of students with disabilities. Therefore, as with student-based programs, it is likely that adaptations and modifications will need to be made to make the program more appropriate and to enhance its effectiveness. Again, school personnel are encouraged to carefully consider the needs of their audience, then thoughtfully review a number of parent programs before selecting the program(s) to be used.

Legal Issues

Substance use in the schools entails a discussion of the legal implications and issues associated when students with disabilities are involved. Two specific legal issues, eligibility for services and disciplinary procedures, are discussed in the following sections.

Eligibility Two questions frequently arise concerning students with disabilities and substance use as it relates to eligibility for special education and related services: 1) Are students with disabilities who are also involved in alcohol or other drug use eligible for special education services?, and 2) Are students who are addicted to alcohol or other drugs considered disabled and, therefore, eligible for special education services? These questions have received considerable attention from federal, state, and local education agencies and by the courts. The answers to these questions are found in the Individuals with Disabilities Education Act of 1990 (IDEA) (PL 101-476), Section 504 of the Rehabilitation Act of 1973 (PL 93-112), and the Americans with Disabilities Act of 1990 (ADA) (PL 101-336).

As far as IDEA and its predecessor, the Education for All Handicapped Children Act of 1975 (PL 94-142), are concerned, students who are addicted to alcohol or other drugs are not entitled to special education services unless they are determined to fall under the category of a disability specifically covered by the act. The Office of Special Education Programs of the United States Department of Education has ruled that a free appropriate public education is not mandated unless it has been determined

Table 8. Encouraging parental involvement

As with any program implementation, the energy and care devoted to planning are the important parts of the process. Done well, it's a very powerful experience for families. Done poorly, parents won't attend, which can create a blaming and hostile relationship between the parent community and the school. Below are some guidelines for implementing a parent education curriculum.

1. Create a plan for outreach and recruitment of the targeted parents.
2. Be creative with your promotional ideas. Use recruitment methods other than promotional flyers, written announcements, and public service announcements. Face to face, personal invitations are essential.
3. Locate all potential community linkages and resources to assist with outreach, instruction, funding, support, and follow-up. Ideas include providing parent support groups, on-site parent resource centers, "hotlines," safe homes for parent communication networks, recreational activities, and Saturday "parent universities."
4. Decide on appropriate ways to evaluate the impact you expect to have.
5. Create a festive, fun atmosphere for the evenings. Interaction, laughter, and refreshments are necessary to build a learning environment and to retain interest.
6. Don't invite the teachers to participate unless they are part of the targeted audience.

From Bickel, A., & Ertle, V. (1991). *Parenting skills curricula: A descriptive guide* (pp. 6–7). Portland: Northwest Regional Educational Laboratory; reprinted by permission.

that the student has one of the disabilities covered by IDEA and is in need of special education and related services. For example, a student who is addicted to alcohol and/or other drugs and who has a learning disability or behavior disorder is eligible for a free appropriate public education. However, a student who is addicted to alcohol and/or other drugs, but is not determined to have a learning disability or behavioral disorder, is not eligible for coverage under the IDEA. However, this second student may be eligible for coverage and protection under other Federal statutes, notably the ADA and Section 504 of the Rehabilitation Act of 1973.

Under Section 504, a student is entitled to certain protections if it is determined that he or she is a "qualified handicapped person." This means that it has been determined that the student: 1) has a physical or mental disability that substantially limits one or more major life activities, 2) has a record of such a disability, or 3) is regarded as having such a disability. If a student needs or is believed to need special education or related services, school districts are obligated to evaluate the student and, if determined to have a disability, provide the individual with a free appropriate public education. Under Section 504, students who are addicted to alcohol and/or other drugs are also considered to have either physical or mental disabilities.

However, this policy has been changed with the enactment of the ADA. Now, schools are no longer required to evaluate or otherwise accommodate a student who is currently engaged in illegal drug use. However, the ADA does not automatically exclude students who are addicted to alcohol from eligibility or accommodation. The specific rationale for this distinction is readily apparent. One might conjecture that the use of illegal drugs is considered by policymakers, as well as the general public, as "bad," but the use of alcohol is still considered more socially acceptable.

While current drug users are excluded from protection under the ADA, students who are no longer currently using and who have either successfully completed a rehabilitation program or are currently participating in one may be eligible for protection if it is determined they are an "otherwise qualified handicapped person." As of 1994, this provision is still so very recent that school districts and the courts have had very little experience implementing its provisions.

Disciplinary Actions Student drug use has focused increased attention on enforcement of strict "zero tolerance" school rules and regulations. For example, current federal policy allows school districts to suspend or, in some cases, expel any student who violates school policies concerning use, possession, or sale of alcohol and/or other drugs on school grounds or at school functions. Are students who are considered to have a disability by the ADA or the IDEA exempt from these sanctions? The specific language in the ADA states that local education agencies may take disciplinary action pertaining to the use or possession of illegal drugs or alcohol against any student with a disability who is currently engaging in the illegal use of drugs or alcohol to the same extent that such disciplinary action is taken against students who do not have disabilities (Kincaid, 1992). This means that school districts may apply standard disciplinary procedures concerning illegal drug or alcohol use to students who are considered to have a disability solely by virtue of an alcohol or other drug addiction.

However, if a student is considered to have a disability because of alcohol or other drug addiction and also has another disabling condition, the due process provisions specified in Section 504 are required. For example, consider the example of a student with mental retardation in whose locker illegal drugs are discovered. This student may be disciplined as all other students would be disciplined only if the school can demonstrate that the student is currently using drugs. If it cannot, the student must be re-evaluated, prior to any disciplinary actions, to determine, among other issues, whether the misbehavior (i.e., possession of illegal drugs) was a manifestation of the primary disability.

Physician-Prescribed Stimulant Medications There continues to be a belief among professionals and the public that students who are diagnosed as ADHD who receive physician-prescribed stimulant medication (e.g., Ritalin) are at great risk for: 1) becoming addicted to their medication or 2) using alcohol or other illegal drugs. Given the increased attention recently given to ADHD, both in terms of the numbers of children and youth identified and the widespread use of stimulant medications to control their behavior, these two questions require some fresh light and a carefully measured response.

While the effectiveness of stimulant medication on the behavior, school performance, and overall adjustment of ADHD students has been extensively examined (see, e.g., Barkley, 1977; Gadow, 1986), few researchers have looked at the long-term effects of using stimulant medications. It is true that children and youth who take stimulant medications may experience mild and transient side-effects such as loss of appetite or insomnia (Gordon, 1991). However, it is not true that taking stimulant medications such as Ritalin will lead to addiction. Russell Barkley, a nationally recognized expert on ADHD, answered this question succinctly when he stated:

> There are no reported cases of addiction or serious drug dependence to date with these medications . . . In fact, there is some clinical evidence to suggest that the children on medication frequently dislike it and wish its discontinuance as soon as possible, especially if they are older children and adolescents. (Barkley, 1990, pp. 589–590)

The same answer can be given to the question of increased likelihood of using alcohol or other illegal drugs. That is, are children and youth who take stimulant medications such as Ritalin more likely to use alcohol and/or other illegal drugs? Again, controlled studies are lacking to answer this question; there are no data to support either a "yes" or "no" response. One could speculate, however, that an ADHD student whose treatment plan included stimulant medication, a structured behavior management and academic program in school, and parent training would be less impulsive, experience more success, and demonstrate more self-control. In other words, a number of the key risk factors for substance use would be reduced.

Conversely, an ADHD student on stimulant medication who does not receive the other necessary components of an effective treatment program will likely continue to experience problems in school, at home, with peers, and in the community—all key risk factors for substance use. In summary, whether either one of these students uses alcohol and/or other drugs as a direct outcome of their use of stimulant medication is a question that cannot be answered at this time. Clearly, more controlled studies are needed to answer this question (Clampit & Pirkle, 1983).

Perhaps a more important issue relating to the use of stimulant medications with ADHD children and youth concerns the mixed messages communicated to all members of society. More children and students receive Ritalin for ADHD in the United States today (between 1% and 2% of the population) than for any other disorder (Barkley, 1990). Legitimate questions have been raised over the years about the prudence of medicating children in an effort to control behavior (Schrag & Divoky, 1975). Prendergast et al. (1990) also articulated a more fundamental contradiction concerning the use of drugs for therapeutic purposes:

> it sends a mixed message about drug use when youths are unnecessarily given them by parents themselves in order to solve problems . . . [it] reflects a tendency to search for simple solutions and quick fixes for difficult, complex problems. It seems that as a society we want things both ways: to blame some drugs for our children's behavior problems and send them off to treatment centers, and to given them other drugs to deal with their behavior problems. In both instances, we are avoiding dealing with the fundamental problems that face us. (p. 23)

CONCLUSIONS

The problem of substance use among children and youth is serious. Students with disabilities are not immune from this problem and may, in some cases, use illegal substances at even higher rates than students without disabilities due to a number of environmental and personal factors. Programs and strategies are now available that show promise in the effort to prevent substance use in students with disabilities. This closing section serves as a summary of those research- and practice-validated principles and strategies that should serve as the foundation on which to build an effective prevention program for students with disabilities.

First, specially designed instruction to meet the unique needs of students with disabilities is critical to the overall success of the prevention effort. As we have seen, few existing programs take into account the learning needs of students with disabilities or incorporate the principles and practices of effective instruction. If program developers fail to recognize this need and continue to market programs designed for the typical student, then teachers and other professionals involved in the education of students with disabilities will need to either develop programs on their own or adapt existing materials as necessary.

Second, programs must actively involve parents in the prevention effort. With many parents of students with disabilities, special recruitment and retention efforts will be required to attract their continued interest and participation. Special educators should not forget that while schools can play a major role in the overall prevention program, ultimately, prevention begins and ends in the home. Third, experience has demonstrated that an effective prevention program involves the entire community. A comprehensive prevention plan enlists the cooperation of education, health, law enforcement, and social services agencies, as well as civic groups, religious groups, the media, and businesses.

Fourth, there is a very big need for well-controlled, long-term research that examines the overall effectiveness of prevention programs for students with disabilities. Although a great deal of activity has occurred in recent years in the area of substance use prevention, there is still much we do not yet know. Unfortunately, one of those unknowns is under what conditions and with whom prevention programs work. In conducting such investigations, researchers, evaluators and practitioners alike should make a special effort to concentrate on the desired outcomes. That is, while it may be nice to know if students know more about substances and their effects or that students' attitudes about substance use have changed for the better or that their self-concepts have improved, the criterion for sucess in this situation must be a change in behavior, that is, students with disabilities should use substances at a lower rate as a result of the prevention program. Finally, an effective prevention program begins early and is continued over a long period of time. One-shot efforts or short-term, low- intensity programs will not be successful with students who require early intervention and high intensity programs in many other areas of learning.

Substantial insight has been gained in terms of how to prevent the use of illegal substances. We also know that substance use prevention programs are a necessary, but insufficient, element in the effort to improve the health of our children and youth. A commitment to healthy living embodies more than just an ability to say "no." It is clear that a comprehensive, multifaceted, and proactive approach is required.

REFERENCES

Allison, K.R., Silverman, G., & Dignam, C. (1990). Effects on students of teacher training in use of a drug education curriculum. *Journal of Drug Education, 20*(1), 31–46.

The Americans with Disabilities Act of 1990, PL 101-336. (July 26, 1990). Title 42, U.S.C. 12101 et seq: U.S. Statutes at Large, 104, 327-378.

Anti-Drug Act of 1988, PL 100-690.

August, G.J., Stewart, M.A., & Holmes, C.S. (1983). A four-year followup of hyperactive boys with and without conduct disorder. *British Journal of Psychiatry, 143*, 192–198.

Austin, G. (1992). *School failure and alcohol and other drug use*. Madison, WI: Wisconsin Clearinghouse.

Bangert-Drowns, R.L. (1988). The effects of school-based substance abuse education: A meta-analysis. *Journal of Drug Education, 18*(3), 243–264.

Barkley, R.A. (1977). A review of stimulant drug research with hyperactive children. *Journal of Child Psychology and Psychiatry, 18*, 137–165.

Barkley, R.A. (1990). *Attention deficit hyperactivity disorder: A handbook for diagnosis and treatment*. New York: Guilford Press.

Benard, B. (1991). *Fostering resiliency in kids: Protective factors in the family, school, and community.* Portland, OR: Northwest Regional Educational Laboratory.

Bickel, A., & Ertle, V. (1991). *Parenting skills curricula: A descriptive guide.* Portland, OR: Northwest Regional Educational Laboratory.

Botvin, G. (1990). *Life skills training.* New York: Smithfield Press.

Botvin, G.J., Baker, E., Renick, N.L., Filazzola, A.D., & Botvin, E.M. (1984). A cognitive-behavioral approach to substance abuse prevention. *Addictive Behaviors, 9,* 137–147.

Brook, J.S., Gordon, A.S., Whiteman, M., & Cohen, P. (1986). Dynamics of childhood and adolescent personality traits and adolescent drug use. *Developmental Psychology, 22,* 403–414.

Bruck, M. (1985). The adult functioning of children with specific learning disabilities: A follow-up study. *Advances in Applied Developmental Psychology, 1,* 91–129.

Clampit, M.K., & Pirkle, J.B. (1983). Stimulant medication and the hyperactive adolescent: Myths and facts. *Adolescence, 18,* 811–822.

Crumley, F.E. (1990). Substance abuse and adolescent suicidal behavior. *Journal of the American Medical Association, 263*(22), 3051–3056.

Delaney, D., & Poling, A. (1990). Drug abuse among mentally retarded people: An overlooked problem. *Journal of Alcohol and Drug Education, 35,* 48–54.

DeMarsh, J., & Kumpher, K.L. (1986). Family-oriented interventions for the prevention of chemical dependency in children and adolescents. *Journal of Children in Contemporary Society, 18,* 117–151.

Edgerton, R.B. (1986). Alcohol and drug use by mentally retarded adults. *American Journal of Mental Deficiency, 90,* 602–609.

Education for all Handicapped Children Act of 1975, 20 U.S.C. §§1232, 1401, 1405–1420, 1453 (1975).

Ellickson, P.L., & Bell, R.M. (1990). Drug prevention in junior high: A multi-site longitudinal test. *Science, 247,* 1299–1305.

Elmquist, D.L. (1991). School-based alcohol and other drug prevention programs: Guidelines for the special educator. *Intervention in School and Clinic, 27*(1), 10–19.

Elmquist, D.L. (1992a). *A systematic review of parent-oriented programs to prevent children's use of alcohol and other drugs.* Unpublished manuscript, Department of Special Education, Utah State University, Logan.

Elmquist, D.L. (1992b). *Development and evaluation of a substance use prevention parent-involvement program for parents of students with mild disabilities.* Unpublished doctoral dissertation, Department of Special Education, Utah State University, Logan.

Elmquist, D.L., Morgan, D.P., & Bolds, P. (1992). Substance use among adolescents with disabilities. *International Journal of the Addictions, 27,* 1475–1483.

Fetro, J.V. (1991). *Step by step to substance use prevention: The planning guide to school-based programs.* Santa Cruz, CA: Network Publications.

Gadow, K.D. (1986). *Children on medication, Volume 1: Hyperactivity, learning disabilities, and mental retardation.* Boston: Little, Brown.

Garfinkel, B.D., Froese, A., & Hood, J. (1982). Suicide attempts in children and adolescents. *American Journal of Psychiatry, 139,* 1257–1261.

Gittelman, R., Mannuzza, S., Shenker, R., & Bonagura, N. (1985). Hyperactive boys almost grown up. *Archives of General Psychiatry, 42,* 937–947.

Gordon, M. (1991). *ADHD/Hyperactivity: A consumer's guide for parents and teachers.* DeWitt, NY: GSI Publications.

Halpern, A.S., Close, D.W., & Nelson, D.J. (1986). *On my own: The impact of semi-independent living programs for adults with mental retardation.* Baltimore: Paul H. Brookes Publishing Co.

Hansen, W.B. (1990). *School-based substance use prevention: A review of the state of the art in curriculum, 1980–1990.* Winston-Salem, NC: Department of Public Health Sciences, Wake Forest University.

Hansen, W.B., & Graham, J.W. (1991). Preventing alcohol, marijuana, and cigarette use among adolescents: Peer pressure resistance training versus establishing conservative norms. *Preventive Medicine, 20,* 414–430.

Hansen, W.B., Graham, J.W., Johnson, C.A., Flay, B.R., & Pentz, M.A. (1988). *Project SMART: A social approach to drug abuse prevention.* Pasadena: University of Southern California Institute for Health Promotion and Disease Prevention.

Hansen, W.B., Johnson, C.A., Flay, B.R., Graham, J.W., & Sobel, J. (1988). Affective and social influences approaches to the prevention of multiple substance abuse among seventh grade students. Results from Project SMART. *Preventive Medicine, 17,* 135–154.

Hartsough, C.S., & Lambert, N.M. (1987). Pattern and progression of drug use among hyperactives and controls: A prospective short-term longitudinal study. *Journal of Childhood Psychology and Psychiatry, 28,* 543–553.

Hawkins, J.D., Lishner, D.M., & Catalano, R.F. (1985). Childhood predictors and the prevention of adolescent substance abuse. In C.L. Jones & R.J. Battjes (Eds.), *Etiology of drug abuse: Implications for prevention* (NIDA Research Monograph No. 56). Rockville, MD: National Institute on Drug Abuse.

Hawkins, J.D., Lishner, D.M., Catalano, R.F., & Howard, M.O. (1985). Childhood predictors of adolescent substance abuse: Toward an empirically grounded theory. *Journal of Children in Contemporary Society, 18,* 11–48.

Heinemann, A.W., Doll, M., & Schnoll, S. (1989). Treatment of alcohol abuse in persons with recent spinal cord injuries. *Alcohol, Health, and Research World,* 1989, *13*(2), 110–117.

Here's looking at you, 2000. (1986). Seattle, WA: Roberts, Fitzmahan, & Associates.

Hopkins, R., Mauss, A., Kearney, K., & Wesheit, R. (1988). Comprehensive evaluation of a model alcohol education curriculum. *Journal of Studies on Alcohol,* 49, 38–49.

Huang, A.M. (1981). The drinking behavior of educable mentally retarded and nonretarded students. *Journal of Alcohol and Drug Education, 26,* 41–50.

Individuals with Disabilities Education Act of 1990 (IDEA), PL 101-476. (October 30, 1990). Title 20, U.S.C. 1400 et seq: *U.S. Statutes at Large, 104,* 1103–1151.

Jaker, G.F. (1985). *Lessons learned: A review of research in drug education.* Anoka, MN: Minnesota Prevention Resource Center.

Jessor, R. (1987). Bridging etiology and prevention in drug abuse research. In C.L. Jones & R.J. Battjes (Eds.), *Etiology of drug abuse: Implications for prevention* (NIDA

Research Monograph No. 56). Rockville, MD: National Institute on Drug Abuse.

Johnson, C.A., Pentz, M.A., Weber, M.D., Dwyer, J.H., Baer, N., MacKinnon, D.P., & Hansen, W.B. (1990). Relative effectiveness of comprehensive community programming for drug abuse prevention with high-risk and low-risk adolescents. *Journal of Consulting and Clinical Psychology, 58*, 447–456.

Johnston, L.D., & O'Malley, P.M. (1986). Why do the nation's students use drugs and alcohol? Self-reported reasons from nine national surveys. *The Journal of Drug Issues, 16*(1), 29–66.

Johnston, L.D., O'Malley, P.M., & Bachman, J.G. (1991). *Drug use among American high school seniors, college students and young adults, 1975–1990. Volume 1, High School Seniors.* Rockville, MD: U.S. Department of Health and Human Services, National Institute on Drug Abuse.

Jones, G.A. (1989). Alcohol abuse and traumatic brain injury. *Alcohol, Health, and Research World, 13*, 104–109.

Jones, R.M., Kline, K., Habkirk, S., & Sales, A. (1990). Teacher characteristics and competencies related to substance abuse prevention. *Journal of Drug Education, 20*, 179–189.

Kincaid, J.M. (1992, May). *School district responsibilities to chemically-dependent students.* Paper presented at the 13th National Institute on Legal Issues of Educating Individuals with Disabilities, San Antonio, TX.

Klitzner, M.D. (1987). An assessment of the nature and effectiveness of federal, state, and local drug prevention/education programs. In U.S. Department of Education & U.S. Department of Health and Human Services (Eds.), *Report to Congress and the White House on the nature and effectiveness of federal, state, and local drug prevention/education programs.* Washington, DC: U.S. Government Printing Office.

Klitzner, M., Gruenwald, P.J., & Bamberger, E. (1990). The assessment of parent-led prevention programs: A preliminary assessment of impact. *Journal of Drug Education, 20*(1), 77–94.

Krishef, C.H. (1986). Do the mentally retarded drink? A study of their alcohol usage. *Journal of Alcohol and Drug Education, 31*, 64–70.

Leone, P.E. (1991). *Alcohol and other drugs: Use, abuse, and disabilities.* Reston, VA: Council for Exceptional Children.

Leone, P.E., Greenberg, J.M., Trickett, E.J., & Spero, E. (1989). A study of the use of cigarettes, alcohol, and marijuana by students identified as "seriously emotionally disturbed." *Counterpoint, 9*(3), 6–7.

Lewis, R.B., & Doorlag, D.H. (1991). *Teaching special students in the mainstream* (3rd ed.). New York: Merrill/Macmillan.

LifeFacts 3—substance abuse. (1990). Santa Monica, CA: James Stanfield.

McIntyre, K., White, D., & Yoast, R. (1992). *Resilience among high-risk youth.* Madison: Wisconsin Clearinghouse.

Minnesota smoking prevention program. (1989). Minneapolis: School of Public Health, University of Minnesota.

Moore, D. (1991). The magnitude of the problem: The scope of prevention and treatment issues for persons with mental retardation or learning disability. In J.S. Lechowicz (Ed.), *Alcohol and other drug abuse: Implications for mental retardation and learning disabilities.* Hempstead, NY: Hofstra University.

Moore, D., & Polsgrove, L. (1991). Disabilities, developmental handicaps, and substance misuse: A review. *International Journal of the Addictions, 26*, 65–90.

Moore, D., & Siegal, H. (1989). Double trouble: Alcohol and other drug use among orthopedically impaired college students. *Alcohol, Health, and Research World, 13*(2), 118–123.

Morgan, D.P. (1992). *RESIST: Resistance education strategies and interventions systematically taught.* Logan: Department of Special Education, Utah State University.

Morgan, D.P., Cancio, E., & Likins, M. (1992). *Preventing substance use: What special educators need to know.* Logan: Department of Special Education, Utah State University.

Moskowitz, J.M. (1989). The primary prevention of alcohol problems: A critical review of the research literature. *Journal of Studies on Alcohol, 50*(1), 54–88.

National Center for Youth with Disabilities. (1990). *Substance use by youth with disabilities and chronic illnesses* (2nd ed.). Minneapolis: Author.

Needle, R., Su, S., Doherty, W., Lavee, Y., & Brown, P. (1988). Familial, interpersonal, and intrapersonal correlates of drug use: A longitudinal comparison of adolescents in treatment, drug-using adolescents not in treatment, and non-drug using adolescents. *International Journal of the Addictions, 23*(12), 1211–1240.

Newcomb, M.D., Maddahian, E., & Bentler, P.M. (1986). Risk factors for drug use among adolescents: Concurrent and longitudinal analyses. *American Journal of Public Health, 76*, 525–531.

Newcomb, M.D., Maddahian, E., Skager, R., & Bentler, P.M. (1987). Substance abuse and psychological risk factors among teenagers: Associations with sex, age, ethnicity, and type of school. *American Journal of Drug and Alcohol Abuse, 13*(4), 413–433.

Office of Substance Use Prevention. (1988). *Quick list: 10 steps to help your child say "no."* Rockville, MD: United States Department of Health and Human Services/Alcohol, Drug Abuse, and Mental Health Administration.

Pandina, R.J., & Schuele, J.A. (1983). Psychosocial correlates of alcohol and drug use of adolescent students and adolescents in treatment. *Journal of Studies on Alcohol, 44*, 950–973.

Prendergast, M., Austin, G., & deMiranda, J. (1990). *Substance use among youth with disabilities* (Prevention Research Update No. 7). Portland, OR: Northwest Regional Educational Laboratory.

Prevention curriculum guide for looking at alcohol and other drugs—special education 7–12. (undated). Kent, OH: Addiction Intervention with the Disabled, Department of Sociology, Kent State University.

Prevention time. (1985). Chesapeake: Southeastern Virginia Planning District Commission.

Project OZ. (1986). *Project OZ: A comprehensive drug education curriculum for learning disabled and behavior disordered populations grades 6–12.* Bloomington, IL: Author.

Rehabilitation Act of 1973, PL 93-112. (September 26, 1973). Title 29, U.S.C. 701 et seq: *U.S. Statutes at Large, 87*, 355–394.

Rogers, T., Howard-Pitney, B., & Bruce, B.L. (1989). *What works? A guide to school-based alcohol and drug abuse prevention curricula.* Palo Alto, CA: Stanford Center for Research in Disease Prevention.

Rundall, T.G., & Bruvold, W.H. (1988). A meta-analysis of school-based smoking and alcohol use prevention programs. *Health Education Quarterly, 15*(3), 317–334.

Schaps, E., DiBartolo, R., Moskowitz, J., Palley, C.S., & Churgin, S. (1981). A review of 127 drug abuse prevention program evaluations. *Journal of Drug Issues, 11,* 17–43.

Schrag, P., & Divoky, D. (1975). *The myth of the hyperactive child.* New York: Pantheon.

Shedler, J., & Block, J. (1990). Adolescent drug use and psychological health: A longitudinal inquiry. *American Psychologist, 45*(5), 612–630.

A special message: A comprehensive drug education curriculum for learning disabled and behavior disordered populations grades 6–12. (1988). Bloomington, IL: Project Oz.

Tobler, N.S. (1986). Meta-analysis of 143 adolescent drug prevention programs: Quantitative outcome results of program participants compared to a control or comparison group. *The Journal of Drug Issues, 16*(4), 537–567.

United States Department of Education. (1989). *What works: Schools without drugs.* Washington, DC: Department of Education.

United States Department of Education. (1990). *Drug prevention curricula: A guide to selection and implementation.* Washington, DC: Department of Education, Office of Educational Research and Improvement.

Utah State Division of Substance Abuse. (1991). *Facts: Substance abuse information for Utah and the nation.* Salt Lake City, UT: Division of Substance Abuse.

Werch, C.E., Young, M., Clark, M., Garrett, C., Hooks, S., & Kersten, C. (1991). Effects of a take-home drug prevention program on drug-related communication and beliefs of parents and children. *Journal of School Health, 61*(8), 346–350.

Chapter Ten

HIV/AIDS Prevention and Education

Christine Y. Mason and Tecla Jaskulski

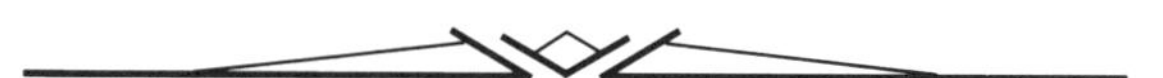

With the exception of the late 1920s and early 1930s, when American eugenicists sought to control the sexuality of people with mental retardation through sterilization (Vitello, 1980), society has virtually ignored the sexuality of and the need for sex education for individuals with developmental disabilities (Crocker, Cohen, Decker, Rudigier, & Harvey, 1989; Gosney & Popenoe, 1929; Hylton, 1990; Jacobs, Samowitz, Levy, Levy, & Cabrera, 1992). Today, informed consent laws and due process procedures protect adults with disabilities against unwanted and unknowing sterilization and sexual exploitation (Macklin & Gaylin, 1981; Reilly, 1991). However, individuals with mental retardation and other developmental disabilities may still be denied privacy, sex education, and opportunities to engage in sexual activities with a partner of their choice.

While sexuality is a normal part of everyday life for most adults, fear, ignorance, denial, and misconceptions have played a large part in the failure of society, professionals, and parents to address basic sex education for people with developmental disabilities (Hingsburger & Griffiths, 1986; Jacobs et al., 1992). Many people have mistakenly thought that individuals with developmental disabilities have no sexual needs or interests; others have assumed that instruction will stimulate experimentation and open a Pandora's box to sexual expression and accompanying problems, such as unwanted pregnancies, sexual disease, and exploitation. Although little formal research has been conducted regarding sexually related concerns for people with disabilities (due partly to the difficulty of gathering such information), anecdotal information discounts these hypotheses and bolsters instead the need for education to reduce the potential for abuse, inappropriate sexual expression, and sexual disease (Kempton, 1990b). Anecdotal information also indicates that learning about human sexuality can both enhance life satisfaction and decrease inappropriate behaviors (including engaging in unexplained aggression that may be the result of sexual frustration or taking sexual advantage of peers who often lack sex education and assertiveness skills) (Monat-Haller, 1992).

With the rapid spread of the acquired immunodeficiency syndrome (AIDS), instruction regarding sexuality and sexual expression has become even more critical. Dramatically adding to the serious consequences of failing to address sexuality, the spread of the human immunodeficiency virus (HIV) has produced another reason to renew efforts to teach youth and adults about their sexuality, appropriate expression of sexual interests, and how to prevent disease and exploitation.

This chapter primarily focuses on HIV/AIDS in the broader contexts of personal safety and sexuality. Also included are strategies for teaching about other sexually transmitted diseases (STDs), assertiveness skills, sexual–social relationships, personal boundaries, and prevention of sexual exploitation and abuse. Although this chapter presents guidelines for school-age students with developmental disabilities (grades K–12), the primary focus is on older youth and adults who may be at particular risk of contracting HIV and the AIDS virus.

HIV/AIDS AND PERSONS WITH DEVELOPMENTAL DISABILITIES

Society cannot assume that the risk of individuals with developmental disabilities acquiring HIV/AIDS is minimal. As summarized by Jacobs and associates (1992) and illustrated in Table 1, these individuals are at risk due to their vulnerability, sexual activity, and overall lack of sex education. In particular, individuals with developmental disabilities lack information on safer sex practices. (The term "safer" is used as the preferred term in AIDS education to reflect the concept that, other than complete abstinence, there are only "relatively safe" sex practices.) To overcome this educational deficit, the National Leadership Forum on HIV/AIDS and Developmental Disabilities, held at the University of San Francisco in 1989, encouraged agencies serving individuals with disabilities to develop policies regarding routine and periodic HIV/AIDS education and prevention (McDaniel & Sells, 1989). In addition to this important forum, other experts in the field of developmental disabilities and HIV/AIDS have urged implementation of effective HIV educational procedures and policies (Crocker et al., 1989; Decker, 1989; Jacobs et al., 1992; Kastner, DeLotto, Scagnelli, & Testa, 1989; Kastner, Hickman, & Bellehumeur, 1989).

Although funding for sex education and HIV/AIDS prevention is an issue, particularly in terms of staff time, organizations providing services to persons with developmental disabilities should address the risk of AIDS as part of their support programs. In a study completed at 10 sites in Indiana and New York, Mason and Jaskulski (1993) found that most sites were able to offer HIV prevention programs by making such programs a priority and rearranging schedules to assure that staff were available and that individuals were able to attend weekly HIV prevention sessions for 8–10 weeks. The

Table 1. Factors that put people with developmental disabilities at risk for contracting HIV/AIDS

1. People with developmental disabilities may have cognitive limitations that impede their decision-making abilities, or they may be accustomed to having others make decisions for them. This can make people with developmental disabilities particularly vulnerable to being persuaded or manipulated into engaging in high-risk behaviors.
2. Some individuals with developmental disabilities are at risk for becoming intravenous drug users and, therefore, may be at risk for contracting HIV infection through needle sharing.
3. People with developmental disabilities may have moved into the community only recently and may not be used to having so much choice about sexual expression.
4. People with developmental disabilities may be limited in their choice of sexual partners, causing them to make decisions out of desperation.
5. People with developmental disabilities might not have the skills required to negotiate safer sex.
6. Like the general population, people with developmental disabilities may have been misinformed about sex by their peers, by television, and by what they have heard on the streets. Comprehensive sexuality training has generally not been effective in this population.
7. People with developmental disabilities often live in settings in which staff, administrators, and parents deny that they are indeed sexual beings.
8. People with developmental disabilities may seek out possibly unsafe sex because they have not had appropriate relationships modeled for them and have received the message that sex is "dirty."
9. Like people without disabilities, people with developmental disabilities may have difficulty forming appropriate sexual relationships, and many will engage in sexual activities in response to peer pressure.
10. People with developmental disabilities are often at risk for sexual abuse, thus increasing their risk for contracting AIDS.

Adapted from Jacobs, Samowitz, Levy, Levy, & Cabrera (1992).

study indicated that it was much simpler to make arrangements for individuals in day programs and sheltered work situations than for those in supported or competitive employment. Needless to say, ways must be found to assure that sex education is available to those individuals who did not receive adequate training in high school or who need updated information.

Incidence of HIV/AIDS Among People with Disabilities

Evaluating the overall impact of HIV/AIDS on persons with developmental disabilities, as well as its overall incidence, has been difficult. While protecting individual rights, policies regarding confidentiality and informed consent have made it impossible to develop precise estimates on the extent of HIV infection among people with developmental disabilities, even more so than among people without disabilities, for two reasons. First, although data based on gender, race, age, and so on are collected by the Centers for Disease Control (CDC), no specific data are collected on the rate of infection of HIV/AIDS among individuals with disabilities. Second, because of previous transgressions regarding informed consent and confidentiality (e.g., sterilization without consent), state and federal policies are very careful to guard the rights of individuals with disabilities, even to the extent of implementing stricter guidelines for individuals with disabilities than for the population as a whole.

In one of the few studies designed to estimate the extent of HIV infection among individuals with developmental disabilities, Kastner, Nathanson, Marchetti, and Pincus (1989) surveyed state mental retardation/developmental disabilities agencies in 1987. Among the 44 states responding to the survey, a total of only 45 adult carriers was reported in 11 states, and all but seven of those infected were reported to be asymptomatic.

A follow-up study (Kastner, Nathanson, & Marchetti, 1992) found that the reported incidence had doubled in a 23-month period and that evidence of underreporting suggests that estimates of between 250 to 500 adults with developmental disabilities who are HIV positive nationwide are realistic. These estimates do not include those who are outside the service system. This is similar to an estimate of over 300 adults with mental retardation now infected with the HIV virus as suggested by Crocker and Cohen (1991). In another survey, data obtained on 67 adolescents and adults with developmental disabilities in Oregon indicated that 39% were known to engage in high-risk behaviors (Hylton, 1990). Furthermore, only 27% of the respondents provided accurate answers to the question, "What can you do to keep from getting AIDS?"

Finally, the National Association of Rehabilitation Facilities (NARF), now the American Rehabilitation Association, conducted a survey among its members in Indiana (79 members) and New York (140 members) (Jaskulski & Mason, 1992). Of 108 agencies, 30% indicated that they were providing services to persons with AIDS, while another 30% reported that they did not know whether they were or not. Current service provision to this population was more frequent in New York than in Indiana (32% vs. 23%). The primary populations served by agencies in both states were adults with mental retardation and other developmental disabilities.

The Impact of AIDS on Related Educational Needs

NARF conducted two surveys to assess the impact of AIDS on related educational needs of adult service providers and the persons they serve. Initially, a mini-survey of the NARF membership was conducted through the organization's weekly vocational newsletter over a 3-week period (NARF, 1989). NARF gathered these responses in order to determine the priority that members gave to NARF's pursuit of HIV education and prevention resources for rehabilitation clients.

Of the first 25 community service providers responding to NARF's initial survey, all but one indicated the need for their clients to receive HIV education. An estimate of the number of adults with mental retardation in their programs who could benefit from such training was over 2,400, or an average of 105 individuals per program. One-fourth of the providers indicated that at least 80% of their clients could benefit from HIV training if it were available. However, despite the reported high level of need for HIV education, respondents also indicated that almost no HIV prevention training was being provided. Although some agencies reported that they were currently offering some training to their clients, none was providing extensive training, and 70% were not providing any training. In addition, over 75% reported that other agencies in their community were offering very little, if any, training to people with disabilities.

GENERAL INFORMATION ON THE EPIDEMIOLOGY OF HIV/AIDS

This section provides basic information on the epidemiology of HIV/AIDS, including how the virus is transmitted and the overall prevalence of the disease in the United States. Additional information on the epidemiology of HIV/AIDS and the status of the epidemic can be obtained through the National Clearinghouse on AIDS and a variety of other sources described in the chapter's appendix.

The HIV virus causes AIDS by gradually destroying the white blood cells (T-helper cell lymphocytes) that fight off disease. Once infected with HIV, a person may not have AIDS or even be aware of the HIV infection for as long as 10 years. Eventually, however, enough T-cells are destroyed to cause the immune system to stop functioning properly. People then begin to have opportunistic diseases identified with HIV infection, such as Kaposi's sarcoma, gynecological conditions in some women (e.g., severe, long-term candidiasis, although such conditions are not necessarily directly related to AIDS), and certain forms of pneumonia.

A diagnosis of AIDS is made on the basis of the presence of AIDS-defining illnesses such as those mentioned above, and/or T-cell counts in the blood that are about one-fifth of normal. Although a few drugs have been developed that can retard the effects of HIV infection and AIDS, cases of survival past 10 years of diagnosis are extremely uncommon. According to an estimate by Callen (1990), of the 1,049 Americans diagnosed with AIDS in 1982, only 25 were still alive as of 1990.

How the AIDS Virus Is Transmitted

Many fears surround AIDS because of its outcome. Along with misinformation on transmission of the disease, these concerns sometimes lead to inordinate fears about the possibility of acquiring AIDS through casual contact. Because HIV requires a moist, temperature-controlled environment, it is fragile outside the human body and does not survive in the air. There are no known cases of HIV infection from sneezing, breathing, or coughing or from touching, hugging, holding, or shaking hands with someone who has HIV/AIDS. Although the virus is present in saliva and tears, the amount present is so minute that no transmission through these fluids has ever been documented.

The primary means of transmission has been through sexual activity (i.e., vaginal, anal, and oral sex). The second most frequent means of transmission has been through direct blood-to-blood contact, usually caused by intravenous drug use and needle sharing. Sexual contact with a current or former injecting drug user involves considerable risk. Other risks include tattooing, ear-piercing, and self-injection of legally prescribed medicines. HIV can also be transmitted from a mother to an unborn child during pregnancy and following delivery through breast milk. Although a problem in the past, since 1985, consistent screening for blood transfusions, organ transplants, artificial insemination, and injection of blood products into the blood has virtually eliminated the risk of HIV transmission from these procedures.

Of particular importance to adults with developmental disabilities and community service providers have been the recent publication of standards and policy clarifications from the Occupational Safety and Health Administration (OSHA) (1992). These standards address safety requirements for infectious waste and prevention of HIV transmission. OSHA has indicated that potential transmission of the virus through blood-soaked materials, including tampons and menstrual pads, as well as sperm-filled condoms, should be avoided by treating these items as potentially infectious, using universal precautions, wearing rubber gloves, and bagging such materials.

HIV/AIDS in the United States

The first case of AIDS in the United States was reported in 1981; that same year, the Centers for Disease Control (CDC) of the U.S. Public Health Service began recording monthly statistics on AIDS, recording 383 cases. As of March 31, 1993, the number of people diagnosed with AIDS had risen to 248,320 (CDC, 1993); on average, someone dies of AIDS in the United States every 7 minutes. In addition, AIDS cases are increasing among people in their 20s, many of whom were probably infected as teenagers (U.S. General Accounting Office, 1990).

The number of individuals infected with HIV (i.e., who are HIV positive) has also risen dramatically. CDC now estimates that approximately one adult male in 100 in the United States is HIV positive, and one adult female in 600 is similarly infected—a total of one million individuals. This number is predicted to rise to 10 million by the year 2,000 (CDC, 1993).

DEVELOPING EFFECTIVE HIV/AIDS PREVENTION AND EDUCATION PROGRAMS

Despite the long-term denial of the sexuality and sexual needs of individuals with developmental disabilities, the seriousness of the AIDS epidemic has prompted many schools and adult service providers to provide HIV/AIDS education to youth and adults with developmental disabilities. Education is increasingly being viewed as an essential component of prevention activities. However, a major concern is the quality of that education—a unit simply covering the topic of HIV/AIDS is inadequate (Acton, 1992; Davis & Lerro, 1991; Mason & Jaskulski, 1993).

Effective HIV/AIDS prevention and education programs for people with mental retardation and other developmental disabilities typically incorporate the following features:

1. Appropriate *behavioral-instructional techniques,* such as those described in the first chapter of this volume (see Chapter 1), are used.
2. *Participants are actively engaged* in the instructional interaction, using such techniques as discussion and role plays, as well as videocassettes and other curricular materials.
3. *Mastery of the knowledge and skills* that are essential in reducing one's risk of HIV infection is promoted.
4. Honest, *frank discussion* is encouraged regarding people's fears, concerns, and attitudes.
5. HIV/AIDS *education is provided in the larger contexts* of sexuality, health, and personal safety.
6. Individuals' abilities to make *informed choices* and to take *personal responsibility* for their actions are supported.
7. HIV/AIDS prevention and education programs are *provided within a framework of organizational policies* that include staff education, confidentiality, nondiscrimination, and appropriate access to HIV testing and counseling.

Recommended Program Components and Initial Steps Toward Development

How should individual schools and adult service providers make decisions about adopting and adapting HIV/AIDS curricula for individuals with disabilities? Recommendations for program development from professional organizations such as the Council on Exceptional Children (CEC) (Byrom & Katz, 1991), the Association for the Advancement of Health Education (AAHE) (1989), and leaders in the rehabilitation field (McDaniel & Sells, 1989) include the following components:

1. ***Collaboration:*** Collaborative efforts need to be developed between health educators and special educators at the state and local lev-

els for implementation in schools and human services agencies.

2. ***Education:*** Among the many practices recommended are: 1) providing education about infectious diseases and the hygienic measures needed in order to reduce their spread; 2) focusing on reducing risk through changes in behavior rather than just on increasing awareness and knowledge levels; 3) providing appropriate risk-reduction training to youth with special needs who are employed in settings where they might be at risk for HIV infection; 4) providing education, where appropriate, to children with infectious diseases about additional control measures that they can practice to prevent transmission of the disease; and 5) incorporating objectives for HIV infection prevention education and health education into students' individualized education programs (IEPs).

3. ***Teacher Training:*** Teacher training and related educational personnel preparation programs should include information on infectious diseases and methods for their management and guidelines for passing this information on to students. Educational personnel should also receive career counseling regarding the level of medical risk in relation to certain infectious diseases and career choices.

4. ***Policies:*** Although policies for implementing HIV/AIDS infection prevention education for children and youth with special needs will be implemented at the local level, they may be modeled after suggestions developed by national experts. These HIV/AIDS educational policies should be placed within the context of policies on sex education, sexual rights, and the realities of sexual behavior for persons with developmental disabilities. In addition, infectious disease policies should address ways to permit personnel who are medically at high risk to work in environments that minimize additional risk.

5. ***Updating Information:*** Provisions should be made for frequent review and revision of HIV/AIDS education and policies to reflect the ever-increasing knowledge being produced through research, case reports, and experience. Recent experience of rehabilitation agencies participating in an HIV/AIDS prevention and education initiative sponsored by the National Association of Rehabilitation Facilities (NARF) (Mason & Jaskulski, 1993) suggest that the following five steps are applicable to developing and carrying out an effective program, regardless of setting:

1. Review existing policies and related education and training programs.
2. Consider needs and priorities specific to the target population, including any special priorities on individuals who appear to be engaging in risky behaviors.
3. Identify appropriate curricula and supplementary resources.
4. Design the plan for implementation, including selection of program participants, scheduling, and lesson plans.
5. Obtain necessary approvals and support.

Recognizing the Sexuality of People with Disabilities Viewing HIV/AIDS prevention and education in the larger context of sexuality education and training in personal living skills will further the gains that can be made in preventing the transmission of HIV/AIDS. Much has been written about the fears regarding sexuality and people with mental retardation (e.g., Hingsburger & Griffiths, 1986; Jacobs et al., 1992). Monat-Haller (1992) explains:

> Acknowledging the existence and development of sexuality in a child with a disability is extremely difficult for parents and for society. There is a great tendency to infantilize the individual with a disability regardless of his or her chronological age. . . . Therefore, as they go through the process of maturation, many individuals with developmental disabilities or mental retardation find themselves in a position where no one in their environment is willing to deal with or even recognize their developing sexuality. (p. xi)

Society's concerns about sexuality and social-sexual issues, along with generic issues of access to education and training that adequately prepare people with mental retardation for adult responsibilities, have resulted in limited access to sexuality education for many individuals. More recently, however, rights to sexuality education and to sexual expression have been articulated in policy statements on mental retardation. Table 2 presents The Arc's (formerly the Association for Retarded Citizens [ARC] of the United States) policy on sexuality as an illustration of the trend toward more progressive policies on sexuality. The Arc's policy statement on sexuality is included in resources on HIV/AIDS prevention and education for parents, board members, and administrators (Davis & Lerro, 1991).

Agency policies need to address the rights of people with mental retardation to receive sexuality education and training in HIV/AIDS prevention. Other policy areas that should be addressed in developing an HIV/AIDS prevention and sexuality education program include staff training on HIV/AIDS; related staff training on blood clean-up and other "universal precautions" to protect against HIV/AIDS and similarly transmitted diseases (e.g., hepatitis); confidentiality, including disclosure of information related to HIV/AIDS; nondiscrimination; and HIV testing and counseling. Resources on policies addressing these areas are included in the appendix to this chapter. Those planning the HIV/AIDS prevention program must also be familiar with applicable federal and state laws, in particular those governing confidentiality and requirements for HIV/AIDS education.

Assessing Individual Needs HIV/AIDS prevention and education must be relevant to the needs and abilities of the target population. Specifically, reviews of various resources on HIV/AIDS education for people with developmental disabilities (e.g., Cowardin & Stanfield, 1990; Hylton, 1990; Kempton, 1990a, 1990b; Levy, Levy, & Samowitz, 1987) indicate that effective programs must assure that learners have some prerequisite skills and an understanding of certain concepts. Programs will be more successful if learning styles, such

Table 2. The Arc policy on sexuality

ISSUE

Sexuality is a natural part of every person's life. Sexuality and sexual expression of people with mental retardation creates diverse reactions. This issue requires respect, understanding, caution, and an awareness of the wide array of human rights. Current social trends make the issue more urgent and complicated. The commitment to full integration into the community has given people with mental retardation new experiences, more risks, and more opportunities to make choices. The ability to make educated choices in the area of sexuality is especially critical.

POSITION

The Arc recognizes and affirms that individuals with mental retardation are people with sexual feelings, needs, and identities, and believes that sexuality should always be seen in the total context of human relationships. Sexuality includes gender identity, friendships, self-esteem, body image, and awareness, emotional development, and social behavior, as well as involvement in physical expressions of love, affection, and desires.

The Arc believes that people with mental retardation have the right on an individual basis to:

- have privacy;
- love and be loved;
- develop friendships and emotional relationships;
- choose friends;
- learn about sex, sexual problems, sexual abuse, safe sex, and other issues regarding sexuality;
- exercise their rights and responsibilities in regard to privacy, sexual expression, and the "pursuit of happiness"; and
- marry and have children.

The Arc supports programs which encourage people with mental retardation to develop expressions of their sexuality that reflect their age and social development, acknowledge the values of their families and are socially responsible. The Arc believes education should be available for people of all ages to assist in and, where appropriate, teach expressions of sexuality and responsible sexual behaviors with respect for the rights of others.

In support of this position, The Arc will advocate that the person with mental retardation be educated and receive proper supports to protect him/herself from abuse, exploitation, unwanted pregnancy and sexually transmitted diseases while safeguarding dignity and rights.

The Arc further advocates that on an individual basis people with mental retardation have the right to receive sex education, to marry, to have children if they so desire, and to receive proper support to assist them in rearing their children. Furthermore, The Arc believes that the presence of mental retardation regardless of severity, must not, in itself, justify either involuntary sterilization or denial of sterilization to those who choose it for themselves.

Adopted by Delegate Body November 10, 1990.

From The Arc. (1990, November 10). *Position statement on sexuality.* Adopted by the Delegate Body on November 10, 1990. Arlington, TX: Author; reprinted by permission.

as individual reading level and ability to generalize, are taken into account and opportunities for practice and peer reinforcement are encouraged. Knowledge and skill levels in sexuality education can be assessed prior to full program design so that remedial education can be provided as needed.

Figure 1 presents a sample assessment from the National Association of Rehabilitation Facilities (NARF) HIV Prevention Project (1989). This assessment should be repeated following the training to provide an indication of the program's success and to highlight any need for remedial instruction. A useful assessment of knowledge, skills, and attitudes is also provided in *Stopping AIDS Through Functional Education (SAFE)* (Hylton, 1990). The *HIV/AIDS Prevention and Education Curriculum Supplement* (Mason & Jaskulski, 1993), a manual for rehabilitation facilities on effective program design and implementation, also provides an assessment of prerequisite skills for

Optional Pre-survey.

Line drawings or pictures from the *Being Me* series (Edwards & Wapnick, 1979), the *LifeFacts* curriculum (Cowardin & Stanfield, 1990), or *Life Horizons I* and *Life Horizons II* sex education materials (Kempton, 1988; 1990) will be helpful in completing this assessment.

For individuals with moderate to severe retardation, identify whether: (Score each correct response with a "+")

____ 1. The learner can identify (name or point to) a picture of:
  ____ a. a penis
  ____ b. a vagina

  (When presented with drawings of a nude male and nude female, the learner can point to or name the above body parts.)

____ 2. The learner can identify (verbally or through pointing) pictures of a couple having sex. (Present several pictures and ask, "Which picture shows a couple having sex?")

____ 3. The learner can identify (name or point to) a condom. (Present several items and ask the learner to point to a condom.)

____ 4. The learner can explain how condoms are used or can simulate putting one on an anatomically correct model.

____ 5. The learner can explain why condoms are used.

____ 6. The learner can explain what to do if he/she does not want to have sex with someone.

____ 7. The learner can explain when to use condoms (prior to oral, anal, or vaginal sex).

____ 8. The learner can describe appropriate places for having sex (in private places, behind closed doors, when alone with one's partner in the bedroom).

____ 9. The learner can explain what he/she would do to initiate sex.

____ 10. The learner can explain what one would do if he/she wanted sex, but his/her partner was not interested.

____ 11. The learner can explain what he/she would do if someone had condoms and wanted to have sex and:
  ____ a. he/she was not interested in sex
  ____ b. the person was a stranger
  ____ c. he/she was interested in sex
  ____ d. was unsure about how he/she felt

____ 12. The learner can explain who might appropriately have sex (people who are in love and have known each other a long time; people who are married).

____ 13. The learner can explain problems with having sex with someone he/she does not know very well (transmission of sexual disease, reputation, vulnerability/exploitation, possible guilt).

Figure 1. The NARF HIV Prevention/Sexuality Information Assessment.

HIV/AIDS prevention and education for individuals who are vulnerable and at risk of being infected with the AIDS virus.

Because HIV infection through unsafe sex, in particular sexual intercourse (anal or vaginal), is likely to be the primary risk, much of the prevention emphasis will be on safer sex techniques of alternatives to intercourse, correct condom use, and abstinence. Students must, therefore, have a basic understanding of body parts, sexual activities, and related considerations of public and private activities. When presented with an array of pictures, slides, video segments, or line drawings, individuals should be able to identify: 1) a penis, vagina, and anus and 2) a couple engaged in sexual intercourse. If the individuals do not have these entry level skills, adaptations, such as additional preliminary instruction in basic sex education, may be necessary.

Determining Critical Concepts to Be Taught

The *Curriculum Supplement* (Mason and Jaskulski, 1993) lists essential skills and knowledge areas (e.g., what to do or say if one does not want to have sex, the importance of limiting the number of one's sexual partners, how to avoid sexual exploitation, and simulated condom use on anatomically correct models). To increase retention and generalization to practical settings, these concepts need to be taught to at least 80% mastery for three consecutive sessions, with assurance of 100% mastery of those concepts and skills that are most relevant to individual circumstances. For example, for an individual who has a known history of previous exploitation and ongoing vulnerability, 100% mastery should be attained on ways to recognize possible exploitation and how to remove oneself from the situation. This instruction could include the use of role plays as well as discussion.

The *Curriculum Supplement* also identifies certain concepts that most individuals with mental retardation who require lower levels of assistance should be capable of learning, such as an understanding of causative relationships (e.g., AIDS is a serious disease that can result in death; AIDS may be prevented through abstinence and safer sex, including mutual masturbation and condom use; risks are involved in needle-sharing and injecting drug use) and knowledge of risk-reducing skills (e.g., where to obtain and how to use condoms and spermicide). The primary difference between concepts listed as "essential" versus those listed as "desirable" is the degree of complexity. For example, the use of spermicide is listed as a desirable, not an essential, concept. For some individuals, spermicide use may be too complex and perhaps confusing. However, it should be noted that experts encourage the use of a spermicide, such as nonoxynol-9, in conjunction with condoms whenever possible, as it serves as a barrier to transmission of HIV and other sexually transmitted diseases.

Because of individual learners' risk factors, some concepts that are listed as "desirable" need to be treated, on occasion, as "essential." For example, an understanding of drug abuse and needle sharing as high-risk behavior is generally considered to be a desirable rather than an essential concept. However, for individuals with greater chance of exposure to injecting drug use (IDU) or to sexual activity with current or former IDUs or their sexual partners, the concept should be viewed as essential. Additionally, if ear piercing is currently a popular fad for a particular age group, it is essential that individuals likely to engage in ear piercing understand risk factors related to needle-sharing for that purpose. (Health professionals recommend that ear piercing be conducted in a physician's office rather than by friends or at specialty stores.)

For all participants, especially those considered to be at higher risk, an individual assessment, based on a pretest of knowledge and on awareness or suspicions of particular risk factors, should be used to determine whether specific concepts or skills need to be treated as essential rather than desirable. The authors recommend that discussions of these concepts be frank in explaining AIDS, the disease, its consequences, how AIDS is contracted and how it may be prevented, and how to obtain HIV testing if an individual has engaged in high risk behaviors. (Authors addressing AIDS and developmental disabilities typically recommend using the term "AIDS" for simplicity of communication [Hylton, 1990; Mason & Jaskulski, 1993].) In addition, instruction should proceed so that each individual is clear about what he or she would do to prevent HIV/AIDS. This may involve individual counseling and joint determination of each person's appropriate course of action (Mason & Jaskulski, 1993).

Some individuals with mental retardation have been identified as being at extremely high risk for HIV/AIDS because of indications that they have been engaging in risky behaviors. Before formal arrangements have been made for the prevention program, staff need to begin prevention and education efforts with anyone suspected of high-risk behaviors. The health belief model developed by Prewitt (1988) will strengthen such a prevention program. This model explains that for programs to be effective individuals must: 1) perceive HIV infection as a personal threat, 2) understand that HIV infection can be prevented, 3) feel able to control their exposure to HIV, and 4) be convinced that they can manage the behavioral changes that may be necessary (Jacobs et al., 1992).

Sensitivity to cultural factors, such as family values and beliefs associated with participants' cultures, will also strengthen prevention programs. For example, it may be particularly difficult in the Latino culture for a woman to ask her partner to wear a condom because asking a man to wear a condom demonstrates sexual experience and knowledge. This challenges a Latino cultural edict for the woman to appear modest and inexperienced. Unfortunately, asking a man to wear a condom in this culture may stigmatize a woman as being "loose" (Turner, Miller, & Moses, 1989). HIV/AIDS prevention and education programs can achieve maximum impact only if they are tailored according to the background and culture of the participants.

Selecting Available Resources Using an instructor's guide and related materials and developing goals and objectives for HIV prevention activities will enhance HIV/AIDS prevention and education curriculum. The objectives of the *SAFE* curriculum (Hylton, 1990) illustrates the kinds of objectives that resources should address, including helping learners to: 1) acquire behaviors needed to protect themselves from HIV infection, 2) overcome unfounded fears about AIDS and HIV, 3) resist the influences of people who engage in high-risk activities, and 4) interact appropriately with people who have HIV infection or AIDS.

The CEC and AAHE developed a checklist for reviewing curricula targeted to special education students (Byrom & Katz, 1991). As illustrated in Figure 2, the CEC/AAHE checklist includes a comprehensive array of skills and content areas that cover such issues as attitudes and personal responsibility, as well as the specifics of HIV transmission. The checklist also covers a review of the actual teaching materials and their appropriateness for teaching individuals with developmental disabilities about HIV infection prevention.

Another consideration in resource selection is the inclusion of multi-media approaches that will engage participants in learning activities and provide varied methods of training for maximum reinforcement. Getting individuals with mental retardation actively involved in their HIV/AIDS prevention and education programs is a critical factor in its effectiveness. The case example on page 171 describes how one agency utilized videotapes, structured discussions, and games to teach HIV/AIDS prevention to individuals with cerebral palsy.

The availability of an instructor's manual or other materials to assist trainers in presenting the program will also facilitate instruction. For example, the Young Adult Institute's training video *AIDS: Training People with Disabilities to Better Protect Themselves* (Levy et al., 1987) comes with a step-by-step instruction manual on how to use the video in combination with guided discussion, practice of correct condom usage, and role plays on practicing safer sex and insisting on condoms. Other materials that can enhance HIV/AIDS prevention and education programs include use of a dildo or anatomical model that includes an erect penis and a supply of latex condoms for participant prac-

HIV prevention training conducted by the United Cerebral Palsy Association of Queens (UCP/Queens), Natalie P. Katz Vocational Center, Jamaica, New York, combined a variety of instructional strategies to keep people interested and to address sensitive subjects. The instructors initiated a discussion of homosexuality and AIDS through the videotape *Seriously Fresh* (Select Media, 1989a), which includes a rap session by Jazzy Jay and covers a variety of HIV-related topics. When one of the characters in the video reveals that he had a homosexual experience and did not use a condom, one participant watching the video asked how he could have done that.

Staff used this question as an opportunity to introduce the topic of bisexuality. They discussed the fact that homosexuals sometimes have heterosexual contacts and that heterosexuals may experiment with homosexuality as a part of exploring their own sexuality. The instructors reinforced the message from the previous week's session: You must always use a condom because you do not know whom your partner may have been with—a homosexual or a heterosexual. The group was very vocal in their approval for this video and asked to see it again.

The movie *Vida* (Select Media, 1989b) was used the following week and group members initiated discussion on oral and anal sex. Staff led the discussion regarding how these activities were practiced by many "normal" individuals as part of their sexuality. The instructors also focused on methods of protection from HIV infection during these activities.

To demonstrate HIV transmission, UCP/Queens used a party game. Each group member was given a set of four index cards; all were blank except for one card marked with the letters "HIV." Staff introduced the activity with the reminder that safer sex precautions must be used whenever you have sex because you have no idea whom your partner may have had sex with. Participants were informed that the game they were about to play would demonstrate how this is true.

Group members were given a few minutes to enjoy refreshments, listen to music, and socialize. When the music stopped, each person was told to exchange one card with his or her partner. The staff then checked all of the cards; if any card in a set was marked "HIV," staff marked all the other cards in that set "HIV." This process was repeated three more times. Members of the group were told to make sure that they chose someone with whom they had not yet spoken. Staff actively encouraged and supervised participants in moving from one partner to another. Conversation between partners seemed stilted initially, but they became more animated as the session progressed.

After the final exchange, group members whose cards were marked "HIV" were asked to raise their hands. Eight of the 12 participants did so. Discussion of the results began spontaneously among group members with statements such as: "I had the virus first, and I infected so-and-so," or "I got the virus from so-and-so." Staff guided this discussion to a conclusion that those who were now "infected" with the virus had not had any contact with the original "infected" person.

tice in using condoms correctly. As noted in the National Association of School Boards of Education guide for policy makers, "education should stress skill development rather than simple presentation of facts" (Fraser & Mitchell, 1988, p. 11). A brief description of available videos and publications from national sources is included in the appendix to this chapter.

Scheduling, Logistics, and Lesson Planning Effective HIV/AIDS prevention and education is based on well-organized scheduling, logistics, and lesson planning. If training of the target group is to be phased in over time, a logical starting point is to begin instruction with those individuals most likely to be engaging in risky behaviors. Another target group would be those who are at significant potential risk because of their living situation or degree of vulnerability and/or dependence on others.

An informal atmosphere is particularly conducive to the kind of sharing and participation that enhances program effectiveness. If possible, sessions should be scheduled in a local community center or agency conference room that program participants associate with pleas-

TITLE: ______
Target student population: ______
______
Publication date: ______
Publisher/source name and address:
______
______
______
Reading level: ______
Cost: ______

CURRICULUM REVIEW

The following list of items is designed as a guide for educators who want to identify and select a quality curriculum that can be used to teach special education students about HIV and AIDS. The items address the essential ingredients of good curriculum as well as special considerations for exceptional learners. Many of the curricula available today are not designed specifically for special education students, but with careful planning, the good ones can be adapted.

To complete the review, put a check mark for each item that is sufficiently and appropriately addressed in the curriculum. Each item should be considered a positive aspect of a curriculum, which means that the higher the number of items checked, the better the curriculum.

I. Goals

___ 1. Are there clearly stated goals?
___ 2. Are the goals appropriate for special education students?
  ___ a. students with cognitive disabilities
  ___ b. students with physical disabilities
  ___ c. students with sensory impairments
  ___ d. students with emotional/behavior problems
___ 3. Are the goals consistent with the Centers for Disease Control guidelines (MMWR Guidelines for Effective School Health to Prevent the Spread of AIDS—see Section VI of this resource book for publication source)

Comments: ______
______
______

II. Objectives

___ 1. Are there clearly delineated learning objectives?
  ___ a. Are there cognitive objectives?
  ___ b. Are there affective objectives?
___ 2. Are the objectives designed to lead to the accomplishment of the goals?

Comments: ______
______
______

III. Concepts

___ 1. Are the concepts clearly identified for the particular ability level and age group?
___ 2. Are all of the relevant concepts addressed?

YOUNG CHILDREN
(Preschool/Primary Grades)
Focus
___ reduction of fear
___ positive feelings about oneself
___ positive foundation about one's body
___ appropriate/inappropriate touching
___ appropriate/inappropriate sharing

(*continued*)

Figure 2. Considerations for evaluating HIV prevention education curriculum and materials for special needs populations. (From Byrom, E. & Katz, G. [1991]. HIV prevention and AIDS education: Resources for special educators, pp. 21–25. Reston, VA: Council for Exceptional Children; reprinted by permission.)

Figure 2. (*continued*)

Content
- ___ body appreciation
- ___ wellness and sickness
- ___ friendships
- ___ family types and roles
- ___ assertiveness
- ___ difference between genders
- ___ serious diseases for children and adults
- ___ avoidances and protection/cautions
- ___ appropriate and inappropriate touching
- ___ scientists are working to solve the problem

CHILDREN
(Late Elementary School Grades)
Focus
- ___ resisting peer pressure
- ___ family values
- ___ body differentiation (pre-puberty/puberty)
- ___ differentiation between fact and fantasy
- ___ sexual feelings
- ___ compassion for people who are ill

Content
- ___ what is HIV infection?
- ___ causes of disease, transmission
- ___ natural sexual feelings
- ___ relationships between body parts and function and body parts and disease
- ___ talking about prevention (playing with needles, saying no, assertiveness)

EARLY ADOLESCENCE
(Middle School/Junior High)
Focus
- ___ protecting self and others from infection
- ___ healthy behaviors (rather than medical aspects)
- ___ establishing a value/belief system
- ___ affirming such belief system
- ___ analyzing opposing views
- ___ respect for others
- ___ peer pressure

Content
- ___ sexuality as a positive aspect of self
- ___ AIDS within the context of sexually transmitted diseases
- ___ discouraging experimentation with and use of drugs and alcohol
- ___ behaviors other than intercourse to express feelings
- ___ process of decision making
- ___ epidemiological information
  - ___ transmission
  - ___ prevalence
  - ___ symptoms
  - ___ medical outcomes
  - ___ treatment
  - ___ prevention
- ___ condoms, how to use properly, limitations
- ___ dangers of sharing needles and syringes for any reason: drugs, steroids, ear pierce, tattoo, razors, and other blood contaminated items
- ___ information on cleaning needles and syringes
- ___ information resources in local community
- ___ testing (promotes testing and posttest counseling)
- ___ information on treatment for drug users

ADOLESCENCE
(High School)
Focus
- ___ coping with disease
- ___ sexually transmitted diseases, including HIV infection and AIDS

(*continued*)

Figure 2. (*continued*)

___ parenting
___ encouraging the delay of sexual intercourse
___ responsibility to the community
___ coping with death and dying
___ attitudes and beliefs impact on decision making

Content

___ transmission modes, specific behaviors described
___ HIV and AIDS and its impact on society
___ manifestations of HIV infection including AIDS
___ testing for HIV infection
___ prevention of HIV infection
___ discussing responsibility with sexual partner
___ assertiveness regarding anxiety and drug usage
___ reduction of feat and myths

Comments: ____________________

IV. Scope and Sequence

___ 1. Will the units of instruction lead to the accomplishment of the objectives?
___ 2. Is the scope and sequence compatible with the developmental characteristics of the target students?
___ 3. Does the curriculum specify prerequisite concepts as well as those to be learned?
___ 4. Does the curriculum provide appropriate learning activities?
___ 5. Do the learning activities promote discussion among students?
___ 6. Do the curriculum segments follow a logical sequence?
___ 7. Does the curriculum address preconceptions, misconceptions, myths, and fears?

Comments: ____________________

V. Evaluation

___ 1. Does the curriculum have an evaluation component, i.e., is there a way to determine whether the curriculum does what it is supposed to do?
___ 2. Does the evaluation measure the extent to which both cognitive and affective objectives are met?
___ 3. Is there an evaluation of the HIV prevention and AIDS education program, i.e., the implementation of the curriculum?
___ 4. Was the curriculum field tested prior to publication and dissemination?

Comments: ____________________

VI. Staff Development

___ 1. Does the curriculum delineate knowledge and skills needed by teachers?
___ 2. Does the curriculum provide suggestions for special educators to work with health educators in teaching special education students about HIV prevention and AIDS?
___ 3. Does the curriculum contain a component that addresses staff development?
___ 4. Do teachers need to be trained to teach about HIV prevention?

Comments: ____________________

VII. Parental and Community Involvement

___ 1. Is the curriculum sensitive to the values of the community in which it will be implemented?
___ 2. Have parents and community representatives reviewed the curriculum?
___ 3. Have the students reviewed the curriculum?
___ 4. Have medical personnel reviewed the curriculum?
___ 5. Have educators reviewed the curriculum?

Comments: ____________________

(*continued*)

Figure 2. (*continued*)

VIII. Interagency Cooperation

___ 1. Does the curriculum contain a component that addresses interagency cooperation?
___ 2. Does the curriculum implementation plan promote interoffice or interdepartmental cooperation?

Comments: ______________________

IX. Presentation and Format

___ 1. Is information presented in an appealing format?
___ 2. Can pages be added or removed, e.g., three-ring binder?
___ 3. Are there worksheets, transparencies, or other materials for teachers included in the curriculum?

Comments: ______________________

Summary

Reviewer's comments: ______________________

Total number of items checked: ______________________

Reviewer's rating: (circle one)

1 2 3 4 5 6 7 8 9 10
poor good

Reviewer: ______________________ Date: __________

MATERIALS REVIEW

The following items are related to instructional materials aimed at teaching special education students about HIV infection prevention. Check all items that apply to the materials being reviewed.

I. Learner Characteristics

___ 1. Are the materials designed to match the instructional or educational level of the target population(s)?
___ 2. Are the materials appropriate for the target students' developmental levels?
___ 3. Are the materials appropriate for learners' needs?
___ 4. Are the materials oriented toward behavior change rather than just information transfer?
___ 5. Are the materials adaptable? Are they designed such that the core information can be extracted and adapted for individual students?
___ 6. Do the materials present a variety of strategies for teaching the same concept?
___ 7. Are there opportunities for repetition and review?
___ 8. Are terminology and vocabulary correct?
___ 9. Is the language appropriate for the target audience?
___ 10. Is the reading level appropriate for the target population?
___ 11. Are the material sensitive to particular features of the target population?
  ___ a. culture?
  ___ b. sexual orientation?
  ___ c. handicapping condition?

Comments: ______________________

II. Orientation

___ 1. Do the materials emphasize responsibility and prevention?
___ 2. Are the materials sensitive to the values of the target community?
___ 3. Do the materials promote compassion for individuals with HIV infection or AIDS?
___ 4. Do the materials emphasize risk behaviors, rather than risk groups?
___ 5. Do the materials use generic references such as "one's partner"—avoiding use of personal pronouns?

(*continued*)

Figure 2. *(continued)*

___ 6. Do the materials have appropriate terminology in referring to people with HIV infection, e.g., "people with AIDS" rather than "AIDS victims"?

Comments: ____

____

____

III. Presentation

___ 1. Are the design and layout of the material appealing?
___ 2. Is there effective use of photographs and illustrations, and, if so, are they appropriate for the target audience?
___ 3. Do the materials support the use of a variety of media?
___ 4. Are the teaching units well organized?
___ 5. Are various methodologies for teaching about HIV prevention described?

Comments: ____

____

____

IV. Content

___ 1. Do the materials support the objectives of the curriculum?
___ 2. Do the materials provide accurate and current information?
___ 3. Are the materials of high interest?
___ 4. Do the materials promote concept development and generalization?
___ 5. Do the materials promote reasoning and decision making?
___ 6. Are complete, understandable directions for use provided?
___ 7. Are supplemental materials suggested?
___ 8. Was the material field tested before publication?

Comments: ____

____

____

Summary

Reviewer's comments: ____

____

____

____

____

____

Total number of items checked: ____

Reviewer's rating: (circle one)

1 2 3 4 5 6 7 8 9 10

poor good

Reviewer: ______________________________ Date: ______________

Note: Permission granted to photocopy curriculum and materials review forms.

ant activities. Many programs have found it helpful to serve refreshments at each session. Other possibilities include incorporating HIV/AIDS prevention training in an evening support group or as part of adult education being provided to people with developmental disabilities at a local community college. Because of the benefits of showing videos on HIV/AIDS prevention, VCR equipment is recommended. In pilot work conducted with sites in New York and Indiana, Mason and Jaskulski (1993) found that videotapes were highly reinforcing and generally ranked as the preferred training activity.

Mason and Jaskulski (1993) advise incorporating HIV prevention recommendations into general sex education/social skills curricula and presenting weekly sessions over a period of 8–10 weeks. In general, training in groups of 6–10 will be effective and coed groups work well for most topics. However, for particular subjects, such as those on menstruation, it may be useful to include a few same-sex only groups.

A difficulty in scheduling for some adults is the conflict with work schedules, especially for those involved in community employment. Because some of these individuals are most likely to be confronted with potentially risky situations, we encourage programs to schedule convenient evening or weekend training opportunities and to conduct vigorous outreach to include employed adults. Special outreach is also essential for adults with developmental disabilities who are not currently in the service system.

Lesson plans will vary according to the curriculum and resources selected. However, including a description of the learning objectives and the measures used to indicate mastery for each lesson will help to ensure the success of the program. Although some published materials include lesson plans, these lessons often need to be adapted for individuals with developmental disabilities so that concepts are reviewed over several weeks. The authors strongly recommend that each session include discussion and other activities that actively involve the participants.

Organizational Preparation

The most significant step an organization can take in preparation for an HIV/AIDS prevention and education program is to make a formal commitment to do so. The commitment entails designation of the single individual who will be responsible for coordinating the program, obtaining necessary approvals from the governing body, and committing the necessary resources for both staff time and supplies. Other initial tasks include: 1) selecting staff to provide the training, 2) purchasing curricular materials, and 3) reviewing agency policies.

Choosing the Appropriate Staff In both school and adult service settings, at least one staff member needs to be identified for direct delivery of HIV/AIDS education curricula. This person(s) should be responsible not only for the presentation of the information, but for assuring that individuals master critical content and thus reduce their risk of becoming infected with or transmitting HIV/AIDS. Although assessing students' mastery of risk reduction is challenging due to concerns about privacy and the nature of sexual and drug-abusing activities, assuring that the student has at least demonstrated a mastery of knowledge-based material and correct condom use on anatomical models should be considered a critical staff responsibility.

If a supervisory staff member assumes responsibility for developing (if needed), reviewing, and updating the agency's HIV/AIDS education and prevention program, then it may be prudent for that same individual to assume primary responsibility for implementation of the program. Many rehabilitation programs have already designated an individual (often a nurse or social worker) to be responsible for sex education and units on communicable disease. In many cases, responsibility for HIV/AIDS prevention education is being added to that person's workload.

Staff providing HIV/AIDS education and training need to be able to handle discussions of sexual issues with relative ease. Teachers and educational administrators, as well as adult service administrators and providers, all need at least an introductory orientation to HIV prevention, education, and policy concerns. Acton (1992) recommends that all agency staff be trained in universal precautions, nondiscrimination, confidentiality, and rights and responsibilities of individuals with HIV/AIDS. (Specific instructor training is discussed in a later section of this chapter.)

Although a single instructor can be used, it is helpful to have at least a two-person team, preferably both a male and female. This is effective for role-play demonstrations and for sharing perspectives in group discussion, as well as for the individual or group sessions that are gender-specific. At a minimum, a trained male instructor needs to be available for one-to-one condom practice with male participants who require individualized instruction and practice.

Purchasing Curricula Many professionals have found that it may be best to purchase several curricula and mix and match according to the unique needs and skills of the individuals served. Curricula can cost from $30 to $900. For $900, several videotapes are available with a fairly comprehensive training package, while the lower priced curricula may focus more exclusively on AIDS or may provide general sex education information without including audiovisual materials. Individual supplementary videos such as those available from Select Media or the Young Adult Institute (see appendix to this chapter) can range in cost from about $30 to $120. A good anatomical model for condom practice may cost $60; however, a dildo, available from "adult" stores in most larger communities for approximately $4–$12, can be used. Using a banana or other objects that do not clearly resemble an erect penis is not recommended because students may not generalize the intended behavior (placing a condom on the penis prior to intercourse).

Reviewing Agency Policies When planning HIV/AIDS education and prevention, agency policies also need to be reviewed. Schools and human services agencies should cover AIDS-related policies and procedures, including the impact of HIV status on insurance coverage and benefits, co-worker expectations, employment, and job accommodations. Efforts should also be made to coordinate with other organizations providing services to the participants. To the maximum extent possible, conflicting messages to participants should be avoided by coordinating efforts.

HIV/AIDS education targeted to students and adults with developmental disabilities requires careful consideration of the organization's overall goals, staff responsibilities, program content, and related activities such as policy development and staff training and eduation. Consistency is an essential element in effective implementation. For example, consistent with its mission, an adult services program might shape its HIV prevention and education component to focus on the goal of preparing individuals with mental retardation to live with maximum safety and independence in the community. Consistent with its emphasis on meaningful employment, a vocationally oriented agency might schedule its HIV education program in ways that do not interfere with time devoted to productive activity.

Consistency within the agency's HIV prevention program can be supported by staff training that includes emphasis on the same messages that are used in client instruction. Staffing patterns can be reviewed to identify those staff most apt to interact with clients in situations where they can reinforce HIV education messages, and these staff can receive additional training in how to handle questions that clients may have. As the program is periodically reviewed, the staff will want to assure consistency with agency policies, or with revisions made to either policies or program components, as appropriate.

Obtaining Community Support If staff plan ahead for anticipated problems or objections to the program that parents, members of the board of directors, or other interested parties may have, then community acceptance can be expedited by preparing alternative solutions for providing information and justifying the need for HIV/AIDS prevention and education. Support from the board of directors or local board of education should be obtained in advance. Parents, board members, and other interested parties should be encouraged to preview materials and to familiarize themselves with applicable laws and policies, including those that require HIV/AIDS instruction. Local resources, such as the health department and Red Cross, can assist in providing information on HIV/AIDS and in gaining community support.

IMPLEMENTATION OF THE PROGRAM

A wide range of techniques in training and education is used to promote HIV/AIDS risk reduction among people with developmental disabilities. These include thorough preparation of instructors, useful behavioral-instructional strategies such as those presented in Chapter 1, and methods for handling sensitive issues. These techniques are described in the following sections.

Preparation of Instructors

Instructors need to be knowledgeable of HIV/AIDS prevention content, effective instructional techniques and materials, applicable laws and policies, and relevant community resources. Inservice or preservice training can enhance familiarity with content, review appropriate teaching strategies, and emphasize procedures for handling sensitive issues. Mason (1992) has developed a program of 1-day inservice training workshops for adult service providers. A self-assessment of each instructor's current knowledge and comfort level is followed by guidelines for enhancing one's comfort with HIV and sex education materials; addressing lesbian, gay, and heterosexual sexuality with the parents of participants; planning the HIV education program and handling the initial implementation; and understanding the essential concepts to cover in HIV prevention. During inservice training, HIV prevention instruction may be simulated through videotapes, role plays, and case scenarios, using material from the Young Adult Institute (Levy et al., 1987), the *SAFE* curriculum (Hylton, 1990), and the NARF *curriculum supplement* (Mason & Jaskulski, 1993). The orientation should also address HIV policies in such areas as confidentiality, staff training, and universal precautions.

Overcoming Staff Discomfort Similar to program participants, instructors are frequently uncomfortable presenting information and encouraging discussion of sexuality. Staff anxiety can negatively influence participants. Overcoming staff discomfort in regard to HIV and AIDS prevention comes with familiarity with the topic. This familiarity can be facilitated by inservice training sessions and assistance from such agencies as the Gay Men's Health Clinic, Planned Parenthood, and American Red Cross (Jaskulski & Mason, 1993). The following case example illustrates how one staff preparation program helps teachers to explore their own feelings about this volatile topic.

Some staff may experience discomfort due to their own fears about contracting the virus. As one becomes familiar with the signs and symptoms of AIDS, a common reaction is to begin to question one's own health. Inservice trainers need to talk about this fear with staff and suggest that some staff may wish to seek HIV testing and counseling. Other staff may be uncomfortable with HIV prevention due to religious or personal values concerning sexual relations between consenting adults or the use of drugs. The concerns also need to be discussed, and guidance should be provided by the agency.

> The Young Adult Institute has designed a series of exercises to "desensitize" staff with regard to teaching about AIDS. Staff who are going to be providing instruction in HIV/AIDS prevention are given practice in the rules of discussion that they will be encouraged to follow when teaching people with developmental disabilities. They are encouraged to try to feel comfortable enough to say anything they want, to have fun with the exercises, to try not to censor themselves, to recognize that they can "pass" if they feel uncomfortable responding to a particular question, and to try not to be judgmental. More serious questions related to the prevention curriculum are intermixed with nonserious and humorous questions, such as asking each person to discuss how their shoes reflect their personality.
>
> To help instructors become more comfortable in discussing sexual matters, they are asked to share information on the sexual climate in which they grew up, including the influence of television and movies, as well as the messages conveyed to them by parents and teachers. The exercise can be repeated with a focus on their attitudes toward the sexuality of people with developmental disabilities, as a background for understanding some of the obstacles they may encounter in teaching risk reduction techniques on safer sex.
>
> Discussions are structured to include use of "street" terms for sexual activities and body parts. Instructors place themselves into small groups and work on developing lists of slang words that are used for specific terms, such as penis or masturbation. Reading back the lists that have been developed further reduces instructor sensitivity and discomfort.

Educating Younger Students Recent studies have reported that a majority of high school students have had sexual relations. Inservice trainers can assist schools and rehabilitation agencies in determining how to provide HIV prevention instruction, even when staff experience personal discomfort and bias. However, for HIV prevention to be effective, it must be realistic and targeted to those at risk. When at least 50% of the students leaving high school have engaged in sexual relations (U.S. General Accounting Office, 1990), merely repeating the message to refrain from sexual activities will not be effective in preventing AIDS. The focus on making sound decisions about sexual activities and the postponement of sexual activities should be presented along with information on abstinence and safer sex techniques, such as condom use and alternatives to intercourse.

Knowledge concerning AIDS is increasing rapidly. Therefore, trainers must stay up-to-date regarding recommended education and training procedures, information on AIDS transmission, and recommendations for AIDS prevention. Agency policies concerning teacher training should be reviewed on an annual basis and revised as appropriate.

Instructional Strategies

The same strategies described in Chapter 1 of this volume should be used to teach HIV/AIDS prevention. For example, with repeated practice, an individual could unroll a condom 5–10 times during a session or have daily practice in condom application until mastery had been achieved. More frequent instruction and practice (daily or twice daily) can be considered if an individual continues to have difficulty learning a task.

Group response and rehearsal, in which the instructor leads a discussion with preplanned questions and expected rote responses are recommended. The correct responses are shaped through modeling. The participant is asked to repeat the correct response and reinforcement is provided, as illustrated in the following example:

Instructor: What is AIDS?
Instructor prompts: AIDS is a disease. You say it.
Participants: AIDS is a disease.
Instructor: That's right.
Instructor: How do you get AIDS?
Instructor prompts: You get AIDS from unsafe sex. You say it.
Participants: You get AIDS from unsafe sex.
Instructor: That's right.
Instructor prompts: You also can get AIDS from other people's blood. How can you get AIDS? Etc.

This approach is particularly helpful in the introduction and explanation of new vocabulary.

Prompting can be used to initiate the correct verbal response, as in the previous example, or the prompting of motor tasks may be involved, such as the sequence of steps to be followed in removing a condom from the package correctly, unrolling it, and preparing to apply it. *Task analysis* can be used to divide the task into small manageable steps. For example, practicing safer sex could be broken down into the following series of tasks following the decision to have sex with a partner: locate a condom (purchase the condom or get one from one's supply), unwrap the condom, unroll the condom, onto the erect penis while holding the tip of the condom to avoid air bubbles (in order to avoid breakage), apply spermicide, have sex, withdraw penis following ejaculation, remove condom being careful to avoid spillage, and discard condom in appropriate container. *Systematic reinforcement* for correct responses, typically through verbal feedback, is an important method of encouraging correct behavior and verbal responses in HIV/AIDS prevention and education programs. *Group reinforcement*, prompted by the instructor as needed, is also helpful, especially in socially sensitive areas like insisting on safer sex even when pressured by one's partner to have unprotected sex.

Generalization of skills is critical in HIV/AIDS prevention and education if the individual is to apply tasks learned in the instructional setting to his or her natural social environment. Generalization can be facilitated by role-play activities and other techniques that transcribe the prevention messages of class to real-life situations. Table 3 presents strategies to promote the generalization of HIV/AIDS prevention skills.

Table 3. Strategies to promote generalization

Practicing the skills in a natural environment: For example, for condom use, a part of the chain of tasks will be to get the condom. If condoms are kept in a drawer by the bed, then individuals having trouble generalizing should practice getting the condom from the drawer.

Practicing the skills with the appropriate individuals: If two clients are sexual partners, then some counseling sessions should be scheduled to include a talk about their decision for safer sex and condom use, including discussions about where condoms are kept and how they should be discarded.

Practicing the skills with several people: If the individual is not in a relationship, but has decided that condom use will be his or her approach to safer sex, role plays could be structured with several other persons playing the role of the hypothetical partner. For example, a discussion about safer sex and the need for condoms could be initiated, with role play of both cooperative and uncooperative partners.

Practicing communication techniques under conditions closely replicating the natural environment: To be most effective, role plays need to prepare people for a variety of circumstances. In addition to role playing interactions with cooperative and uncooperative partners, role plays of interactions with individuals who either want to have sex when you do not want to or you do want to have sex and the other person does not should be included as strategies for generalization.

Role plays for a variety of situations: Further preparation for actual events includes role plays of such situations as:

1. You and your partner want to have sex and you cannot locate a condom.
2. Your partner wants to have sex just one time without a condom.
3. You tear the condom getting it out of the package.
4. You do not want to have sex with the other person, even though that person has a condom.
5. Semen spills as the condom is removed from the penis. (The "spill" situation can be practiced with water and an anatomically correct model.)

Handling Sensitive Issues

Some of the participants are likely to be uncomfortable with the content being covered, especially those who are sexually inexperienced or who have been taught that sex should not be discussed openly. Reassuring participants that while some discomfort is natural, it is okay in the privacy of the classes to talk about sexuality, will facilitate group interaction and learning. Stressing that whatever is discussed in the sessions is confidential and not a subject for casual conversation outside the program, at work, or around the community, will help participants feel more comfortable and will reinforce appropriate behavior. See the following case example for an illustration of how to deal with this type of situation.

During the first session of classes on HIV/AIDS prevention training for adults with mental retardation, one of the participants, a young man named Jim, bolted from the room. One of the instructors talked with Jim after the session and learned that he was extremely uncomfortable with the subject of sexuality, especially any graphic references to body parts or sexual activity. The instructor explained to Jim that the classes were very important and that although they would like his participation, training could be provided to him privately if necessary. Jim was also reassured that anything discussed in class was confidential and that everyone's privacy would be respected.

After a few sessions on a one-to-one basis, during which the instructor covered the information that had been presented in the group, Jim resumed the group training. He reentered the group feeling more comfortable with the subject matter and less embarrassed by the discussions. By the end of the program, Jim was able to participate in discussion on a limited basis.

If an individual refuses to participate, whether due to discomfort or other personal reasons, the availability of alternative programs can be critical, especially if that individual is involved in risky behaviors. Arrangements might be made for individualized instruction or possibly for participation in an HIV/AIDS education program being offered through another community agency. Gay and lesbian individuals may be more comfortable with HIV/AIDS prevention programs sponsored by gay and lesbian organizations, with support from their mental retardation service agency as appropriate.

Discussions of HIV/AIDS prevention frequently precipitate other concerns that instructors must be prepared to address. It is not uncommon for one or more participants to reveal that he or she has been a victim of sexual abuse, including incest. Instructors must be familiar with appropriate specialized resources in the community for individual follow-up and counseling and with laws governing reporting requirements in cases of suspected abuse.

Some individuals are vulnerable to sexual exploitation and unprotected sex because they lack assertiveness skills (see chap. 11, this volume). If individuals have difficulty expressing their preferences regarding television programs, recreational activities, or even likes and dislikes in food or clothing, then it is doubtful that they will be able to let others know their preferences regarding sexual activities. If general assertiveness skills are lacking, the authors recommend training in assertiveness over a wide area, including practice of assertive social–sexual behaviors as a part of the training.

The Young Adult Institute (YAI) (Levy et al., 1987), *SAFE* (Hylton, 1990), and *Circles* (Walker-Hirsch & Champagne, 1988) programs all include segments on insisting on safer sex. Vignettes in the SAFE and YAI videos illustrate situations in which both men and women refuse to engage in sex without a condom, even though it is difficult for them to do so. *LifeFacts 2: Sexual Abuse Prevention* (Cowardin, Stanfield, & Downer, 1990) includes lessons on self-assertion and the right of mutual respect as part of curriculum on self-protection strategies.

Promoting Condom Use Lack of access to condoms can be a barrier to effective risk reduction, especially if policies prevent condoms from being made available through the program. Participants who are sexually active need to know how to obtain condoms, which ones to select, and how to maintain an adequate supply. Planned Parenthood organizations and other family planning service agencies in many communities provide condoms at low cost, as do special projects in some cities. To promote appropriate condom use, participants can be furnished with a wallet-size card identifying the preferred type of condom (latex) and the recommended spermicide (nonoxynol-9). The card can then be presented to the pharmacist, rather than trying to rely on ever-changing packaging or other clues which may not assure purchase of condoms effective in HIV prevention.

Recommending HIV Testing and Counseling Group discussions and individual sessions may lead to recognition that HIV testing and counseling is needed for a particular individual. A diagnosis of HIV positive is made through two tests, the ELISA and the Western Blot; the latter is a more definitive test. Testing and counseling services are offered at no cost, usually anonymously, at health centers throughout the United States. Programs should be aware of such resources and be prepared to support the testing and counseling process. Testing must always be accompanied by counseling; the availability of counseling should be verified before making arrangements for testing.

Staff may find it necessary or useful to provide consultation to the local testing and counseling center(s) regarding an individual's ability to give informed consent and to recommend effective counseling and communication techniques for the individual being tested. Such consultation may be particularly critical if the person is indeed HIV positive. Under most state laws, testing and counseling centers are not authorized to provide results to agencies without the consent of the individual. Thus, a situation could arise in which the only counseling an HIV positive individual receives is from an HIV testing center. Equally critical, the program must have clear policies regarding confidentiality and disclosure. As discussed in various resources on policy (e.g., AAHE, 1989; Crocker et al., 1989; Davis & Lerro, 1991; McDaniel & Sells, 1989; Rennert, Parry, & Horowitz, 1989, 1991), agencies are advised to avoid any disclosure of HIV status without the individual's consent and to scrupulously maintain confidentiality on issues that would potentially stigmatize the person as likely to be HIV positive (e.g., discussing the individual's use of AZT or another medication associated with HIV/AIDS).

EDUCATION ON SEXUALITY AND OTHER SEXUALLY TRANSMITTED DISEASES

A wide range of curricula are available on sexuality and on related personal safety issues, including materials appropriate for students of various ages and for people with various levels of skills. As indicated in Table 4, sexuality needs to be broadly addressed, including exploration of personal responsibility and awareness of appropriate norms (see chap. 11, this volume, for additional information). Sexuality education needs to be individualized, as well as provided nonjudgmentally and with the same candor that characterizes effective HIV/AIDS education. As with HIV/AIDS curricula, the authors recommend that programs on sexuality education be adapted to reflect individual values, beliefs, preconceived attitudes or fears, and individual living situations (Hingsburger, 1988).

Sex and Personal Safety

Parents have a strong interest in personal safety issues, particularly those that relate to sexuality. For example, a recent survey on the safety concerns of parents of children with disabilities found that 100% of the parents of elementary school children and 75% of the parents of adolescents identified stranger recognition, caution in public bathrooms, saying "no" to physical approaches, and knowledge of private body parts as important skills (Collins, Wolery, & Gast, 1991; see also Table 2 in chap. 2 of this volume). Fears of sexual victimization appear to be borne out by statistics on the experiences of people with disabilities, indicating that from 70%–90% of the population is victimized in some way during their lives (Kempton, 1990b). Sobsey (1994) estimates that 15,000–90,000 people with developmental disabilities are raped each year in the United States alone.

Table 4. Objectives for sex education instruction

The student will:
Understand and appreciate his or her own sexuality
Know basic male and female anatomy and male-female roles in the reproductive process
Understand that no one has the right to do something sexual to him/her or anyone else without permission
Understand the responsibilities of parenting
Understand that birth control methods should be used unless children can be provided for and are wanted
Understand his or her role in protecting personal health and the health of others
Know the resources available for persons who have been sexually abused or have contracted a sexually transmitted disease
Understand the social–sexual values of society
Recommended teacher qualities:
Comfort with one's own sexuality
Comfort with the language of sex, both technical and slang
Acceptance and tolerance of the feelings, attitudes, and values of others
Honesty and directness in manner and speech
Sense of humor

From Sparks, S., & Caster, J. (1989). Human sexuality and sex education. In G. Robinson, J. Patton, E. Polloway, & L. Sargent (Eds.), *Best practices in mild mental retardation* (pp. 294–295). Reston, VA: Council for Exceptional Children, Division on Mental Retardation; reprinted by permission.

Teaching people with developmental disabilities about avoiding or coping with sexual abuse requires a great deal of sensitivity on the part of the instructor. Available resources to assist instructors in these areas are presented in the appendix to this chapter. Common themes in these resources are determining boundaries, knowing what is appropriate within boundaries, and what to do to avoid abuse if and when it occurs.

The concept of boundaries is the central focus of the Circles program (Walker-Hirsch & Champagne, 1988). In the Circles series, the following concepts are taught:

1. You are the most important person in your world—you are the center of your circle, no one touches you unless you want to be touched, and you do not touch anyone unless she or he wants to be touched.
2. There are very few people it is appropriate for you to hug—mother, father, siblings, boyfriend, or girlfriend.
3. There are a few more people to whom you give "far away" hugs, such as your best friend on special occasions.
4. You shake hands with acquaintances once you know their names.
5. You wave to children when you know their names, wave to your friends when you see them and it is not convenient to be closer to them, and you wave to your friends when it would be wrong to interrupt them, such as at work.
6. You talk to community helpers only about business, and you do not touch strangers —strangers do not touch you.
7. For circle relationships to change, you and the other person must agree to the change.

The *Life Horizons II* curriculum (Kempton, 1990b) presents guidelines on preventing and coping with sexual abuse, including boundaries for appropriate public and private behaviors as well as how to reinforce personal boundaries or handle inappropriate touching by others. A series of rules summarizing the lessons on sexual abuse covers rules to avoid abuse (do not forget house safety rules, do not approach strangers, do not respond to strangers, do not accept presents or money as bribes, do not go anywhere with a stranger, do not give out personal information to strangers, and do not walk alone in lonely places or at night); what to do when approached (learn how to say no, know right from wrong feelings, tell someone you can trust, get away); and what to do if you are abused (if you aren't hurt and you know the molester, tell someone you trust; if this person doesn't believe you, tell someone else; if you are hurt by a molester, use a phone or a taxi or stop a policeman or passerby to ask for help) (Kempton, 1990b, p. 108).

As with education on the prevention of HIV/AIDS, teaching individuals to generalize lessons on personal safety to real-life situations is the ultimate educational goal. Although role plays and repetition are valuable, practicing skills (with prompts as needed) to the point of mastery is a first step to preventing abuse and using good judgment in real-life settings. To facilitate generalization, Kempton recommends that instructors set up a testing situation to see if personal safety training has been generalized, such as having an "actor" who is not known to the participants approach them in a community setting, try various techniques (e.g., offering them a ride in a car), note reactions of participants, and provide additional instruction as necessary.

Explaining Sexuality

Although sexuality education provides information about the body and the physical expressions of sexuality, teaching about relationships and the ability to express feelings is also essential. Several curricula are available that provide information on such areas as grooming, friendship, dating, feeling attraction, forming long-term relationships, marriage, and having children. Some of these also cover anatomy, hygiene, masturbation, sexual intercourse, homosexuality, pregnancy, birth control, STDs, and illegal sexual activity (e.g., see Edwards & Wapnick, 1979).

It is important for sexuality instruction to address the concept of romantic attraction and the realities of dating. Some curricula combine the subject of dating with discussions of boundaries and assertiveness similar to the information presented in HIV/AIDS prevention and education programs. For example, the *LifeFacts 1* (Stanfield & Downer, 1989) lesson on dating covers saying "no" to a date if the person does not agree with what the date is doing or wants to do, what to do when someone breaks a date, and how to tell if someone loves you. *Life Facts 1* provides a format for instruction in this area using a combination of role play, discussion, and audiovisual materials.

Training for parents can help garner support for sexuality education. Pedler and Hingsburger (1990) recommend group training designed to help reduce or relieve parental anxieties regarding their children's evolving sexuality and to foster acceptance of their sexuality; to learn that sexuality is part of being human, whether people do or do not have a disability; and to build realistic goals for their child's sexual behavior.

Other Sexually Transmitted Diseases

In addition to HIV/AIDS, other sexually transmitted diseases are included in most curricula on sexuality for people with developmental disabilities (Sparks & Caster, 1989). These diseases include gonorrhea, herpes, syphilis, and chlamydia. Typically, information on STDs covers the disease itself, that is, how to recognize its symptoms, how it is transmitted, related dangers and outcomes, treatment, and prevention. The *Life Horizons I* curriculum (Kempton, 1990a), for example, uses discussion and a series of slides to illustrate the sores (chancres) caused by syphilis, the discharge from the penis associated with gonorrhea, herpes sores on both men's and women's genitals, and condoms that can be used to protect against STD infection.

Although many programs are beginning to focus on HIV/AIDS education, training on preventing infection with other STDs must continue to be emphasized, especially among young adults living in the community. STDs are currently at near epidemic levels among the general population of American teenagers and young adults, with one in every seven teenagers currently infected, and 85% of reported STDs occurring in people ages 15–30 (Quackenbush & Sargent, 1990). Consistent and correct condom use (with spermicide if possible) also reinforces prevention of HIV infection. As individuals with developmental disabilities assume more responsibility for living and working in the community, they must also assume responsibility for expression of their own sexuality. Presenting concrete information on STDs is recommended, not only because it will help individuals avoid behaviors that can lead to STDs, but also because such education will teach individuals how to recognize their own STDs if they should become infected, thus expediting appropriate treatment and preventing transmission to sexual partners.

Related Disease Prevention

Education on STD prevention, including HIV/AIDS risk reduction, is frequently related to the understanding of disease prevention in general. In *Teaching AIDS: A Resource Guide on Acquired Immune Deficiency,* Quackenbush and Sargent (1990) recommend that the basics on communicable diseases should be taught before teaching about AIDS. The *Life Horizons* curriculum (Kempton, 1990a, 1990b) segment on sexual and reproductive health provides extensive information on personal health care, before addressing AIDS and other STDs.

The concept of universal precautions, which focuses on proactive risk reduction regarding contact with blood and other body fluids that might contain HIV, hepatitis, or other bloodborne diseases, may be included effectively in training programs on health, sexuality, and HIV/AIDS. The *SAFE* curriculum (Hylton, 1990) uses the example of a young woman with a developmental disability who works in a hospital where she might be exposed to blood. A video illustration of correct universal precautions procedures is combined with lecture and discussion in this segment.

CONCLUSIONS

The need for HIV/AIDS prevention and education for people with mental retardation and other developmental disabilities is not likely to diminish. Despite a few encouraging developments in research on the virus and on the treatment of the disease, there is little optimism that a vaccine to prevent HIV infection will be readily available in the near future. In the meantime, the rate of increase has not slowed, with the greatest increases occurring among the heterosexual population. Young adults are especially vulnerable because of their sexual activity and their failure to practice safer sex. It is particularly discouraging to note that many younger people are not practicing safer sex even when they are relatively well-informed about HIV transmission and the reasons for condom use and other safer sex behaviors.

Individuals with developmental disabilities are not immune to the risk factors affecting the general population and may have vulnerabilities that increase their overall risk. Also, individuals with developmental disabilities are becoming increasingly more concerned about HIV/AIDS. Even in small rural midwestern communities, Mason and Jaskulski (1993) found that program participants were aware of at least one local resident who had died of AIDS and that it was something that could affect them.

Several barriers to providing effective HIV/AIDS prevention and education and to related sexuality education persist, but they are weakening. Progressive policies are being written by various agencies including The Arc and the federal Health Care Financing Administration (HCFA). Although many family members have previously been reticent to address sexuality for their sons and daughters with disabilities, the AIDS epidemic has heightened concerns and renewed interest. Family members are increasingly recognizing that knowledge regarding sexuality and its responsibilities is a plus rather than a negative in promoting personal safety. Commitments among schools and adult service agencies to provide HIV/AIDS prevention and education are also increasing, as are state and local mandates to provide such programs to individuals with developmental disabilities.

In summary, it is reasonable to expect that as the AIDS epidemic continues to increase, more people with developmental disabilities will be infected. Assuring reduction in the transmission of HIV is one of the most pressing priorities facing society today. To date, HIV has not spread to an epidemic level within the population of those with developmental disabilities. However, it is a crisis waiting to happen.

Lack of knowledge regarding sexuality and sexually transmitted diseases places many people with developmental disabilities at a disadvantage. Societal attitudes and behaviors toward the sexuality of this population, the vulnerability of many individuals, and the lack of explicit materials that use simple language further increase the probability that people with developmental disabilities will be at risk for contracting AIDS. For HIV prevention and instruction to be effective, barriers and prejudices must be erased and replaced with competent, effective instruction tailored to the individual. Resources such as those listed in the appendix are available that include information on how other agencies have designed and carried out effective programs. Our challenge is to determine that appropriate instruction in HIV/AIDS prevention—and related sexuality, personal safety, and assertiveness training, as needed—is available to people with developmental disabilities. Until a "cure" or vaccine for HIV/AIDS is found, education is literally a life-saving measure.

REFERENCES

Acton, G. (1992). Comprehensive sexuality policy, procedures, and standards. In A. Crocker, H. Cohen, & T. Kastner (Eds.), *HIV infection and developmental disabilities: A resource for service providers* (pp. 133–140). Baltimore: Paul H. Brookes Publishing Co.

The Arc. (1990, November 10). *Position statement on sexuality.* Adopted by the Delegate Body on November 10, 1990. Arlington, TX: Author.

Association for the Advancement of Health Education. (1989). *Summary of the national forum on HIV/AIDS prevention education for children and youth with special education needs.* Reston, VA: Author.

Byrom, E., & Katz, G. (1991). *HIV prevention and AIDS education: Resources for special educators*. Reston, VA: Council for Exceptional Children.

Callen, M. (1990). *Surviving AIDs*. New York: HarperCollins.

Centers for Disease Control. (1993, March). *HIV/AIDS surveillance report*, 1–18.

Collins, B.C., Wolery, M., & Gast, D.L. (1991). A survey of safety concerns for students with special needs. *Education and Training in Mental Retardation, 26*(3), 305–318.

Cowardin, N., & Stanfield, J. (1990). *LifeFacts 1: Sexuality.* Santa Barbara, CA: James Stanfield.

Cowardin, N., Stanfield, J., & Downer, A. (1990). *LifeFacts 2: Sexual Abuse Prevention*. Santa Barbara, CA: James Stanfield.

Crocker, A.C., & Cohen, H.J. (1991). *Guidelines on developmental services for children and adults with HIV infection*. Silver Spring, MD: American Association of University Affiliated Programs.

Crocker, A.C., Cohen, H.J., Decker, C.L., Rudigier, A.F., & Harvey, D.C. (1989). Special section: Public policy affirmations affecting the planning and implementation of developmental services for children and adults with HIV infection. *Mental Retardation, 27*(4), 255–262.

Davis, S., & Lerro, M. (1991). *The HIV guide: Resources for board members and administrators*. Arlington, TX: The Association for Retarded Citizens of the United States.

Decker, C.L. (1989). Protection of persons with HIV infection: Concluding remarks. *Mental Retardation, 27*(4), 253–254.

Edwards, J., & Wapnick, S. (1979). *Being me: A social/sexual training guide for those who work with the developmentally disabled.* Austin, TX: PRO-ED.

Fraser, K., & Mitchell, P. (1988). *Effective AIDS education: A policymakers guide*. Alexandria, VA: National Association of State Boards of Education.

Gosney, E.S., & Popenoe, P. (1929). *Sterilization for human betterment: A summary of results of 6,000 operations in California*. New York: Macmillan.

Health Care Financing Administration. (1991). *ICF/MR instructor's manual (Draft).* Baltimore: Author.

Hingsburger, D. (1988). Clients and curriculum: Preparing for sex education. *Psychiatric Aspects of Mental Retardation Reviews, 7*(3), 13–17.

Hingsburger, D., & Griffiths, D. (1986). Dealing with sexuality in a community residential service. *Psychiatric Aspects of Mental Retardation Reviews, 5*(12), 63–67.

Hylton, J. (1990). *SAFE: Stopping AIDS through functional education*. Portland, OR: CDRC Publications, Oregon Health Sciences University, Child Development & Rehabilitation Center.

Jacobs, R., Samowitz, P., Levy, J.M., Levy, P.H., & Cabrera, G. (1992). Young Adult Institute's comprehensive AIDS staff training program. In A.C. Crocker, H.J. Cohen, & T.A. Kastner (Eds.), *HIV infection and developmental disabilities: A resource for service providers* (pp. 161–170). Baltimore: Paul H. Brookes Publishing Co.

Jaskulski, T., & Mason, C. (1992). AIDS policies and education: What are vocational and residential rehabilitation providers doing? *American Rehabilitation, 19*(3), 12–19.

Kastner, T.A., DeLotto, P., Scagnelli, B., & Testa, W.R. (1989). Proposed guidelines for agencies serving persons with developmental disabilities and infection with HIV. *Mental Retardation, 28*(3), 139–145.

Kastner, T.A., Hickman, M.L., & Bellehumeur, D. (1989). The provisions of services to persons with mental retardation and subsequent infection with human immunodeficiency virus (HIV). *American Journal of Public Health, 79*(4), 491–494.

Kastner, T.A., Nathanson, R., & Marchetti, A. (1992). Epidemiology of HIV infection in adults with developmental disabilities. In A.C. Crocker, H.J. Cohen, & T.A. Kastner (Eds.), *HIV infection and developmental disabilities: A resource for service providers* (pp. 127–132). Baltimore: Paul H. Brookes Publishing Co.

Kastner, T.A., Nathanson, R., Marchetti, A., & Pincus, S. (1989). HIV infection and developmental services for adults. *Mental Retardation, 27*(4), 229–232.

Kempton, W. (1990a). *Life horizons I: The physiological and emotional aspects of being male and female for persons with developmental and learning disabilities* (new ed.). Santa Barbara, CA: James Stanfield.

Kempton, W. (1990b). *Life horizons II: The moral, social and legal aspects of sexuality.* Santa Monica, CA: James Stanfield.

Levy, P.H., Levy, J.M., & Samowitz, P.M. (1987). *Training video and manual: AIDS, training people with disabilities to better protect themselves*. New York: Young Adult Institute.

Macklin, R., & Gaylin, W. (Eds.). (1981). *Mental retardation and sterilization: A problem of competency and paternalism*. New York: Plenum.

Mason, C. (1992, August). *HIV/AIDS prevention and education curriculum supplement: A manual to assist facilities*. Washington, DC: National Association of Rehabilitation Facilities.

Mason, C., & Jaskulski, T. (1993). *HIV/AIDS prevention and education curriculum supplement: A manual to assist facilities*. Washington, DC: National Association of Rehabilitation Facilities.

McDaniel, R.H., & Sells, N.N. (1989). *AIDS/HIV policy development guidelines for rehabilitation organizations: A report from the 1989 national leadership AIDS/HIV forum*. San Francisco: University of San Francisco, Rehabilitation Administration.

Monat-Haller, R.K. (1992). *Understanding & expressing sexuality: Responsible choices for individuals with developmental disabilities*. Baltimore: Paul H. Brookes Publishing Co.

National Association of Rehabilitation Facilities. (1989). *1989 NARF education needs analysis survey.* Washington, DC: Author.

Occupational Safety and Health Administration, U.S. Department of Labor. (1992). *Enforcement procedures for the occupational exposure to bloodborne pathogens standard, 29 CFR 1910.1030* (OSHA Instruction CPL-2.44C). Washington, DC: OSHA Publications Office.

Pedler, B., & Hingsburger, D. (1990). Sexuality: Dealing with parents. *The Habilitative Mental Healthcare Newsletter, 9*(4), 29–34.

Prewitt, V. (1988, August). *The health belief model and AIDS education: A content analysis of education literature*. Paper presented at the Second International Conference on AIDS Education, Charleston, SC.

Quackenbush, M., & Sargent, P. (1990). *Teaching AIDS: A*

resource guide on acquired immune deficiency syndrome (3rd ed.). Santa Cruz, CA: Network.

Reilly, P. (1991). *The surgical solution: A history of involuntary sterilization in the United States.* Baltimore: Johns Hopkins University Press.

Rennert, S., Parry, J., & Horowitz, R. (1989). *AIDS and persons with developmental disabilities: The legal perspective.* Washington, DC: American Bar Association, Commission on Mental & Physical Disability Law.

Rennert, S., Parry, J., & Horowitz, R. (1991). *AIDS/HIV and confidentiality: Model programs and procedures.* Washington, DC: American Bar Association, Commission on Mental Disabled and Center on Children and the Law.

Select Media. (1989a). *Seriously fresh: For teenagers* [Videotape]. New York: Select Media Educational Film & Video.

Select Media. (1989b). *Vida* [Videotape]. New York: Select Media Educational Film & Video.

Sobsey, D. (1994). *Violence and abuse in the lives of people with disabilities: The end of silent acceptance?* Baltimore: Paul H. Brookes Publishing Co.

Sparks, S., & Caster, J. (1989). Human sexuality and sex education. In G. Robinson, J. Patton, E. Polloway, & L. Sargent (Eds.), *Best practices in mild mental disabilities.* Reston, VA: Council for Exceptional Children, Division on Mental Retardation.

Stanfield, J., & Downer, A. (1989). *LifeFacts 1. Sexuality: Essential information about life . . . for persons with special needs.* Santa Monica, CA: James Stanfield.

Turner, C., Miller, H., & Moses, L. (Eds.). (1989). *AIDS, sexual behavior, and intravenous drug use.* Washington, DC: National Academy Press.

United States Department of Labor, Occupational Safety and Health Administration. (1992). *Enforcement procedures for the occupational exposure to bloodborne pathogens standard, 29 CFR 1910.1030* (OSHA Instruction CPL 2-2.44C). Washington, DC: OSHA Publications Office.

United States General Accounting Office. (1990, May). *Report to the Chairman, Committee on Governmental Affairs, U.S. Senate. AIDS education: Public school programs require more student information and teacher training* (GAO/HRD-90-103). Gaithersburg, MD: Author.

Vitello, S.J. (1980). The legislative and judicial history of sterilization of mentally retarded persons in the United States. In National Institute of Mental Retardation (Ed.), *Sterilization and mental handicap: Proceedings of a symposium sponsored by the National Institute on Mental Retardation and the Ontario Association for the Mentally Retarded* (pp. 33–37). Downsview, Ontario, Canada: National Institute on Mental Retardation.

Walker-Hirsch, L., & Champagne, M. (1988). *Circles: Safer Ways: Communicable diseases and casual contact and sexually transmitted diseases, AIDS, and intimate contact.* Santa Monica, CA: James Stanfield.

Appendix

A number of organizations provide useful information and materials relating to HIV/AIDS prevention and education for people with developmental disabilities. Some of these organizations are presented here. Every effort has been made to ensure that information provided in this appendix is current at the time of publication.

Policies

The Benefits of Rehabilitation for People with HIV/AIDS: A Manual to Assist AIDS Service Organizations, Rehabilitation Providers, and Rehabilitation Counselors. (1994).

American Rehabilitation Association
1910 Association Drive
Reston, VA 22091
(800) 368-3513
COST: $25 members, $35 nonmembers postpaid

AIDS/HIV and Confidentiality: Model Policy and Procedures. Rennert, S., Parry, J., & Horowitz, R. (1991).

Commission on Mental and Physical Disability Law
American Bar Association
1800 M Street, N.W., Suite 200
Washington, DC 20036
(202) 331-2282
COST: $25; $5.00 S/H

AIDS and Persons with Developmental Disabilities: The Legal Perspective. Rennert, S., Parry, J., & Horowitz, R. (1989).

Commission on Mental and Physical Disability Law
American Bar Association
1800 M Street, N.W., Suite 200
Washington, DC 20036
(202) 331-2282
COST: $15; $5.00 S/H

AIDS/HIV Policy Development Guidelines for Rehabilitation Organizations: A Report from the 1989 National Leadership AIDS/HIV Forum, McDaniel, R.H., & Sells, N.N. (1989).

Rehabilitation Administration
2130 Fulton Street
San Francisco, CA 94117
(415) 666-6333
COST: $5 postpaid

HIV/AIDS: A Legal, Policy and Practical Guide for Human Service Providers in New York. (1991).

Legal Action Center
153 Waverly Place
New York, NY 10014
(212) 243-1313
COST: $15.00

HIV Infection and Developmental Disabilities: A Resource for Service Providers. Crocker, A.C., Cohen, H.J., & Kastner, T.A. (1992).

Paul H. Brookes Publishing Co.
P.O. Box 10624
Baltimore, MD 21285-0624
(410) 337-9580
COST: $47.00 (Cite Stock No. 0832)

The HIV Guide: Resources for Board Members and Administrators. Davis, S., & Lerro, M. (1991).

The Arc
P.O. Box 300649
Arlington, TX 76010
(817) 261-6003
COST: $6.00

Staff Guide to Control of Infectious Disease for the Special Needs Population in Residential Sites and Day Programs. Prepared by Developmental Disabilities Community Nurses Coalition of Boston, Massachusetts. (December, 1989).

The Arc
P.O. Box 300649
Arlington, TX 76010
(817) 261-6003
COST: $4.00

Videos

Working Beyond Fear. This 40-minute video provides a clear, overall introduction to AIDS: what it is, its medical symptoms, how it is—and is not—spread, and how people can prevent exposure to the virus. (American Red Cross; contact your local chapter, Cite Stock No. 329529)

Don't Forget Sherrie. This award winning video uses an excellent cast, a rhythmic musical score, and a realistic script to tell the story of a young African-American man who is worried because his former girlfriend has died of AIDS. (American Red Cross; contact your local chapter, Cite Stock No. 329533)

Sex, Drugs & HIV. Provides peer support for negotiating strategies for safer sex and abstinence, and promotes understanding for people who are HIV positive or who have AIDS. This is a very direct and straightforward film about AIDS for teenagers. (Select Media)

Seriously Fresh: For Teenagers. During basketball practice, four fun-loving, fast-talking teens discuss with candor and humor everything from cars to girls, pipes to needles, and condoms to AIDS. Each confronts his own vulnerability to HIV transmission. (Select Media)

Select Media
Educational Film & Video
33 West 17th Street, 9th Floor
New York, NY 10011
(212) 727-7507

AIDS: Training People with Disabilities to Better Protect Themselves. This unique, state-of-the-art training video and manual provides comprehensive step-by-step instruction on how to teach people with disabilities about the hazards of AIDS and how to better protect themselves. (Young Adult Institute)

Young Adult Institute
Education & Training Dept.
460 West 34th Street
New York, NY 10001
(212) 563-7474

Teaching People with Developmental Disabilities

HIV/AIDS Prevention and Education Curriculum Supplement: A Manual to Assist Facilities. Mason, C. & Jaskulski, T. (1993).

American Rehabilitation Association
Publications Department
1910 Association Drive
Reston, VA 22091
COST: $25 members, $35 nonmembers postpaid

SAFE: Stopping AIDS Through Functional Education. Hylton, J. (1990).

CDRC Publications
CDRC/OHSU
P.O. Box 574
Portland, OR 97207-0574
COST: $75 postpaid [make check payable to Child Development and Rehabilitation Center]

Life Horizons I: The physiological and emotional aspects of being male and female for persons with developmental and learning disabilities (New ed.). Kempton, W. (1990). COST: $399

Life Horizons II: The moral, social and legal aspects of sexuality for persons with developmental and learning disabilities. Kempton, W. (1990). COST: $399

Circles I: Intimacy and Relationships. Champagne, M., & Walker-Hirsch, L. (1993). COST: $599

Circles II: Stop Abuse. Champagne, M., & Walker-Hirsch, L. (1986). COST: $399

Circles III: Safer Ways. Walker-Hirsch, L., & Champagne, M. (1988). COST: $399

LifeFacts 1: Sexuality. Cowardin, N., & Stanfield, J., New Edition. (1990). COST: $199

LifeFacts 2: Sexual Abuse Prevention. Cowardin, N., Stanfield, J., & Downer, A. (1990). COST: $199

LifeFacts 3: Substance Abuse. Cowardin, N., & Stanfield, J. (1989). COST: $199

Curriculum Available From:
James Stanfield Publishing Co.
P.O. Box 41058-C
Santa Barbara, CA
1-800-421-6534

Training Video & Manual, AIDS: Training people with Disabilities to Better Protect Themselves. Levy, P.H., Levy, J.M., & Samowitz, P.M. (1987).

Young Adult Institute
460 West 34th Street
New York, NY 10001
(212) 563-7474
COST: $145; specify ½″ VHS or ¾″ VHS; $4 S/H

Human Immunodeficiency Virus and Developmental Disabilities: A Leader's Guide for a Workshop. Kastner, T., Grosz, J., Harvey, D.C., Hopkins, K.M., Murphy, A., Nathanson, R., & Rudigier, A.F. (1991).

American Association
of University Affiliated Programs
for Persons with Developmental Disabilities
8630 Fenton Street, Suite 410
Silver Spring, Maryland 20910
(301) 588-8252

Understanding & Expressing Sexuality: Responsible Choices for Individuals with Developmental Disabilities. Monat-Haller, R.K. (1991).

Paul H. Brookes Publishing Co.
P.O. Box 10624
Baltimore, MD 21285-0624
(410) 337-9580
1-800-638-3775
COST: $25.00 (Cite Stock No. 0735)

HIV Prevention and AIDS Education: Resources for Special Educators. Byrom, E., & Katz, G. (1990).

The Council for Exceptional Children (CEC)
1920 Association Drive
Reston, VA 22091
(703) 620-3660
COST: $5.00

Other Agencies

The National Association of Protection & Advocacy Systems (NAPAS), with a grant from the AIDS Prevention & Services Program of the Robert Wood Johnson Foundation, has developed a series of AIDS Technical Reports:

AIDS Resource Manual: A Guide for Advocates in Mental Health and Developmental Disability Services. (130 pages). COST: $35.

AIDS Technical Reports: Series 1–5 (Entire Series). COST: $40.

1. *HIV Education for People with Mental Disabilities*. COST: $10.
2. *HIV Liability & Disability Service Providers: A Background & Checklist for Advocates*. COST: $10.
3. *Strategies for Implementing AIDS Guidelines in Developmental & Mental Health Services: A Background & Checklist for Advocates*. COST: $10.
4. *HIV & Mental Health Institutions*. COST: $10.
5. *Building Coalitions to Provide Legal Advocacy Services: Utilizing Existing Disability Models*. COST: $10.

Chapter Eleven

Crime Prevention and Personal Safety

Dick Sobsey

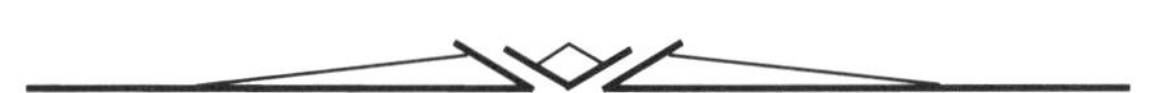

All of us, not just people with disabilities, are vulnerable to violence and other crimes. Although steps can be taken to reduce individual risk, no amount of preventive behavior can ever eliminate risk entirely. Too much emphasis on reducing risk can intrude on other aspects of our lives. The primary responsibility for crime lies with the offenders, not the victims. Environmental factors beyond the victim's control can play a powerful role. People who have offenses committed against them should never be blamed for failure to prevent their own victimization. Like other citizens, individuals with disabilities can learn to take positive steps that reduce their risk of victimization; however, no amount of training can provide an absolute safeguard, and risk reduction procedures should not be allowed to become so intrusive that they interfere with other aspects of community adjustment.

Furthermore, not all aspects of risk reduction can be accomplished by training individuals to avoid or resist victimization. Other important aspects of reducing crimes against people with disabilities involve selecting and training staff, reforming legislation, implementing safeguards within agencies, implementing generic crime prevention efforts, and changing public attitudes that encourage violence against people with disabilities (Waxman, 1991). Although primary emphasis in this chapter is placed on training the individual with a disability to enhance personal safety, other approaches to crime prevention are also addressed, as successful attempts to reduce victimization must combine personal safety education with other essential components.

This book emphasizes health and safety in community settings; therefore, crimes against people with disabilities that occur in these settings are stressed in this chapter. It would be a grave error, however, to misconstrue this emphasis as suggesting that people with disabilities experience greater risk in community, as opposed to institutional, settings. In fact, there is strong evidence that the opposite is true. The

Portions of the material presented in this chapter were developed as part of a research project funded by the Social Sciences and Humanities Research Council of Canada (Project 410-91-1665). This chapter was written at The Donald Beasley Institute while the author was a Roy McKenzie Foundation Visiting Professor of Mental Retardation in the Department of General Practice, University of Otago Medical School, Dunedin, New Zealand. The author gratefully acknowledges the support of these agencies. The opinions expressed are solely those of the author and not necessarily those of the supporting agencies.

work of several researchers suggests that institutional environments are associated with much more frequent violence than community alternatives (e.g., Blatt & Brown, 1986; Rindfleisch & Rabb, 1984; Sobsey & Doe, 1991; Sobsey & Mansell, 1990; Sullivan, Vernon, & Scanlan, 1987). Also, anthropological analyses of abuse suggest that embeddedness in the community and attachment to family and friends are powerful deterrents to abuse, whereas isolation from the mainstream of society facilitates abuse (Korbin, 1987).

This chapter presents basic information about teaching people with developmental disabilities to protect themselves from crime. Because little has been written on this topic and less has been validated, the strategies presented here must be viewed as preliminary suggestions in a developing field of instruction. In this chapter, emphasis is placed on prevention of child abuse, physical assault, sexual assault, and other violent crimes. That emphasis results partly from research suggesting that people with disabilities are more likely to be victims of such violent crimes (Carmody, 1991) and that these crimes typically have the most devastating effects on their victims.

TERMINOLOGY

Three terms used in this chapter need some explanation. Some people feel that the word *victim* stigmatizes the individuals who have it applied to them. There is good cause for this concern, as some approaches to crime and crime prevention focus on the characteristics of victims and seem to blame them for the crimes committed against them, viewing them as provoking the crime through intention or incompetence. Victim blaming is said to result from an individual's need to maintain his or her view of life as fundamentally just, creating a need to believe that those who suffer somehow deserve it (Lerner & Simmons, 1966). It is also said to stem from a need to maintain one's own feelings of safety by distancing oneself from those who are victimized (Williams, 1976). In either case, *victim*, as used here, only refers to an individual who is offended against and does not imply that he or she bears any responsibility for the offense.

The term *vulnerable* is also used in this chapter. It is used to indicate an individual who is more likely to be victimized. Vulnerability may result in part from disability (e.g., if the ability to defend oneself, get help, or escape is impaired), situational factors (e.g., being isolated from potential sources of help), or from a number of other sources (e.g., cultural attitudes that dehumanize disability and thereby disinhibit abuse).

Finally, the term *community-based crime prevention* requires explanation. This book is about community-based curriculum and instruction, teaching people needed skills for community living, and providing instruction in community environments. The term *community-based* has the same meaning in this chapter, but also carries a second implication. While the philosophical and procedural bases for community-based instruction were being developed among educators (e.g., Brooks & Baumeister, 1977; Brown et al., 1983), the concept of community-based crime prevention was also developing in the field of law enforcement (see, e.g., National Advisory Commission on Criminal Justice Standards & Goals, 1973; Trojanowicz, Trojanowicz, & Moss, 1975). Community-based crime prevention is based on an ecological model of human interaction similar to that of community-based instruction. It suggests that crime can best be understood within such a model, and prevention is best achieved by building communities that deter crime and integrating law enforcement with the communities it is intended to protect. For example, community constable programs, neighborhood watch programs, employment programs, social services, and crime resistant community planning and architectural design represent some specific applications of community-based crime prevention (National Advisory Commission on Criminal Justice Standards & Goals, 1973).

As used in this chapter, the terms community-based crime prevention and personal safety skills are intended to encompass both meanings of "community-based." They refer to skills that are functionally relevant to and can be taught within community settings. They also refer to skills that are consistent with crime-resistant communities and integrated law enforcement strategies.

Advocates of community-based crime prevention and law enforcement believe that communities have an essential role, along with police, in protecting themselves (e.g., Trojanowicz et al., 1975). They argue that even the best-staffed police force with the most modern equipment is powerless to control crime without community support. Community involvement should not be interpreted as the vigilantism of the old west where people "took the law into their own hands," but rather cooperative efforts between community members and a police force that represents and protects community interests. Driving while intoxicated, speeding, spousal abuse, child abuse, and abuse of people with disabilities are all crimes that have been tolerated in varying degrees by at least some segments of the community. If community attitudes permit these infractions or leave these problems entirely for the police to control, law enforcement can be expected to have little success in eliminating any of these crimes.

Both community-based crime prevention and community-based instruction depend on the existence of functioning communities. Traditional communities were small and people got to know each other. Even in large cities, neighborhoods often functioned like communal villages. In the last half of the nineteenth and twentieth centuries, increasing industrialization, urbanization, suburbanization, and geographical mobility have eroded traditional communities and shifted our focus away from families and communities to larger social units such as agencies and government. For people with disabilities, these shifts often meant institutionalization. For law enforcement, these changes meant a move away from greater reliance on community resources to greater reliance on police and other external agencies while crime increased. With continued erosion of traditional community relationships and the increasing difficulty of developing new ones, building and maintaining stable communities may be among the major challenges for community-based educational programs (Biklen, 1983; Shearer, 1986).

VULNERABLE VICTIMS OF CRIME

The fact that people with developmental disabilities are more likely to be victimized than people without disabilities has been recognized for some time. For example, von Hentig (1967) identified people with "mental defects" among four frequently victimized groups in one of the first systematic attempts to study crime by examining its victims. Subsequent studies of child abuse, sexual assault, and other crimes suggest that most people with disabilities will become crime victims at some time during their lives. For example, in a survey of women with disabilities (Stimpson & Best, 1991), 73% reported that they had been victims of violence.

Although numerous studies report similarly high rates of victimization among people with disabilities (e.g., Gil, 1970; Sobsey & Doe, 1991; Sullivan et al., 1987), precise figures are unknown because uniform crime reports do not code information regarding the disability status of victims, and arrests and convictions in these cases appear to be extremely rare. Sobsey and Doe (1991) reported convictions in 8% of the reported cases they studied, while Stimpson and Best (1991) reported 6%. Even these conviction figures are probably high estimates, as there is an indeterminate number of crimes known only to the perpetrator and the victim.

People with all types of developmental, sensory, and physical disability appear to have increased risk; however, no conclusive patterns have emerged from research to suggest that a particular severity level is associated with higher risk than another. Nevertheless, it appears that people with cognitive impairment, especially those with combined physical and cognitive impairment, are among those at greatest risk (Mullan & Cole, 1991; Sobsey & Doe, 1991). Even if precise figures were available regarding the numbers of crimes committed against people with disabilities, statistics can do little to describe the nature of the offenses or their impact on the lives of people with disabilities and their families.

Child Abuse

During the 1970s, many people became more aware of the extent of child abuse in our society and the harm that it does. During the 1980s and continuing into the 1990s, focus has shifted from awareness to prevention and treatment of child abuse. Child abuse can refer to neglect of children or to their physical, psychological, or sexual maltreatment. It is typically perpetrated by parents or other people in positions of authority, but strangers, other children, or anyone who can exert power over a child can be an offender.

Children with disabilities have been identified as frequent victims of child abuse for many years. Hawkins and Duncan's (1985) study of child abuse reported that 9% of the abused children studied had developmental disabilities; many more than would be expected by chance. West, Richardson, LeConte, Crimi, and Stuart (1992) reported 34%. Other estimates have been much higher. For example, Chotiner and Lehr (1976) reported a Denver Department of Welfare study that found 70% of abused children had disabilities.

Crimes Against People with Disabilities

The relationship between abuse and disability is complex. The traditional explanation for the association between abuse and disability has been the dependency-stress theory. It postulates that increased dependency of children with disabilities causes increased stress for their parents, and this increased stress leads to abuse. Research on this theory has not only failed to support it (Benedict, Wulff, & White, 1992), but it has provided strong contradictory evidence (Sobsey, 1990).

Some disabilities are caused by childhood abuse and the number in this category grows as better diagnostic techniques emerge (e.g., Dykes, 1986; McCelland, Rekate, Kaufman, & Persse, 1980). Familial use of alcohol and other drugs may result both in disability and abuse (O'Sullivan, 1989). These factors contribute to the association between abuse and disability but are not sufficient to explain the strength of the relationship.

Attachment between caregivers and children has been identified as a deterrent to abuse (Youngblade & Belsky, 1989), but attachment formation may be discouraged between children with disabilities and their parents (Blacher, 1984). For example, infants with disabilities often require special medical care and are placed in "isolettes" during their early days of life, while other children are being held by their parents. Families of children with disabilities may also become isolated from the community, and family isolation has consistently been associated with increased incidence of abuse (Smith, 1984).

Many people with disabilities live outside their natural homes, and, as discussed earlier in this chapter, much of the abuse of people with disabilities is associated with these out-of-home placements (Sobsey & Doe, 1991). These placements rarely provide the opportunity for the development of strong attachments between caregivers and the children they care for. They are often isolated from the community and typically have other attributes associated with risk. For example, evidence suggests that some offenders enter employment in service-providing institutions as a deliberate method for accessing victims (Sobsey & Doe, 1991).

Some people with disabilities have impaired abilities to recognize danger, fend off an attack, seek help, or escape from a dangerous situation. Learned helplessness, as a result of previous abuse experiences, can also weaken their natural self-protective responses. Even when individuals with disabilities are capable of protecting themselves, the belief by potential offenders that they are "easy prey" increases their risk.

Beliefs and attitudes that permeate society appear to contribute to abuse of people with disabilities in many other ways. Normal inhibitions that deter abuse in most people must be overcome by the person who commits violence. This disinhibition is often accomplished through a cognitive distortion process. For example, people who would have difficulty hurting an individual child face-to-face under normal conditions may find it easier to detonate a bomb that kills many children when the enemy is characterized as "the great Satan" or as "inhuman terrorists." Many cultural images of people with disabilities also disinhibit violence in offenders. Those who abuse people with disabilities may characterize them as menaces who provoke abuse, inhuman or worthless and, therefore, unworthy of protection or remorse, or as being incapable of understanding what is happening to them and insensitive to pain, therefore, not really suffering from the abuse.

WHO COMMITS CRIMES AGAINST PEOPLE WITH DISABILITIES?

No simple description fits all of the people who exploit or abuse people with disabilities. Sobsey and Doe (1991) found that 44% of the offenders in 166 cases of child sexual abuse or sexual assault were people who came in contact with the victim primarily through special services for people with disabilities. Many were paid caregivers (27.7%). Another 5.4% were specialized transportation providers, 4.3% were specialized foster parents, and 6.5% were other people with disabilities. The remaining 56% of offenders were members of the victims' natural family (16.8%), casual acquaintances (15.2%), generic service providers such as baby-sitters (9.8%), strangers (8.2%), dates (3.8%), and step-family members (2.2%).

Research suggests that the majority of abusers are male, but a significant minority are female. For example, Marchetti and McCartney (1990) reported a rate of abusive caregivers about three times higher among males than females. Sobsey and Doe (1991) found that less than 10% of those committing sexual offenses against people with disabilities are female.

Some of the individuals who commit particularly severe violent offenses appear to exhibit stereotypical characteristics. They appear to be intimidated by authority figures or anyone they see as possessing the power to defend themselves, yet they seek positions of authority and desire control over others, particularly those they view as defenseless. Some show difficulty controlling impulsive behavior and often exhibit demeaning attitudes toward people with disabilities. These attitudes can be hostile, but may appear to be very caring while engendering greater dependency and exerting greater control.

Gary Heidnik provides a good example of such a stereotypical offender (Englade, 1988). He failed in his bid to become a military policeman and trained as a nurse instead. He believed his role in life was to care for people with disabilities. In the process, he abducted them, chained them up, tortured them, and murdered them. Psychological and presentencing reports suggested that he was afraid of people whom he felt were his equals and needed to control those he viewed as most vulnerable. Most offenders against people with disabilities, however, do not exhibit such clear patterns of personality or behavior.

Andre Rand and Daniel Siebert were also prototypical offenders (Newton, 1990). Rand abducted his last victim, a 12-year-old girl with Down syndrome, from her Staten Island neighborhood and brought her back to the deserted ruins of Willowbrook, where he had previously worked as an attendant, to kill her. Siebert was so anxious to work as an art teacher at the Alabama School for the Deaf and Blind that he volunteered to work for free. He then raped and murdered two of his students.

DANGEROUS EDUCATIONAL PRACTICES

Before an effective crime prevention training program for people with disabilities can be developed, some of the traditional educational practices that appear to have contributed to their victimization must be examined. The first step in changing our educational practices for teaching people to resist crime must be to stop training them to be victimized. These dangerous educational practices include the following:

1. Teaching people to be too compliant
2. Teaching people to generalize compliance across trainers
3. Using too much physical prompting as instruction

4. Teaching dysfunctional sex education
5. Responding with intrusive control procedures to problem behavior, without adequate analysis of the function that the behavior serves for the individual
6. Teaching behavior that is not appropriate to the individual's chronological age (Sobsey & Mansell, 1992).

Compliance Training

It is ironic that in a world that offers assertiveness training to people who already have the power to make decisions for themselves, people with disabilities are often taught to be more compliant. However ironic this emphasis on compliance may seem, it is nonetheless consistent with the well-demonstrated social control function of special education curricula (Tomlinson, 1982). Winett and Winkler (1972) were among the first to identify that for students with disabilities, "good" behavior is typically defined as being passive and docile while responding to others' demands.

Although compliance training may have functional value for service providers who "manage and control" people with disabilities, it is not particularly functional for many people with disabilities who are likely to be victimized if they are too compliant. People who are taught to be docile to their caregivers often generalize this docility to those who exploit and abuse them. It many cases, generalization is not required because some caregivers and abusers are the same individuals. Too much compliance is cited as a contributing risk factor in the sexual abuse or sexual assault of 24% of victims with cognitive disabilities (Sobsey, 1994a). Even when compliance is not a stated curriculum goal, a long list of special education curricula objectives such as, "when asked to do _____, the student will do _____ on 9 out of 10 trials for 3 consecutive days," may have the same effect.

Teaching generalization of compliance across trainers creates a further problem. Not only are students taught to do whatever they are told, they are taught to do it regardless of who gives the order. Curricula that specify that students must demonstrate mastery by "performing for three different trainers including one that they have never seen before" and apply this standard to objectives like undressing and handing over possessions are obvious correlates to vulnerability and victimization.

Intrusive Physical Prompting

Self-protection curricula emphasize people's right to determine who touches them and who may enter the personal space that surrounds them (e.g., Champagne & Walker-Hirsch, 1982). More often, however, people's educational experiences contradict this principle. Widespread use of physical prompting procedures encourages students to accept being touched and controlled. It may also prevent them from developing a sense of personal space (i.e., recognition of when traditional conventions of social distance are violated) that is critical to self-protection. While physical prompting has appropriate uses, care must be exercised to avoid overuse and misapplication. If and when physical prompts are used, they should be used with the cooperation of the student; they should not be used to overpower the student. Failure to develop a sense of personal space makes it difficult for people to recognize early signs of intrusive behavior by offenders. Their lack of response to mild intrusions often signals offenders to proceed with more severe offenses.

Dysfunctional Sex Education

Most people with disabilities do not receive any formal sex education. Unfortunately, those who do receive it are often given information in a dysfunctional manner. Sex education programs that are provided are often so inexplicit or incomplete that they create misunderstandings about sexuality that leave people vulnerable to exploitation. Teachers often focus on the biological and hygienic aspects of sex and fail to address fundamental social and emotional issues. Sometimes these omissions result from the trainer's discomfort in addressing these issues. Other times they result from unclear or restrictive policies that make it difficult to provide clear answers to the questions of greatest practical importance to the students. (See chap. 8, this volume, for more on sex education for people with disabilities.)

Invalid Behavioral Intervention

Responding to behavior problems with intrusive programs before knowing the function of the behavior also increases the risk of victimization. Noncompliant, aggressive, self-injurious, and sexually inappropriate behavior are often the result of victimization and may serve as the victim's only means of communicating distress. When such behavior is suppressed by behavioral intervention, those who apply it may unknowingly become accomplices to the offender. If the "treatment" succeeds, the victim is stripped of his or her last means of defense. As a result, learned helplessness develops and the victimized individual is often more acquiescent to future abuse.

Teaching Age-Inappropriate Behavior

Teaching skills, encouraging behavior, and having expectations that are appropriate for individuals significantly younger than the student learning them also helps to foster abuse. These practices encourage learners to act like children and allow potential offenders to view them as vulnerable. Learning behavior that is inappropriate to the student's age also interferes with developing social relationships with peers that can help to keep the student safe.

The problems associated with traditional approaches to special education suggest that community-based instructional methods have some general advantages in reducing risk of victimization, regardless of the specific topic of instruction. Because community-based instruction is typically less *command* driven and more *context* driven, it tends to require less focus on compliance. Teaching in community settings requires that teacher–student interactions are normalized, thus, physical prompting is minimized. Finally, as the community provides exposure to a great variety of people, events, and other stimuli, discriminating functional and dysfunctional cues for behavior must be part of every learning opportunity. Thus, the normalization effects of community-based instruction help develop behavior appropriate to self-protection. The following sections discuss appropriate elements of an effective community-based crime prevention curriculum.

DEVELOPING A CRIME PREVENTION AND RESPONSE CURRICULUM FOR PEOPLE WITH DISABILITIES

Expert rankings suggest that training people with disabilities is among the most useful methods of preventing victimization. Rankings of potential training components for sexual abuse or assault prevention by 112 experts suggested the following priorities for program components:

- Assertiveness
- Sex education
- Personal rights
- Personal safety
- Social skills
- Choice making
- Communication training (Sobsey, Mansell, & Wells, 1991)

These components were identified primarily as methods of preventing sexual offenses; therefore, three additional curriculum components are discussed in this chapter:

- Self-defense
- Personal property protection
- Money management

Assertiveness and Personal Rights

Much has been written about teaching people with disabilities to increase their compliance (e.g., Burgio, Jones, & Willis, 1988; Schoen, 1983, 1986; Singer, Singer, & Horner, 1987). For some individuals with cognitive disabilities, increased compliance may be useful. As discussed in the last section, however, for many others, too much compliance increases the chance that they will be assaulted, robbed, or exploited. These individuals need to become more assertive. Assertiveness training programs have been developed and adapted to meet the needs of young adults with physical disabilities (Starke, 1987), elderly people with physical disabilities (Ruben, 1984), psychiatric in-patients (Katz, 1986; Zappe & Epstein, 1987), people who are blind or who have visual impairments (Ruben, 1984), and people with mental retardation (Bregman, 1984, 1985).

People cannot assert their rights unless they know what their rights are. Unfortunately, many people with disabilities are unaware of their rights either because these rights have been chronically denied or because they simply have not been informed of them. Learning about rights has little value unless a person also learns how to exercise them. For example, unless one knows how to get assistance, knowing that one has a right to personal security does not always help if that right is being violated.

It is important that teaching people about rights and their limits includes frequent opportunity and encouragement to apply what they are learning. The rights of people with disabilities are fundamentally the same as those of any other citizen. Several advocacy organizations have prepared statements of rights for people with disabilities; typically, they emphasize the rights that are the most frequently violated for this group. One example is a booklet prepared by the Ohio Legal Rights Society (Crossmaker, no date) that stresses the right to safety, respect, consensual sexual relationships, control over one's own money, liberty, treatment, freedom from unwanted or intrusive intervention, freedom from restraint, the right to refuse or accept medication, and freedom from coercion and abuse. Although the booklet is intended for people residing in institutions, it is easily applied to community settings. It also provides information useful for teaching people to identify abuse and to seek assistance.

Sex Education

Sex education is essential to preventing sexual abuse of children and sexual assault of adults with disabilities (Sobsey, 1994b), but it is important for other reasons as well. As adolescents approach adulthood, knowledge of human sexuality and its social and emotional context is important for normal social interaction. Individuals should have the knowledge required to make or participate in, to the greatest extent possible, their own decisions regarding sex and to protect themselves against unwanted pregnancies and sexually transmitted diseases.

Some people feel that sex education should be withheld from people with more severe disabilities, possibly because they fear that teaching about sexuality may encourage these people to become sexually active and therefore more vulnerable to exploitation. Others may consider people with disabilities to be asexual beings (Sobsey & Mansell, 1990). These beliefs continue to be reflected in some state laws that prohibit sex with an individual (usually the prohibition is specific to females) with a cognitive disability. Restrictive or unclear agency guidelines about sexual activity for people with disabilities may also make it difficult to determine if and when training should be initiated, who should be responsible for training, and what should be included in training.

Despite such restrictions, a lack of education in sexuality increases one's risk for abuse. Muccigrosso (1991) cited figures indicating that 90%–99% of people with developmental disabilities are sexually exploited, in part because they are not appropriately knowledgeable about sexuality. Segal and Craft (1983) pointed out that because of their learning difficulties, people with cognitive disabilities usually need more help understanding their feelings, and those without education are likely to be exploited unless instruction is provided. Sex offenders often exploit their victims' lack of sexual knowledge and rationalize their abuse as being educative (Sobsey & Mansell, 1990). Thus, the real question is not whether or not sex education should occur, but, who should provide it? Should sex education be provided by caring and competent people, or should it be left to those who want to exploit the vulnerable person?

Many programs have been developed for teaching people with cognitive disabilities about various aspects of sexuality. Table 1 lists some of these topics. Readers interested in more detailed information on appropriate sex education curriculum for individuals with developmental disabilities should see Chapter 10, "HIV/AIDS Prevention and Education," this volume.

Table 1. Sex education program components

Anatomy, physiology, and vocabulary
Maturation and body changes
Birth control
Sexually transmitted disease prevention
Masturbation
Responsibility for sexual behavior
Marriage and long-term relationships
Heterosexual behavior
Homosexual behavior
Social and emotional aspects of sexuality
Pregnancy and parenting
Appropriate and inappropriate sexual behavior
Preventing exploitation, abuse, and assault
Personal hygiene
Sexual lifestyle choices

On first consideration, the community may not seem like the appropriate setting for learning about sexuality, but this is only partly true. Some aspects of sexuality are private and should be taught privately. However, community environments provide a rich source for learning about a variety of relationships and behaviors from a wide range of models. For individuals to learn how environment, relationship, and interaction influence sexual behavior, they need both private and community-based instruction.

Sex education should not be broken down into artificially separate units such as sexual hygiene, biology, and abuse prevention. It is essential that social skills training, hygiene, abuse prevention, and many other areas are integrated to achieve a comprehensive and effective curriculum. For example, the prevention of sexually transmitted diseases (see chap. 8, this volume) requires elements of social skills training, general sex education, and abuse prevention because a significant number of people with disabilities contract sexually transmitted diseases in assaultive or exploitive encounters that allow little opportunity for hygienic protection.

Personal Safety

Teaching self-defense skills to people with disabilities has been recommended as a means to ensure personal safety (e.g., see Aiello, 1984–1986; Pava, Bateman, Appleton, & Glasscock, 1991). Nevertheless, it remains a controversial topic. In fact, teaching self-defense to any potential crime victim is a debatable strategy for many of the same reasons. Several questions regarding the value of self-defense training have been raised. First, is self-defense training likely to be adequate to overcome a potential offender? Offenders are typically bigger and stronger than the people they choose to victimize. They are almost always more experienced in the use of violence and less inhibited about hurting another human being. These advantages are often difficult to overcome, even for the individual with considerable competence in self-defense. For people with significant physical or developmental disabilities, the disadvantage is likely to be even greater.

Second, if attempts at self-defense skills prove inadequate, might the offender respond with even more extreme brutality? In some cases, this seems to be true, although the frequency of such events is unknown. What frightens away one attacker may only provoke another (New Zealand Police, 1991a).

Third, might teaching people to defend themselves create a false sense of security, encouraging them to take greater risks and discouraging them from involvement with other more valuable risk-reduction programs? Finally, might the individuals taught self-defense skills to protect themselves use these skills aggressively to victimize others? For example, teaching eye-jab, earclap, and kicking techniques to individuals who already exhibit aggression may create more problems than it solves.

These questions raise valid concerns, and good self-defense programs address them in a number of ways. These programs carefully select candidates on the basis of individual goals and expectations. They do not promote self-defense as a sole solution to self-protection; instead it is presented as a component of a total personal security program that encourages students to avoid, rather than seek, physical confrontation. Good self-defense programs also teach decision-making skills to assist individuals to determine if and when to fight back.

Furthermore, advocates of teaching self-defense suggest that it can be valuable in increasing self-esteem and overcoming the effects of learned helplessness. Knowledge that potential victims have the ability to defend themselves and an increased self-confidence acquired through training may also deter offenders. In consideration of all of these factors, self-defense training is probably a valuable component of community-based personal safety skills training for at least some individuals with disabilities (Aiello, 1984–1986; Rinear, 1985).

While 88.4% of experts ranked physical self-defense training as a useful strategy for people with disabilities to prevent sexual abuse or assault, 7.1% felt it would provide no significant benefit and another 4.5% felt that it would actually increase risk (Sobsey et al., 1991). Even for the majority who felt that physical self-defense would be useful, they generally assigned a low priority to this component, indicating that other training components would be more helpful in preventing abuse.

Experts in personal security often recommend self-defense training as part of a total personal security package. Recommended strategies often focus on learning simple methods of breaking free or temporarily disabling the offender to permit escape (Bodnar & Hodge, 1989; New Zealand Police, 1991a). These experts point out that "no matter how many precautions you take, you may someday be faced by a would-be attacker" (Alberta Solicitor General, 1987, p. 16) and "the choice of whether to resist or not can only be made by you" (New Zealand Police, 1991a, p. 7).

In teaching self-defense skills to people with disabilities, individualization is essential. Every student must learn to recognize appropriate conditions for the use of various self-defense techniques, but those techniques will vary across individuals. For example, an individual who can run or move quickly in a wheelchair might learn to strike and flee if attacked, but an individual with limited mobility will have little use for this strategy.

Social Skills and Communication Training

Social skills and communication training are essential elements of abuse prevention (Sobsey, 1994b). People who are isolated are typically among those individuals chosen by offenders for victimization and exploitation. Therefore, active friendships and community relationships can serve as powerful deterrents to abuse. Experts ranked friendship interaction skills as the highest teaching priority for social skills training components of sexual abuse prevention programs. Skills relating to family interaction, dating, client–service provider relationships, and stress management, respectively, also were ranked as useful (Sobsey et al., 1991).

Friendship and healthy social interactions contribute to abuse prevention in many ways. They prevent isolation and provide a source of advice and protection. They teach people about healthy and supportive relationships and provide alternatives to exploitative ones. They build self-esteem, which appears to improve resistance to abuse. Access to appropriate social and sexual relationships is a critical factor in personal safety, and teaching individuals how to develop such relationships allows them to take advantage of that access.

Great care must be taken in teaching people to build friendships. Many people will need instruction and assistance, but too much intervention is intrusive. The goal of instruction should be to foster friendships through developing skills that provide opportunities for informal social interaction. Teaching potential leisure skills often allows for inclusion in activities that provide such opportunities (Dattilo, 1991).

Communication impairment was cited as a contributing factor in 18.3% of 119 cases of sexual abuse and assault against people with developmental disabilities reported to the University of Alberta Abuse & Disability Project (Sobsey, 1994a). Experts ranking communication components indicated that expressing feelings, general communication enhancement, rejecting and protesting, and describing experiences, respectively, were important components of communication training for reducing risk of abuse. Aiello (1984–1986) also points out that communication skills are critical to stopping victimization and minimizing the harmful effects of abuse if it does occur. Docherty (1989) points out that some people with disabilities are more limited in communication by restrictive policies than by their own skill limitations. An environment that permits and encourages communication is essential both to learning communication and to using the skills that have been learned.

Teaching communication skills to people with disabilities has been a major curriculum area in special education. The complexities of pragmatics, semantics, and modes of communication as they are applied to individuals with great differences in cognitive, receptive, and expressive skills (e.g., see Reichle, York, & Sigafoos, 1991) go beyond the scope of this chapter, yet are essential to every aspect of community life. Some of the communication functions most relevant to crime prevention and personal safety skills include being able to protest against mistreatment, getting the attention of people who can help, seeking advice, being able to tell what has happened, and demonstrating all of the functions required for developing positive social interactions. Telephone use and writing skills are also important. Learning to use a pay telephone, keeping a coin available to do so in an emergency, and knowing when and how to call 911 are extremely valuable (Crime Prevention Tips for the Disabled, no date; see also chap. 2, Figure 5, this volume, for a detailed lesson plan for teaching this skill).

Personal Property Protection and Money Management

Traditionally, people with disabilities have had little personal property to protect. For example, Barron (1981) provides a typical description of traditional institutional life where people worked long hours for a few cents per week. Even this trifle was often withheld for petty infractions such as failing to say "thank you" or reaching out to accept payment with the left, rather than the required right, hand. Residents were routinely searched for such contraband items as coins or breadcrusts, which were then confiscated from them. Even clothing belonged to the institution rather than to the individual. Under these conditions, it was often impossible for people to develop a concept of ownership or how to care for and protect their possessions. Ironically, the lack of these skills was often used as a rationale for continued denial of personal possessions, and the lack of possessions made it impossible for individuals to learn how to care for them.

Functional experiences with money provide the best opportunities for community-based instruction (Ford et al., 1989). At the same time that students are learning to use money in restaurants or stores, they should also be learning how to keep their money safe and protected. As greater numbers of people with disabilities are allowed more normal lives in the community, understanding ownership rights and responsibilities becomes essential. The number and type of possessions, as well as the degree of independence and control, will vary across individuals and settings. Therefore, training must be individualized, but the principles remain the same.

Home Security Whether individuals with disabilities live independently in their own home or apartment, with their natural family, or in a group living facility, it is their home and they should exercise some control over and responsibility for it. Learning to travel independently in the community should include training in how to lock and unlock the door and safely keep a key to the house. They should also understand and take part in basic home security programs. Police and home security experts advise that all doors and windows need to be secured with appropriate locks (e.g., Bodnar & Hodge, 1989; New Zealand Police, 1991b). However, unless the people living there can operate them, they become prisoners in their own home, dependent on others to allow them to come and go. In some communities, home intruder alarms may be advisable. Again, people with disabilities must be taught to operate them or they become dependent on others to do so.

Personal Possessions People with disabilities also have a right to privacy, as well as secure places for storing their possessions. In group living situations, this may require a lock on the door to their room or a lockable drawer or closet. The use of identifying marks engraved, branded, or written in indelible pen can be useful in helping individuals to identify their own property; discourage others from taking their possessions; and recover items that have been stolen, misplaced, or accidentally appropriated. Marking can be done in unobtrusive ways (e.g., ultraviolet ink), but more obvious marking will be a greater deterrent to theft and more useful in helping individuals to recognize their own property (New Zealand Police, 1991b).

People with developmental disabilities should be taught to recognize the markings of their own items. In implementing marking programs, it is important to consider aesthetics, style, and neatness to ensure that markings do not stigmatize the owner. Engraved nameplates and personalized automobile registration plates are examples of how markings can be used to enhance the perception of status, while having a name scrawled on the back of one's jacket may be stigmatizing. Some items are particularly high risk for theft (e.g., bicycles, cassette players, food items, money). These should be marked, if possible, and each individual should be taught to keep these items in his or her personal possession, in a secure place, or with a trusted associate.

Money Money is probably one of the most difficult things for any individual to keep track of or protect. Nevertheless, using money is an extremely important skill that is functionally required in a great variety of community environments. Before people can learn how to protect their money, they must learn how to use it and understand its value. These skills are basic to money usage programs. Once they have learned these skills, they should be taught to keep their money in a safe place and to carry only relatively small amounts adequate for their immediate needs. They must also learn not to let people know when they are carrying larger sums of money. Some people with developmental disabilities can learn to use checks or credit cards. For these individuals, the risk associated with larger sums of cash is reduced. However, other risks associated with checks and credit cards need to be considered, and these risks may be greater for individuals with only partial mastery of how to use such noncash alternatives.

Responding to Crime

In spite of the best prevention efforts, crime still occurs and all members of the community need to be prepared to recognize and report crime, work with law enforcement professionals, and serve as witnesses in criminal proceedings. Learning about one's rights is essential to recognizing when an offense has been committed. If people with disabilities believe they have been victimized, they must know whom to tell. Many offenders try to manipulate their victims, convincing naive individuals to keep quiet by telling them that disclosure will have dire consequences. It is essential that people with disabilities know several people whom they can go to and trust with a disclosure.

Such a trusted person may assist the individual in seeking help from the appropriate authorities and may even assist him or her in giving a statement. It is important, however, to let each individual give a statement as independently as possible. Otherwise, the police may feel the individual is being unduly influenced by the support person or that the individual would be unable to tell the story independently and, therefore, be unable to testify in court.

Learning the location of the community police station, block parent or neighborhood watch houses, and neighbors and merchants who can be trusted can be extremely valuable if a crisis occurs. Some people with disabilities are fearful of police and having a brief social introduction can help develop a positive relationship. Such an introduction also helps law enforcement officers to become more knowledgeable about the individuals with disabilities whom they serve. This knowledge can be very useful if an individual with a disability needs assistance from (or could provide assistance to) the police in the future.

In many cases, the testimony of the crime victim is essential to successful prosecution, and the deterrent effect of such prosecutions is essential to law enforcement. Therefore, offenders who prey on people with disabilities are unlikely to be stopped unless an individual with a disability can give testimony against them. Unfortunately, the law, until recently, showed far more concern for protecting society from the "menace" presented by people with disabilities than for protecting people with disabilities from being victimized by others (Robb, 1990). While the courts have made some accommodations for children who give evidence, the same accommodation has generally not been available to adults with disabilities who have similar needs (Coles, 1990). To give evidence in court, an individual with a disability may be required to do more than just give a valid account of events. Such an individual may have to demonstrate a knowledge of the abstract meaning of truth, the significance of an oath, and the meaning and consequences of perjury (Robb, 1990). The individual must also be prepared for cross-examination.

Although it is important not to try to teach people with developmental disabilities exactly what to say in court (this may invalidate their testimony), many useful things about the process of being a witness should be explained to them. They should be taught the function of the court, who the various people are who have roles in the proceedings, and how to answer concisely. They should also be reassured that it is okay to say, "I don't know," when they cannot answer a question and to feel free to take their time in answering (Harvey & Watson-Russell, 1986).

INSTRUCTIONAL METHODS

The instructional methods used to teach personal safety and crime prevention skills should be similar to the methods used in other community-based instructional programs (Falvey, 1989). Both content and instructional delivery must be individualized to suit each student. Age-appropriate, functional activities should be used as the context for teaching functional skills.

Teaching within the context of the student's natural activities and routines is desirable and should be used when appropriate; however, this is not typically adequate for teaching some crime prevention skills for three important reasons. First, natural opportunities for using some of these skills (e.g., fighting off an attacker) are dangerous and undesirable events. Second, emergencies occur infrequently, yet functional mastery of the required skills is essential when crises occur. Natural opportunities for practice simply may not occur often enough to learn the skills required. Third, it would be unacceptably intrusive to try to teach all of these skills (e.g., sex education) within natural activities.

Because natural opportunities will not always be adequate or appropriate for learning all of these skills, training should be supplemented with verbal instruction, general-case simulation training, and repeated distributed trials of component skills. Instruction must make the best use of natural community environments, but should also integrate other instructional settings as needed (Baine, 1991). When relying on simulation, verbal instruction, and other alternatives, it is essential that instruction be explicit and, whenever possible, students must be given the opportunity to practice in natural activities or under the most natural conditions that can be provided. Realistic visual aids and other instructional resources can be used to help with this process. Careful assessment is also necessary to ensure that the skill will be functional for the student if required. Whenever natural opportunities do occur for teaching personal safety or crime prevention skills, they should be utilized as incidental teaching times.

Traditional training of self-protection skills to people with developmental disabilities has often depended solely on classroom instruction and been evaluated largely by students' verbal responses in a training environment. This raised the question about whether academic gains would translate to functional behavior in critical situations. Multiple-environment instruction has been recommended as a means of combining thc advantages of community-based teaching with those of other instructional environments (Baine, 1991). This type of instruction is especially relevant when the situations in which functional self-protection behavior should naturally occur are both infrequent and hazardous.

Haseltine and Miltenberger (1990) provide an example of effective multiple-environment instruction for teaching self-protection skills to men and women with developmental disabilities. They combined traditional small-group instruction, audiovisual aides, modeling, rehearsal, role playing, and *in situ* simulation to teach skills required to identify potential abduction situations. *In situ* situations used to determine generalization from the training environment to the natural community environment were a critical aspect of this training. These simulations minimized the risks experienced by students, while ensuring that the essential mastery of material in the training environment translated to functional behavior in the community.

In situ probes during baseline used a confederate who approached and then solicited the student in a public place (Haseltine & Miltenberger, 1990). If the student refused to go with the confederate or failed to respond for 15 seconds, a second request followed. Most subjects complied with the confederate's request during baseline. In training, they were taught to say "no," get away from the solicitor, and inform a trusted friend or authority figure. *In situ* testing after training and in 1- and 6-month follow-up sessions indicated that 9 out of 10 students carried out these behaviors when encountering a solicitation in the community. While there was some concern that the simulations or other aspects of training might produce emotional or behavioral side effects (e.g., excessive fear of strangers, nightmares, preoccupation with personal safety issues), no adverse effects were observed in a social validation survey of caregivers given before and after training.

Community-based instruction also has important implications for program planning. The objectives taught must be ecologically valid, reflecting the requirements of the students and the community. The dangers that people face and the appropriate methods of self-protection depend on the environment and how they interact with it. Direct assessment of the individual in the environment or an ecological inventory of environmental requirements (see chap. 2, this volume, section on "Identifying Safety Skills for Instruction") can help to ensure that instructional planning addresses relevant skills (Baine, 1991).

OTHER CRIME PREVENTION STRATEGIES

Every crime can be viewed as an interaction involving an offender and a victim that takes place within an environment that can encourage or deter the crime and within a culture that helps shape and give meaning to the environment and the interaction. Crime prevention can be accomplished by intervening to make the victim better able to avoid, escape, or deter the crime. It can also be accomplished by decreasing the offender's capacity or inclination to commit the offense. The environment can be altered to provide greater protection and less risk, and cultural attitudes and beliefs can be influenced to increase safety. Although the primary focus of this chapter has been on teaching the individual to prevent personal victimization through community-based instruction, it is essential that any program undertaken combine crime prevention strategies that are directed toward eliminating potential offenders, safeguarding environments, reducing opportunities for crimes to take place, and adjusting cultural influences on crime.

Community Inclusion

As previously discussed, there is evidence to clearly suggest that community environments are safer than institutional alternatives. Thus, a simple strategy for reducing the risk of crime for people with disabilities is community inclusion. It is important to remember, however, that geographical relocation does little to reduce risk unless it is accompanied by meaningful social integration. For example, a group home on a busy street can be as socially isolated as the back wards of an institution.

Community-based residences must interact with their neighbors and communities for effective risk reduction. Participation in community activities, the establishment of friendship networks, and the identification of common goals are essential for meaningful social inclusion. One of the best ways that people with disabilities and the residences that serve them can accomplish active participation in the community is to identify services that the group home and its residents can provide for the larger community. For example, group homes can make an excellent contribution to a neighborhood watch or block parent program. Because at least some of the residents and staff are almost always present in many group homes, they are likely to observe events that other members of the community may miss and are available to provide assistance when needed. Having neighborhood organizational meetings at the group home can be a good first step toward generating community interaction.

Staff Screening and Training

Unfortunately, paid caregivers are among the most frequent perpetrators of crimes against people with disabilities. There is evidence that some people take jobs as caregivers of vulnerable populations primarily as a means of accessing victims (Sobsey & Mansell, 1990). Police checks should be conducted for all applicants for jobs that entail working with vulnerable people. People with current charges or previous convictions for violent or sexual offenses should be eliminated. Careful reference checks should also be conducted to prevent staff who were "encouraged" to leave one agency because of inappropriate behavior from moving on to other human services agencies. Staff should be well-trained in clear procedures for recognizing and reporting abuse. Training should also prepare staff for responding appropriately to the physically or sexually aggressive behavior that some people with disabilities might exhibit.

Administrative Reforms

Policy must be written and implemented that ensures that offenses are reported to the appropriate authorities and properly investigated. Several court decisions holding agencies responsible for assaults committed by their residents or staff have established a responsibility to control known risk and to maintain safety levels that meet general community standards (LeGrand, 1984). Thus, agencies must take responsibility for maintaining reasonable levels of safety in the services that they provide and establishing procedures for monitoring and controlling risks.

Cultural Attitudes and Beliefs

The role of cultural attitudes and beliefs in increasing risk of victimization of individuals with disabilities is a complex one, but it cannot be underestimated. Waxman (1991) suggests that "as the incidence of anti-disability violence continues in seclusion and also becomes more overt, social psychological research on disabled victims of violence must shift" (p. 196) to a focus on the underlying cultural beliefs. Waxman identifies a fundamental inconsistency in our society's willingness to identify crimes directed toward a person's race, gender, religion, or sexual preference as "hatred," and to consider crimes against people with disabilities as being somehow explainable by the so-called "abuse-provoking characteristics" or "vulnerability" of these individuals. Videocassettes with titles such as *Children Who Invite Child Abuse* (no date) or scholarly articles entitled *Abuse-Provoking Characteristics of Institutionalized Mentally Retarded Individuals* (Rusch, Hall, & Griffin, 1986) lend powerful support for this view.

Such attitudes were powerfully illustrated when five New Jersey high school boys, including the twin co-captains of the football team, were charged with sexually assaulting a young woman with mental retardation with a broomstick and miniature baseball bat while eight others, including the son of a police lieutenant, watched and cheered ("Five accused," 1989). Fellow students voiced concern and dismay that the lives and future careers of these boys could be damaged by this unfortunate incident. Concern for the victim of the attack was apparently less popular, particularly after threats (including at least one death threat), property vandalism, and physical attacks were reported by schoolmates who failed to stand behind the accused students. One of these fellow students, a young man, is quoted in the Associated Press story as saying, "These kids are really not bad kids at all." A female student, apparently having a little more empathy for the victim suggested, "You've got to have sympathy for both sides."

Such views encourage offenders who use them to disinhibit and rationalize their violence toward people with disabilities (Sobsey & Mansell, 1990). Changing such culturally pervasive attitudes is fundamental to reducing the risk of victimization for people with disabilities. Until such attitudes are changed, no amount of personal safety instruction can be expected to provide completely adequate protection. However, as long as such attitudes promote violence against people with disabilities, personal safety skills training will remain essential.

LANA: CASE EXAMPLE OF A COMPREHENSIVE INDIVIDUALIZED CRIME PREVENTION PLAN

The following case example illustrates how a comprehensive individualized crime prevention plan can be sensitively implemented to reduce an individual's risk of exploitation and abuse.

Lana is a 16-year-old student in a special classroom for students with mental retardation who require high levels of assistance in a general junior high school in a small suburban community. Next fall she is scheduled to advance to a much larger consolidated high school with a number of vocational program options. Although Lana's mental retardation has been diagnosed as moderate to severe, it is not immediately obvious to most observers. She is an attractive young woman with no physical abnormalities, who responds socially to others and uses speech with only minor difficulties. More careful observation is required before it becomes apparent that although her articulation is only slightly impaired, she often uses vocabulary that she does not understand and frequently responds without really understanding what she has heard.

A few months ago, Lana's mother and teacher expressed concerns that she might be vulnerable to sexual exploitation or assault. They requested consultation to help address their concerns. Her mother suggested that "Lana will do anything to please her friends at school," and her teacher suggested that the other "kids act like they are her friends, but they can be cruel; they laugh at her and they just want to use her." Her mom worried aloud, "She likes babies, but she couldn't take care of one. If she gets pregnant, I'm the one who will have to care for her child, and I'm just too old and tired to care for more babies." National media coverage of a trial of several high school students alleged to have participated in a group sexual assault of a young woman a few years older than Lana with a somewhat milder disability had done nothing to ease their suspicions. Her mother felt that sending Lana to a residential institution might be the only way to protect her from her being abused.

Neither Lana's mother nor teacher were sure about how much Lana knew about sexuality or exploitation. Neither knew for certain if Lana was already sexually active or exactly what kind of relationships she had with the other adolescents that she called her friends. Lana's mother said that she had tried to discuss her concerns about this topic with her daughter, but that Lana seemed confused, and she sometimes thought that Lana was deliberately lying to her.

Assessment Initial assessment was informal. The consultant spent time with Lana in private discussions in her office, as well as at Lana's school, and in the community leisure environments where Lana and her friends spent time together. Several initial assessment sessions were devoted primarily to desensitizing Lana and her friends to the consultant's presence and establishing a relationship of trust. Some of Lana's friends were also interviewed. This phase of the assessment revealed that Lana's peers really were her friends. They realized that she was different in some ways, that she needed help with many activities, and that she sometimes responded without really understanding, but they valued her company and were willing to help. One young man whom Lana had referred to as her "boyfriend" indicated that he liked Lana and didn't mind going out with her and a group of others, but didn't really want to be her boyfriend and hoped she could understand that. Observation of her activities revealed only a few areas of concern.

(*continued*)

When Lana's primary peer group was not present, she would talk to and interact with other people she didn't know well. Her conversation or manner at these times was slightly inappropriate. She appeared to be too informal, affectionate, or personal for strangers or casual acquaintances. For example, sometimes she would stand too close, put her hands on people's arms, shoulders, or backs or talk about personal details of her life. These behaviors occurred with people of both genders and often resulted in people avoiding her because this made them feel uncomfortable. Some seemed to perceive this behavior as an attempt to be seductive. When her friends or even very casual acquaintances discussed sex, Lana was anxious to join in the conversation. Sometimes she would use more explicit language than the others and often her comments were off topic or raised doubts that she understood what she was saying or what was being said to her. Often her comments evoked smiles and sometimes laughter from others, and Lana seemed to enjoy the attention. This behavior had the potential to result in ridicule and possibly in sexual exploitation.

Lana sometimes kept secrets from her teacher, mother, and even her close friends. She indicated that she kept secrets when she is afraid that others would worry or disapprove, and sometimes when she is afraid that she will not be allowed to do things. Once she bought candy and brought it to school to give to a boy she liked, but after she told her teacher, the teacher would not allow her to give it to the boy and insisted that she share it with the entire class. This incident had been very upsetting to Lana, and after it occurred she kept more secrets.

Lana was assessed to determine her knowledge of sex education and personal safety skills, her individual rights, and her level of self-esteem. These revealed that Lana knew very little about sexuality and lacked some knowledge of personal safety. Her self-esteem was somewhat low and she was confused about her personal rights.

Instruction A program was developed for Lana that included individual, group, and community-based instruction. Personal safty and sex education were combined and taught primarily to a group of young women who were about Lana's age. One of the programs used was the *Circles* program (Champagne & Walker-Hirsch, 1982). This program teaches the concepts of privacy, intimacy, and social distance using concentric circles as a visual aid to help participants categorize the relationships they have, and learn the kinds of behavior that are appropriate to use with people in various categories. Lana and the other students enjoyed watching the videotapes that are included with this program, featuring a young woman who looked about the same age as Lana explaining and acting out social behavior.

Lana learned the information quickly, but observation, reminders, and some follow-up in the community were a necessary supplement to ensure generalization to the community. Lana was instructed to "think of her circles" in conjunction with her social skills training, before she began interacting with others. If Lana's interactions with others in the community seemed inappropriate, the consultant used this same phrase as a stimulus prompt to remind her to think about her actions (see Page, 1991). This was less intrusive than using a response prompt (telling her specifically what to do or not to do) and was easier to fade so that she could become more independent.

After a few weeks, no more prompting from the consultant was required, and she was able to monitor and regulate her own behavior. She was now repeating the prompt silently to herself and, although she occasionally would repeat it out loud, this did not prove disruptive. Social validation data collected from some of her friends and high school staff indicated that she continued to act appropriately after the consultant was no longer present.

A key element of Lana's program was motivation. She responded well to praise, and care was taken to ensure that she was frequently praised for her progress. When error correction was necessary, it was presented as informational feedback and not as criticism or punishment. Rather than focusing on her failures, she was typically praised for the things she had done right and told how she might do even better next time. Sometimes, in private, after an interaction in the community, her consultant would role play the interaction with her so that she could rehearse improvements. Lana usually thought that this was fun. Another important aspect of motivation for Lana resulted from her participation in developing the risk-reduction plan. Lana clearly indicated two goals: she wanted more friends and she wanted to be more like the other girls she associated with. These goals were incorporated in the program, and she was frequently reminded that the skills she was working on would help achieve these goals.

A multi-unit sex education program was also used with the same group of young women. Some of the women in Lana's group used *Blissymbols* (semantically based icons), so a program with both Blissymbols and English text was selected. Lana could read some of the English text herself, but found the illustrations and her teacher's verbal instruction more useful. Sexual abuse was covered in one unit of this program (see Ludwig & Hingsburger, 1993), but not until after 14 previous units on other aspects of sexuality had been completed. Although Lana had been told about many aspects of sexual abuse covered in this unit, she lacked the basic understanding of sexuality that is a prerequisite to understanding sexual abuse.

Lana had been very confused about her emerging sexuality. Although she had been involved in some minor petting and auto-erotic stimulation and had heard her schoolmates talking about sex, she was not sure about many of the details of sexual behavior. She was even more uncertain about the feelings that went along with it. In their efforts to protect Lana from abuse, her parents and teachers had inadvertently encouraged her to believe that all sexual interactions were abusive. Sometimes Lana thought that she wanted to become more sexually active, and then she thought this meant that she wanted to be abused. This belief left her vulnerable to abuse and also left her feeling that she was a bad person. Now, through sex education, she was beginning to understand that sexuality could be a good or bad thing and that eventually she would have to make her own choices. She was willing to wait a while and to discuss her choices with others, as long as she knew that she would be in control of her own life.

Because sexual behavior is private, it is not normally a suitable area for community-based assessment or instruction. However, some aspects of her learning could be observed and evaluated in community activities. Observation during interactions with her friends indicated that Lana's discussion of sexuality had become more cautious and appropriate to the situation.

Friendships were another important aspect of Lana's risk-reduction plan. Lana had already begun to form friendships, and careful observation during community leisure activities revealed a few areas of intervention to help strengthen those relationships. For example, Lana was often late meeting her friends, and she sometimes failed to respect their privacy when they wanted to do things alone. With a little prompting she improved in these areas.

The woman who worked with Lana on this program needed to be careful about establishing boundaries in her own relationship with Lana. It was important to spend time gaining Lana's confidence and trust, but it was also important to avoid building dependence and friendship because her time in these roles would be limited. Therefore, the consultant used her interactions with Lana to build and support Lana's friendships with others and thus avoid competing with these friendships. Community-based assessment and instruction often made this easier, as Lana's friends were almost always present.

In spite of these efforts, special care had to be taken as the consultant withdrew from her involvement. Lana was sorry to see her go, and the feeling was mutual. They discussed the termination, stressing that it signaled Lana's success with the program. Lana was allowed to call her once or twice a week after they stopped spending time together.

The consultant also worked with Lana's family, teacher, and friends. Lana's mother and teacher needed to accept legitimate risks for Lana. When they understood that some of their attempts to protect her were isolating her from her friends and depriving her of important information about sexuality and that these things were actually increasing her risk, they became more supportive of her adolescent development. Two of Lana's best friends knew about her program and helped provide her with guidance for more appropriate social behavior.

Lana's risk-reduction program cannot guarantee that she will never be abused or exploited. Unfortunately, none of us can be guaranteed that degree of safety. However, Lana's program has improved her understanding of abuse and what she can do to avoid it. It has strengthened her friendships with others and reduced the isolation that put her at risk for abuse. Lana exhibits less of the slightly inappropriate social behavior that might have signaled her vulnerability to potential offenders. Considering all of these changes, her chances of avoiding abuse or exploitation are now significantly better.

CONCLUSIONS

People with disabilities, like other community members, can contribute to their own personal safety as well as to the safety and welfare of the whole community. The curriculum focus and instructional methods associated with community-based instruction are natural choices for teaching community-based crime prevention to people with disabilities. Nevertheless, the application of these principles to this topic is new, and future research is required to develop and refine effective procedures.

Skills that help people reduce their risk of victimization can help manage their risks, but these cannot be taught in isolation. As personal risk-management achieves greater recognition as essential curriculum content, it must also be integrated into all areas of the curriculum rather than being treated as a separate area of instruction. Instructional procedures also need to evolve. Future programs should be aimed at improving personal safety for all citizens by combining training for people with disabilities with training for other members of the community whenever possible.

With the general trend toward community-based instruction, more effective personal safety training programs can be expected to follow naturally for two important reasons. First, community-based instruction fosters community involvement and helps combat the isolation that puts people at greater risk. Second, the inherent need for self-monitoring and self-regulation in community-based instruction requires learners to make their own decisions and discourages the passive responding that has characterized much of the segregated special education that has typically been delivered in the past.

REFERENCES

Aiello, D. (1984–1986). Issues and concerns confronting disabled assault victims: Strategies for treatment and prevention. *Sexuality and Disability, 7*(3/4), 96–101.

Alberta Solicitor General. (1987). *Personal safety: A guide to sexual assault prevention.* Edmonton, Alberta, Canada: Author.

Baine, D. (1991). Selecting instructional environments for students having severe multiple handicaps. In D. Baine (Ed.), *Instructional environments for learners having severe handicaps* (pp. 1–14). Edmonton, Alberta, Canada: Vector.

Barron, D. [Assisted by E. Banks]. (1981). *A price to be born. Twenty years in a mental institution.* Leeds, England: Leeds University Printing.

Benedict, M.I., Wulff, L.M., & White, R.B. (1992). Current parental stress in maltreating and nonmaltreating families of children with multiple disabilities. *Child Abuse & Neglect, 16,* 155–163.

Biklen, D.P. (1983). *Community organizing: Theory and practice.* Englewood Cliffs, NJ: Prentice Hall.

Blacher, J. (1984). Attachment and severely handicapped children: Implications for intervention. *Journal of Developmental and Behavioral Pediatrics, 5*(4), 178–183.

Blatt, E.R., & Brown, S.W. (1986). Environmental influences on incidents of alleged child abuse and neglect in New York State psychiatric facilities: Toward an etiology of institutional child maltreatment. *Child Abuse & Neglect, 10*(2), 171–180.

Bodnar, M., & Hodge, M. (1989). *Personal security.* Wellington, New Zealand: GP Books.

Bregman, S. (1984). Assertiveness training for mentally retarded adults. *Mental Retardation, 22*(1), 12–16.

Bregman, S. (1985). Assertiveness training for mentally retarded adults. *Psychiatric Aspects of Mental Retardation Reviews, 4*(11), 43–48.

Brooks, P.H., & Baumeister, A.A. (1977). A plea for consideration of ecological validity in the experimental psychology of mental retardation. A guest editorial. *American Journal of Mental Deficiency, 81,* 407–416.

Brown, L., Nisbet, J., Ford, A., Sweet, M., Shiraga, B., York, J., & Loomis, R. (1983). The critical need for nonschool instruction in education programs for severely handicapped students. *Journal of The Association for the Severely Handicapped, 8*(3), 72–77.

Burgio, L.D., Jones, L.T., & Willis, K. (1988). Increasing retarded adults' compliance with occupational and household tasks with a guided compliance and verbal praise procedure: A preliminary investigation. *Behaviour Change, 5*(3), 128–136.

Carmody, M. (1991). Invisible victims: Sexual assault of people with an intellectual disability. *Australia and New Zealand Journal of Developmental Disabilities, 17,* 229–236.

Champagne, M.P., & Walker-Hirsch, L.W. (1982). Circles: A self-organization system for teaching appropriate social/sexual behavior to mentally retarded/developmentally disabled persons. *Sexuality and Disability, 5*(3), 172–174.

Children who invite child abuse. The early years: Sensory problems [Videocassette]. (no date). Eugene, OR: Eugene Public Library, Audio-visual Department.

Chotiner, N., & Lehr, W. (1976). *Child abuse and developmental disabilities: A report from the New England regional conference.* Boston: New England Developmental Disabilities Communication Center.

Coles, W. (1990). Sexual abuse of persons with disabilities: A law enforcement perspective. *Developmental Disabilities Bulletin, 18*(2), 35–43.

Crime prevention tips for the disabled. (no date). Forestville, MD: Prince George's County Police and Office for Coordination of Services to the Handicapped.

Crossmaker, M. (no date). *Abuse and neglect: Awareness and reporting for individuals labeled as mentally ill.* Columbus: Ohio Legal Service.

Dattilo, J. (1991). Recreation and leisure: A review of the literature and recommendations for future directions. In L.H. Meyer, C.A. Peck, & L. Brown (Eds.), *Critical issues in the lives of people with severe disabilities* (pp. 171–193). Baltimore: Paul H. Brookes Publishing Co.

Docherty, J. (1989). *Indicators of abusive residential care facilities.* Toronto, Ontario, Canada: James Docherty & Associates.

Dykes, L.J. (1986). The whiplash shaken infant syndrome: What has been learned? *Child Abuse & Neglect, 10*(2), 211–221.

Englade, K. (1988). *Cellar of horrors: The true story.* New York: St. Martins.

Falvey, M. (1989). *Community-based curriculum: Instructional strategies for students with severe handicaps* (2nd ed.). Baltimore: Paul H. Brookes Publishing Co.

Five accused of sex attack on retarded girl. (1989, May 26). *Edmonton Journal* (Associated Press Wirestory).

Ford, A., Schnorr, R., Meyer, L., Davern, L., Black, J., & Dempsey, P. (Eds.). (1989). *The Syracuse community-referenced curriculum guide for students with moderate and severe disabilities.* Baltimore: Paul H. Brookes Publishing Co.

Gil, D.G. (1970). *Violence against children: Physical abuse in the United States.* Cambridge, MA: Harvard University Press.

Harvey, W., & Watson-Russell, A. (1986). *So, you have to go to court.* Toronto, Ontario, Canada: Butterworths.

Haseltine, B., & Miltenberger, R.G. (1990). Teaching self-protection skills to persons with mental retardation. *American Journal on Mental Retardation, 95,* 188–197.

Hawkins, W.E., & Duncan, D.F. (1985). Children's illnesses as risk factors for child abuse. *Psychological Reports, 56,* 638.

Katz, G. (1986). Group assertive training with psychiatric inpatients. *Psychiatric Journal of the University of Ottawa, 11*(2), 62–67.

Korbin, J.E. (1987). Child abuse and neglect: The cultural context. In R.E. Helfer & R.S. Kempe (Eds.), *The battered child* (pp. 23–41). Chicago: The University of Chicago Press.

LeGrand, C. (1984). Mental hospital regulation and the safe environment. *Law, Medicine, & Health Care, 12,* 236–242.

Lerner, M.J., & Simmons, C.H. (1966). Observer's reaction to the innocent victim: Compassion or rejection. *Journal of Personality and Social Psychology, 4*(2), 203–210.

Ludwig, S., & Hingsburger, D. (1993). *Being sexual: An illustrated series on sexuality and relationships. Unit 15: Sexual abuse.* East York, Ontario, Canada: Sex Information and Education Council of Canada.

Marchetti, A.G., & McCartney, J.R. (1990). Abuse of persons with mental retardation: Characteristics of the abused, the abusers, and the informers. *Mental Retardation, 6,* 367–371.

McCelland, C.O., Rekate, H., Kaufman, B., & Persse, L. (1980). Cerebral injury in child abuse: A changing profile. *Child's Brain, 7*(5), 225–235.

Muccigrosso, L. (1991). Sexual abuse prevention strategies and programs for persons with developmental disabilities. *Journal of Sexuality and Disability, 9*(3), 261–272.

Mullan, P.B., & Cole, S.S. (1991). Health care providers' perception of the vulnerability of persons with disabilities: Sociological frameworks and empirical analyses. *Journal of Sexuality and Disability, 9*(3), 221–241.

National Advisory Commission on Criminal Justice Standards and Goals. (1973). *A national strategy to reduce crime* (Publication No. 2700–00204). Washington, DC: U.S. Government Printing Office.

New Zealand Police, Crime Prevention Section. (1991a). *Your personal and practical guide to crime prevention: Vol. 1. Personal protection.* Wellington, New Zealand: Author.

New Zealand Police, Crime Prevention Section. (1991b). *A practical guide to crime prevention: Your home and possessions.* Wellington, New Zealand: Author.

Newton, M. (1990). *Hunting humans: The encyclopedia of serial killers (Vol. 2).* New York: Avon.

O'Sullivan, C.M. (1989). Alcoholism and abuse: The twin family secrets. In G.W. Lawson & A.W. Lawson (Eds.), *Alcoholism and substance abuse in special populations* (pp. 273–303). Rockville, MD: Aspen.

Page, A.C. (1991). Teaching developmental disabled people self-regulation in sexual behavior. *Australia and New Zealand Journal of Developmental Disabilities, 17*(1), 81–88.

Pava, W.S., Bateman, P., Appleton, M.K., & Glasscock, J. (1991, December). Self-defense training for visually impaired women. *Journal of Visual Impairment and Blindness,* 397–401.

Reichle, J., York, J., & Sigafoos, J. (1991). *Implementing augmentative and alternative communication: Strategies for learners with severe disabilities.* Baltimore: Paul H. Brookes Publishing Co.

Rindfleisch, N., & Rabb, J. (1984). How much of a problem is resident mistreatment in child welfare institutions? *Child Abuse & Neglect, 8,* 33–40.

Rinear, E.E. (1985). Sexual assault and the handicapped victim. In A.W. Burgess (Ed.), *Rape and sexual assault* (pp. 139–145). New York: Garland.

Robb, J. (1990). The dilemma of the disabled sexual abuse victim. *Developmental Disabilities Bulletin, 18*(2), 1–12.

Ruben, D.H. (1984). Comparison of two analogue measures for assessing and teaching assertiveness to physically disabled elderly: An exploratory study. *Gerontology and Geriatrics Education, 5*(1), 63–71.

Rusch, R.G., Hall, J.C., & Griffin, H.C. (1986). Abuse-provoking characteristics of institutionalized mentally retarded individuals. *American Journal of Mental Deficiency, 90*(6), 618–624.

Schoen, S.F. (1983). The status of compliance technology: Implications for programming. *Journal of Special Education, 17*(4), 483–496.

Schoen, S.F. (1986). Decreasing noncompliance in a severely multihandicapped child. *Psychology in the Schools, 23*(1), 88–94.

Segal, S., & Craft, A. (1983). Sexuality and mental retardation: A review of the literature. In A. Craft & M. Craft (Eds.), *Sex education and counselling for mentally handicapped people* (pp. 1–37). Tunbridge Wells, Kent, England: Costello.

Shearer, A. (1986). *Building community with people with mental handicaps, their families, and friends.* London: Campaign for People with Mental Handicaps.

Singer, G.H., Singer, J., & Horner, R.H. (1987). Using pretask requests to increase the probability of compliance for students with severe disabilities. *Journal of The Association for Persons with Severe Handicaps, 12*(4), 287–291.

Smith, S.L. (1984). Significant research findings in the etiology of child abuse. *Social Casework, 65*(6), 337–346.

Sobsey, D. (1990). Too much stress on stress? Abuse and the family stress factor. *Quarterly Newsletter of the American Association on Mental Retardation, 3*(1), 2, 8.

Sobsey, D. (1994a). Sexual abuse of individuals with intellectual disability. In A. Craft (Ed.), *Practice issues in sexual and learning disabilities.* London: Routledge.

Sobsey, D. (1994b). *Violence and abuse in the lives of people with disabilities: The end of silent acceptance?* Baltimore: Paul H. Brookes Publishing Co.

Sobsey, D., & Doe, T. (1991). Patterns of sexual abuse and assault. *Journal of Sexuality and Disability, 9*(3), 243–259.

Sobsey, D., & Mansell, S. (1990). The prevention of sexual abuse of people with developmental disabilities. *Developmental Disabilities Bulletin, 18*(2), 51–66.

Sobsey, D., & Mansell, S. (1992). Teaching people with disabilities to be abused and exploited: Part I: Blaming the victim. *Active Treatment Solutions, 3*(4), 1, 7–11.

Sobsey, D., Mansell, S., & Wells, D. (1991, March 31). *Sexual abuse of children with disabilities and sexual assault of adults with disabilities: Prevention strategies* (Report to Family Violence Prevention Division, National Health Research and Development Program, Health and Welfare, Canada). Edmonton, Alberta, Canada: University of Alberta.

Starke, M.C. (1987). Enhancing social skills and self-perceptions of physically disabled young adults: Assertiveness training versus discussion groups. *Behavior Modification, 11*(1), 3–16.

Stimpson, L., & Best, M.C. (1991). *Courage above all: Sexual assault against people with disabilities.* Toronto, Ontario, Canada: DisAbled Women's Network.

Sullivan, P.M., Vernon, M., & Scanlan, J.M. (1987). Sexual abuse of deaf youth. *American Annals of the Deaf, 132*(4), 256–262.

Tomlinson, S. (1982). *A sociology of special education.* London: Routledge & Kegan Paul.

Trojanowicz, R.C., Trojanowicz, J.M., & Moss, F.M. (1975). *Community based crime prevention.* Pacific Palisades, CA: Goodyear.

von Hentig, H. (1967). *The criminal and his victims.* Hamden, CT: Archon Books.

Walker-Hirsch, L. (1986). *Circles: Stop abuse.* Santa Monica, CA: James Stansfield.

Waxman, B.F. (1991). Hatred—The unacknowledged dimension in violence against disabled people. *Journal of Sexuality and Disability, 9*(3), 185–199.

West, M.A., Richardson, M., LeConte, J., Crimi, C., & Stuart, S. (1992). Identification of developmental disabilities and health problems among individuals under child protective services. *Mental Retardation, 30,* 221–225.

Williams, K.M. (1976). The effect of victim characteristics on the disposition of violent crimes. In W.F. McDonald (Ed.), *Criminal justice and the victim* (pp. 177–213). Beverly Hills: Sage.

Winett, R.W., & Winkler, R.C. (1972). Current behavior modification in the classroom: Be still, be quiet, be docile. *Journal of Applied Behavior Analysis, 5,* 499–504.

Youngblade, L.M., & Belsky, J. (1989). *Topics in Early Childhood Special Education, 9*(2), 1–15.

Zappe, C., & Epstein, D. (1987). Assertiveness training. *Journal of Psychosocial Nursing and Mental Health Services, 25*(8), 23–26.

Index

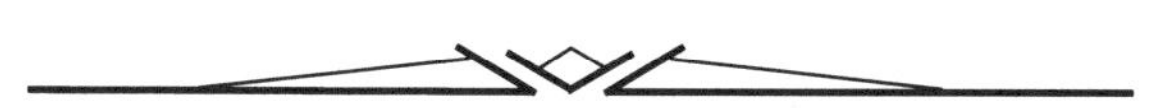

Page numbers followed by t *and* f *denote tables and figures, respectively.*